DEJA REVIEW™
Pathology

NOTICE

Medicine is an ever-changing science. As new research and clinical experience broaden our knowledge, changes in treatment and drug therapy are required. The authors and the publisher of this work have checked with sources believed to be reliable in their efforts to provide information that is complete and generally in accord with the standards accepted at the time of publication. However, in view of the possibility of human error or changes in medical sciences, neither the authors nor the publisher nor any other party who has been involved in the preparation or publication of this work warrants that the information contained herein is in every respect accurate or complete, and they disclaim all responsibility for any errors or omissions or for the results obtained from use of the information contained in this work. Readers are encouraged to confirm the information contained herein with other sources. For example and in particular, readers are advised to check the product information sheet included in the package of each drug they plan to administer to be certain that the information contained in this work is accurate and that changes have not been made in the recommended dose or in the contraindications for administration. This recommendation is of particular importance in connection with new or infrequently used drugs.

DEJA REVIEW™
Pathology

Second Edition

Jessica L. Davis, MD

Resident, Department of Pathology
University of California, San Francisco
San Francisco, California;
Oregon Health & Science University
School of Medicine
Portland, Oregon
Class of 2010

Emily E. King, MD, MPH

Resident, Department of Pathology
Brigham and Women's Hospital
Boston, Massachusetts;
Oregon Health & Science University
School of Medicine
Portland, Oregon
Class of 2010

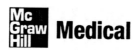

New York   Chicago   San Francisco   Lisbon   London   Madrid   Mexico City
Milan   New Delhi   San Juan   Seoul   Singapore   Sydney   Toronto

The McGraw·Hill Companies

Déjà Review™: Pathology, Second Edition

Copyright © 2010, 2007 by The McGraw-Hill Companies, Inc. All rights reserved.
Printed in the United States of America. Except as permitted under the United States
Copyright Act of 1976, no part of this publication may be reproduced or distributed in
any form or by any means, or stored in a data base or retrieval system, without the
prior written permission of the publisher.

Déjà Review™ is a trademark of the McGraw-Hill Companies, Inc.

1 2 3 4 5 6 7 8 9 0   DOC/DOC   14 13 12 11 10

ISBN 978-0-07-162714-6
MHID 0-07-162714-6

This book was set in Palatino by Glyph International.
The editor was Kirsten Funk and Karen G. Edmonson.
The production supervisor was Catherine H. Saggese.
Project management was provided by Arushi Chawla, Glyph International.
RR Donnelley was printer and binder.

This book is printed on acid-free paper.

Library of Congress Cataloging-in-Publication Data

Davis, Jessica, 1983-
    Deja review. Pathology / Jessica Davis, Emily King.—2nd ed.
        p. ; cm.—(Deja review)
    Other title: Pathology
    Rev. ed. of: Deja review / Sarah Kott Galfione, Kenny delBarco
Kronforst, Julia Conlon. c2007.
    Includes index.
    ISBN-13: 978-0-07-162714-6 (pbk. : alk. paper)
    ISBN-10: 0-07-162714-6 (pbk. : alk. paper)   1. Pathology—Examinations, questions, etc.
2. Physicians—Licenses—United States—Examinations—Study guides.   I. King, Emily,
1982- II. Galfione, Sarah Kott. Deja review.   III. Title.   IV. Title: Pathology.   V Series:
Deja review.
    [DNLM: 1. Pathologic Processes—Examination Questions.   QZ 18.2 D262d   2010]
    RB119.G25   2010
    616.07076—dc22
                                                                                        2010017288

McGraw-Hill books are available at special quantity discounts to use as premiums and
sales promotions, or for use in corporate training programs. To contact a representative
please visit the Contact US pages at www.mhprofessional.com

To my family, Matthew, Christina, Jon, Mom, and Dad, whose love and encouragement are ever present, allowing me to take on new challenges knowing they are always there to support me. To my friend, Emily, thank you for tackling this adventure with me—may we collaborate again together.
—Jessica

To my family and friends without whose patience, support, and understanding my contributions to this edition would not have been possible. And especially to Jessica, it has been wonderful having a friend for a collaborator, your work ethic and enthusiasm motivate me often, thank you.
—Emily

Contents

Faculty Reviewer

Terry K. Morgan, MD, PhD
Department of Pathology
Assistant Professor of Pathology and
    Obstetrics & Gynecology
Director of Placental Pathology and the
    Cytopathology Fellowship Program
Heart Research Center Scientist
Oregon Health & Science University
Portland, Oregon

Student Reviewers

Pete Pelletier, M(ASCP)
University of Utah
School of Medicine
Class of 2010

Robert Nastasi
SUNY Upstate Medical University
Class of 2009

Sheree Perron
Eastern Virginia Medical School
Class of 2010

Preface

The *Déjà Review* series is a unique resource that has been designed to allow you to review the essential facts and determine your level of knowledge on subjects tested on Step 1 of the United States Medical Licensing Examination (USMLE). This second edition of *Déjà Review: Pathology* is designed for the students as a compact yet high-yield review of major pathophysiologic and histopathologic concepts which make up a large percentage of USMLE Step 1 questions and which will contribute to overall mastery of this subject matter.

ORGANIZATION

There are multiple ways of approaching the broad topic of pathology. We have included chapters on broad topics which inherently fall under the domain of pathology: biochemistry, microbiology, and chromosomal/genetic disorders. The chapter on radiology has been expanded, and we have emphasized the inherent overlap between these two specialties. For the remaining chapters, we have attempted to integrate two organizational approaches in this second edition: organ system based and process based. As in the first edition, chapters are organized by organ system. New in this second edition, chapters are further subdivided by process (ie, neoplastic, inflammatory, infectious). We believe that this organizational approach will appeal to many different learning preferences.

The question and answer format has several important advantages:

- It provides a rapid, straightforward way for you to assess your strengths and weaknesses.
- It serves as a quick, last-minute review of high-yield facts.
- It allows you to efficiently review and commit to memory a large body of information.

At the end of each chapter, you will find clinical vignettes that expose you to the prototypic presentation of diseases classically tested on the USMLE Step 1. These board-style questions put the basic science into a clinical context, allowing you apply the facts you have just reviewed in a clinical scenario.

Of note, eponymous disease names and physical examination findings are intentionally printed in the nonpossessive form (ie, Hodgkin lymphoma, Trousseau sign) to reflect current medical terminology implemented in the *AMA Manual of Style*, 10th edition. Please be aware that this recommendation may not yet be completely adopted by other review resources, medical textbooks, other medical professionals, or your classmates. It is our opinion that the majority of medical students will still encounter possessive eponyms on a daily basis and should be aware of the reasoning behind this change for the second edition.

HOW TO USE THIS BOOK

This text was assembled with the intent to represent the core topics tested on course examinations and USMLE Step 1. Remember, this text is not intended to replace comprehensive textbooks, course packs, or lectures. It is simply intended to serve as a supplement to your studies during your pathophysiology and histopathology course work and Step 1 preparation. You may use the book to quiz yourself or classmates on topics covered in recent lectures and clinical case discussions. A bookmark is included so that you can easily cover up the answers as you work through each chapter. The compact, condensed design of the book facilitates portability and will allow you to review this material practically anywhere you wish.

However you choose to study and whatever your learning style, we hope you find this resource helpful throughout your preparation for course examinations and the USMLE Step 1.

Jessica and Emily

Acknowledgments

We would like to acknowledge **Dr Terry Morgan** for his advice and support. We would also like to acknowledge the faculty in the Department of Pathology at Oregon Health & Science University whose enthusiasm for pathology has encouraged and motivated us throughout medical school and especially in the preparation of this second edition. Special thanks also to **Charles Fredman** for assistance preparing the digital images featured in this edition.

We would also like to acknowledge and give special thanks to **Sarah Galfione, Kenny Kronforst,** and **Julia Conlon,** the authors of the first edition of *Deja Review: Pathology,* for beginning this project of building a comprehensive and thorough review of a large and complicated subject matter. We hope our additions and revisions will only improve the framework they created.

CHAPTER 1

General Concepts in Pathology

Define *pathology:*	The study of suffering (from the Greek *pathos*), or the study of functional changes in cells, tissues, and organs that underlie disease
Define *homeostasis:*	State of internal equilibrium at which normal physiologic demands of a cell are met; pathophysiology results when stimuli (ie, cell injury) sufficiently disrupt homeostasis.
What are some mechanisms of cell injury?	Altered physiological stimuli; reduced oxygen supply; microbial infection; metabolic alteration; cumulative aging
What are the ways that cells adapt to stress?	Hyperplasia; hypertrophy; atrophy; metaplasia
Define *hyperplasia:*	An increase in number of cells as an adaptive response to stress, usually resulting in increased volume of an organ or tissue. Cells must be capable of mitotic division (eg, prostate).
Define *hypertrophy:*	An increase in cell size due to synthesis of cellular structural components as an adaptive response to stress, usually resulting in increased size of an organ or tissue. Does not require mitotic division (eg, myocardium).
Define *atrophy:*	Reduction of cell size due to loss of structural components of the cell. An attempt by the cell to reduce demand to match reduced supply. The entire tissue/organ diminishes in size when enough cells are involved.

Give examples of physiologic atrophy:	Loss of certain embryologic structures (eg, digit web-space, umbilicus); uterus returning to nongravid state after parturition
What are some causes of pathologic atrophy?	Hypoxia, loss of innervation, disuse, and aging
What is the process of reversible change that occurs when one adult cell type is replaced by another adult cell type?	Metaplasia
What are the hallmarks of reversible cell injury?	Reduced oxidative phosphorylation, adenosine triphosphate (ATP) depletion, cellular swelling, ion efflux, and water influx
When does irreversible cell injury occur?	This is highly variable and largely dependent on the cell/tissue type. Continued insult can eventually lead to irreversible cell injury but the threshold at which irreversible cell injury occurs is different in different tissue types. Irreversibly injured cells invariably undergo cell death.
Define *karyolysis:*	Dissolution of the nucleus (karyo- = nucleus, -lysis = to break apart)
Define *karyorrhexis:*	Nuclear fragmentation (karyo- = nucleus, -rrhexis = rupture)
Define *pyknosis:*	Nuclear shrinkage and condensation
What are the two main types of cell death?	1. Apoptosis 2. Necrosis
Define *apoptosis:*	A process of cell death by which a cell activates enzymes ("caspases") that degrade the cell's own DNA and proteins (ie, "programmed cell death") while maintaining an intact plasma membrane. The entire cell is then phagocytized.
Define *necrosis:*	A process of cell death by lysosomal enzymatic digestion and loss of plasma membrane integrity

What are the key differences between apoptosis and necrosis?

Apoptosis may be physiologic or pathologic whereas necrosis is always pathologic; due to loss of plasma membrane integrity, necrosis often elicits inflammation in adjacent tissue; in necrosis, lysosomal enzymes may come from the dead cells (ie, autolysis) or from leukocytes.

Describe the steps of apoptosis:

Cell shrinkage, chromatin condensation and fragmentation, formation of *apoptotic bodies*, phagocytosis by macrophages.

What are the three pathways which may initiate apoptosis?

1. Intrinsic (mitochondrial) pathway
2. Extrinsic (death receptor-initiated) pathway
3. Cytotoxic T-lymphocyte mediated pathway; all three converge on executioner caspases to initiate the execution phase of apoptosis

What are the examples of triggers of apoptosis via the intrinsic pathway?

Lack of hormonal or growth factor stimulation, DNA damage leading to p53 activation

What are the examples of triggers of apoptosis via the extrinsic pathway?

Tumor necrosis factor (TNF) receptor ligands (ie, TNF-α), FAS receptor ligands (ie, FasL)

What are the key steps in the intrinsic pathway of apoptosis?

Loss of anti-apoptotic molecules (ie, Bcl-2) and gain of pro-apoptotic molecules (ie, Bak, Bax, Bim) in the mitochondrial membrane, increased mitochondrial membrane permeability and release of cytochrome *c*, activation of caspase-9

What are the key steps in the extrinsic pathway of apoptosis?

Creation of a death domain by ligand binding of TNFR1 or FAS and adaptor proteins. The death domain then cleaves and activates pro-caspase 8 (ie, creating caspase 8).

What are the key steps in the cytotoxic T-lymphocyte (CTL) mediated pathway of apoptosis?

CTLs secrete perforin allowing entry of granzyme B and activation of executioner caspases. CTLs also secrete Fas ligand to initiate the extrinsic apoptotic pathway.

What are the key steps in the execution phase of apoptosis?

Activated caspase-9 or activated caspase-8 lead to cascade and activation of caspase-3 and/or caspase-6 (executioner caspases), disruption of cytoskeletal components or cell replication machinery, and changes to cell surface molecules which facilitates phagocytosis.

What are the histologic features of necrosis?

Increased cytoplasmic eosinophilia, vacuolated cytoplasm, nuclear changes (karyolysis, pyknosis, or karyorrhexis), calcification, and inflammation in adjacent tissue

Give examples of histologic patterns of necrosis:

Liquefactive necrosis, coagulative necrosis, and caseous necrosis

In which type of necrosis is normal tissue architecture rapidly transformed into a liquid mass due to autolysis and heterolysis?

Liquefactive necrosis

Give examples of liquefactive necrosis:

Pancreatitis, bacterial abscess, central nervous system (CNS) infarction, gastric ulcer, and fungal infection

What is the common pattern of necrosis observed in ischemic and infracted tissue?

Coagulative necrosis, except for CNS ischemia/infarction

Describe the appearance of coagulative necrosis:

The tissue has a firm texture, general tissue architecture is maintained, and "ghost" outlines of necrotic, anucleated cells may be present for weeks before undergoing phagocytosis.

Describe the appearance of caseous necrosis:

The tissue has a soft "cheesy" appearance, general tissue architecture is obliterated, and "ghost" outlines of anucleated cells may be present.

When is caseous necrosis likely?

Tuberculosis or fungal infection and at the center of malignant tumors

Define *fat necrosis*:

Fat degradation with possible saponification most commonly due to release of enzymes from the pancreas

When does one see fat necrosis?

Acute pancreatitis, ruptured ulcer, penetrating trauma, and subcutaneous infection

What is surgical necrosis?

A synonym of gangrenous necrosis which is generally used to describe a limb which has lost blood supply and undergone coagulative necrosis

Define *dystrophic calcification*:

Local deposition of predominately calcium salts in injured or necrotic tissue in the setting of otherwise normal calcium levels

Define *metastatic calcification*:

Local or wide deposition of predominately calcium salts in otherwise normal tissue in the setting of hypercalcemia

What are the histologic features of dystrophic and metastatic calcification?

Amorphous, basophilic granules in intracellular, extracellular, or in both locations. Over time, ossification may occur at sites of dystrophic calcification.

Define *hypoxia*:

A state of reduced oxygen availability (ie, poor hemoglobin saturation, inadequate ventilation, hemolysis)

Define *ischemia*:

A state of significantly reduced blood flow (ie, thrombotic occlusion, trauma), which leads to tissue damage if not reversed

What are the early consequences of ischemic injury?

Transient shift to anaerobic glycolysis; disturbed ionic and fluid balance; inhibited beta-oxidation of fatty acids

What are the late consequences of ischemic injury?

Lysosomal activation; leakage of proteins into serum (creatine kinase [CK], troponin, myoglobin, cellular enzymes)

Which injures tissues faster, ischemia or hypoxia?

Ischemia. In hypoxic tissues, anaerobic glycosis can continue whereas in ischemic tissues anaerobic glycolysis stops when substrates are depleted or when there is accumulation of excessive waste products due to the impaired blood flow.

Why does reperfusion injury occur?

When blood flow is restored, cells that survived the initial ischemia may now be damaged or irreversibly injured by processes initiated by oxygen free radicals, inflammatory cells, or activation of the complement pathway.

What is the process by which lysosomes digest material from the extracellular environment?

Heterophagy

What is autophagy?

Lysosomal digestion of a cell's own components

What are the three types of intracellular accumulations?

1. Excess of a normal cellular constituent
2. Abnormal substance
3. Pigments (exogenous or endogenous)

How do intracellular accumulations of protein appear?

Generally as discrete eosinophilic cytoplasmic droplets, vacuoles, or aggregates

Which cell type scavenges for exogenous pigments?

Macrophages

What is the most common exogenous pigment?

Carbon or coal

When a person gets a tattoo, where does the pigment go?

The pigment is ingested by dermal macrophages, usually without an inflammatory response.

Give examples of endogenous pigments:

Lipofuscin, hemosiderin, melanin, hematin, bilirubin

Iron is stored in cells in the form of which pigment?

Hemosiderin

What color does hemosiderin stain?

Blue with the Prussian blue histochemical stain and yellow-brown with hematoxylin-eosin (H&E) stain

What pigment is derived from hemoglobin but contains no iron?

Bilirubin

Define *jaundice*:

Excess of bilirubin within cells and tissues

What is the only endogenous brown-black pigment and how is it formed?

Melanin; it is formed during the oxidation of tyrosine to dihydroxyphenylalanine (DOPA) by tyrosinase in melanocytes.

Define *inflammation*:

Biologic response to a perceived injurious agent that results in vascular changes which allow fluid and leukocytes into extravascular tissue.

What is acute inflammation?	Early and immediate response to injury lasting for a short duration
What features and cell type typically characterize the acute phase of inflammation?	Hyperemia (rubor), pain (dolor), heat (calor), edema/swelling (tumor); polymorphonuclear (PMN) leukocytes
What is edema?	Excess transudative or exudative fluid in the interstitial space or a body cavity
Define _transudate:_	A clear, extravascular, low-protein, low-cellularity fluid usually due to changes in hydrostatic or osmotic pressure. Specific gravity is <1.012.
Define _exudate_:	A clear to cloudy extravascular, high protein, high-cellularity fluid usually due to changes in capillary permeability. Specific gravity is >1.012.
What is the term for an exudate rich in neutrophils and parenchymal cell debris?	Pus (purulent exudate)
What is the term for an acute inflammatory process where there is an overlay of fibrin and debris on a mucous membrane?	Pseudomembrane formation
What are the key steps in acute inflammation?	Vasodilation, increased vascular permeability and exudation into extravascular tissues, intravascular stasis, and leukocyte margination
What causes vasodilation and increased vascular permeability in acute inflammation?	Inflammatory mediators such as histamine, nitric oxide, bradykinin, interleukin-1, tumor necrosis factor, and interferon-γ
Which two vasoactive amines are among the first mediators to be released in acute inflammation? Why?	1. Histamine 2. Serotonin These are the first to be released because they are present in preformed stores in mast cells, basophils, and/or platelets.
What are the steps of leukocyte extravasation?	1. Margination, rolling, and adhesion to endothelium 2. Transmigration across endothelium (leukocyte diapedesis) 3. Migration toward a chemotactic stimulus in tissues

Which cell surface molecule families play a role in leukocyte adhesion?

Selectins (P-selectin, E-selectin on endothelial cells, and L-selectin on leukocytes), immunoglobulins (ICAM-1 and VCAM-1 on endothelial cells), and integrins (on leukocytes)

What are the common chemotactic agents?

Bacterial products, complement (especially C5a), leukotrienes, cytokines (interleukin-8)

What is the major pathway by which chemotactic agents cause leukocyte movement?

Chemotactic agents bind seven-transmembrane G-protein-coupled receptors leading to activation of effector and second messenger molecules which ultimately induced cytoskeleton component polymerization and contraction.

What are the three stages of phagocytosis?

1. Recognition and attachment
2. Engulfment
3. Killing and degradation

What enzymes or molecules are involved in O_2-dependent phagocytosis?

Nicotinamide adenosine dinucleotide phosphate (NADPH) oxidase, H_2O_2 activity, superoxide radicals, NADPH oxygenase

What enzymes or molecules are involved in O_2-independent phagocytosis?

BPI (bactericidal permeability increasing protein), lactoferrin, lysozyme, major basic proteins, defensins

What is the role of the complement system in inflammation?

The complement system is a part of the innate and adaptive immune system by contributing to mediation of vascular permeability and vasodilation, leukocyte adhesion and chemotaxis, and phagocytosis.

Which complement cleavage product is a powerful chemoattractant?

C5a

Which two components of the complement system act as opsonins to coat bacteria?

1. C3b
2. iC3b

*"Be covered"

What is the role of the kinin system in inflammation?

The kinin system serves to produce bradykinin which mediates vascular permeability and vasodilation.

Which neutrophil storage structure may contain lactoferrin, lysozyme, and collagenase?

Specific granules

*Think Specific are Smaller than azurophil

| Which neutrophil storage structure may contain myeloperoxidase, defensins, and elastases? | Azurophil granules |

Table 1.1 Mediator Associations

Action	Mediator
Vasodilation	NO
Increased vascular permeability	Vasoactive amines, bradykinin
Pain	Bradykinin and prostaglandins
Chemotaxis, leukocyte activation	Leukotriene B4 and C5a
Tissue damage	NO, O_2 metabolites
Leukocyte adhesion and transmigration	Selectins, ICAM, CD31
Fever	IL-6, IL-1, TNF

Abbreviations: NO, nitric oxide; ICAM, intercellular adhesion molecule, IL, interleukin; TNF, tumor necrosis factor.

What are the four patterns of acute inflammation?	1. Serous inflammation 2. Fibrinous inflammation 3. Suppurative inflammation 4. Ulcerative inflammation
What are the four possible outcomes of acute inflammation?	1. Complete resolution 2. Fibrosis 3. Abscess formation 4. Chronic inflammation
What is chronic inflammation?	A complex process lasting weeks to months of variable degrees of concurrent active inflammation, tissue destruction, and attempts at tissue repair.
What are some causes of chronic inflammation?	Persistent infections, prolonged exposure to toxins, autoimmune diseases
What cell types are present in chronic inflammation?	Mononuclear cells predominate: macrophages/monocytes, lymphocytes, plasma cells

How do macrophages accumulate at the site of chronic inflammation?

1. Continued recruitment
2. Local proliferation
3. Immobilization at the target site by cytokines and oxidized lipids

What is a focal collection of epithelioid-macrophages surrounded by a rim of lymphocytes and plasma cells?

A granuloma

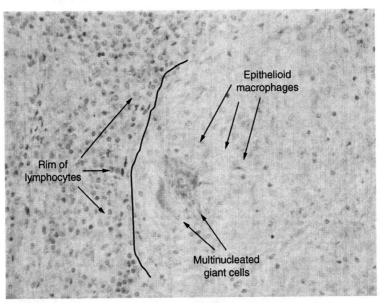

Figure 1.1   Granuloma with epithelioid macrophages, multinucleated giant cells, and rim of lymphocytes. (Reproduced, with permission, from OHSU.)

Name two types of granulomas:

1. Foreign-body granuloma
2. Immune granuloma

Give an example of a foreign body granuloma:

A nonabsorbable suture left in the body over a long time

What is the prototype of the immune granuloma?

A granuloma with central caseous necrosis (ie, tuberculosis).

What is granulomatous inflammation?

A pattern of chronic inflammation defined by the presence of granulomas.

What is granulation tissue?

It is a specialized type of connective tissue which replaces a fibrin clot during wound healing. Angiogenesis, fibroblasts producing extracellular matrix, and some inflammatory cells are present. Granulomas are not present in granulation tissue.

What are mediators of angiogenesis?

Basic fibroblast growth factor (bFGF), vascular endothelial growth factor (VEGF), vascular permeability factor (VPF)

What are the steps in wound healing and repair?

Acute inflammation, formation of granulation tissue, re-epithelialization collagen accumulation, regression of vascular channels, replacement of granulation tissue with scar, and wound contraction

How long does it take for an inflammatory exudate to be removed?

36 hours to 3–4 weeks

What is the sequence of scar formation?

1. Acute inflammation and fibrin clot formation.
2. Granulation tissue produced by fibroblasts and endothelial cells replaces fibrin clot.
3. Fibroblasts lay down vertically oriented collagen fibers at the wound margin.
4. Wound space is completely filled with granulation tissue.
5. Progressive re-epithelialization, devascularization, and collagen deposition over next 2 to 3 weeks results in a dense, white scar.

How does granulation tissue become a "scar"?

Proliferating fibroblasts in the granulation tissue lay down collagen which accumulates in the location of the eventual scar.

Define *"healing by primary intention"*:

A technical description that indicates that wound edges have been mechanically brought together. Fibrin clot will occupy the small residual space and initiate steps of wound healing.

Define *"healing by secondary intention"*:

A technical description that indicates that wound edges (usually of a large skin defect) are separated and that wound healing will require more extensive granulation tissue growth and repair. Subsequently, more wound contracture is likely to occur.

What is the ultimate source of strength for the healed wound?

Collagen

What might inhibit wound healing?

Secondary infection, foreign body acting as a nidus for inflammation, protein depletion, vitamin C deficiency, hydrocortisones, and ischemia

Define *neoplasm*:

Neo- = new, -plasia = growth. This term can be applied to any mass, benign or malignant.

Are most neoplasms monoclonal or polyclonal?

Monoclonal since they arise from proliferation of a single cell. Malignant neoplasms are monoclonal proliferations of a single cell that inherited or acquired genetic alterations which cause phenotypically malignant behavior.

What are subclones?

Tumor cells that develop over time within a monoclonal neoplasm and have additional mutations which confer a growth advantage

What are the general characteristics of a benign tumor?

Slow growth, noninfiltrative, no metastasis

What are the general characteristics of a malignant tumor?

Rapid growth, infiltrative/invasive, metastasis

What is an important determinant of tumor growth potential?

Degree of vascularization (ie, blood supply)

Define *dysplasia*:

A process wherein nuclear features of malignancy are observed but general architectural features are benign

Define *anaplasia*:

Lack of differentiation (almost always indicative of malignancy)

What does the suffix -sarcoma indicate?

A malignant neoplasm of mesenchymal origin, including bone and soft tissue

What is a carcinoma?

A malignant neoplasm of epithelial origin

What does the suffix -oma generally imply about a neoplasm?

Most commonly this indicates a benign neoplastic process (eg, hemangioma, lipoma, fibroma); however, there are notable malignant exceptions including, melanoma, hepatoma, mesothelioma.

What is a tumor that arises from germ cells and contains cells from more than one germ layer?

Teratoma

What are the most common locations for cancer in women?	Skin, breast, lung, colon, uterus
What are the most common locations for cancer in men?	Skin, prostate, lung, colon
What are the most common cancers in young children?	Acute leukemia, neuroblastoma, retinoblastoma, rhabdomyosarcoma
What cancer causes more deaths than any other cancer?	Lung cancer
What is a familial cancer syndrome?	An inherited susceptibility to malignancy, typically involving a mutation in either an oncogene (autosomal dominant) or tumor suppressor gene (autosomal recessive)
Give an example of a familial cancer syndrome:	Familial adenomatous polyposis coli
What is xeroderma pigmentosa?	Autosomal recessive syndrome of defective deoxyribonucleic acid (DNA) repair causing increased skin cancers
What are paraneoplastic syndromes?	Unexplained symptom complexes that sometimes accompany certain cancers
Give an example of a paraneoplastic syndrome:	Cushing syndrome, resulting from ectopic hormone production of corticotrophins (ACTH) by small cell lung carcinoma
What lung cancer is associated with syndrome of inappropriate antidiuretic hormone (SIADH)?	Small cell carcinoma of the lung
What is a Virchow node?	Left (usually) supraclavicular lymph node metastasis from an abdominal malignancy
What is a Trousseau sign?	Migratory venous thrombosis most often associated with pancreatic and bronchogenic carcinomas
What is the "guardian of the genome" and how do mutations affect its function?	p53, a tumor suppressor gene which normally serves to arrest the cell cycle and induce apoptosis under condition of DNA damage. When mutated, this function is lost and cells with DNA damage will continue to divide and proliferate, possibly acquiring mutations which confer malignant behavior.

Where is the p53 gene located?	Chromosome 17
What tumors are associated with Epstein-Barr virus?	1. African form of Burkitt lymphoma 2. Posttransplant B-cell lymphomas 3. Hodgkin lymphoma 4. Nasopharyngeal carcinomas
What is human T-cell leukemia virus type 1 associated with?	Adult T-cell leukemia/lymphoma, seen most often in Japan and the Caribbean, and a demyelinating disorder called tropical spastic paraparesis
What staging system is used to describe most cancers in the United States?	TNM staging (*T*umor size, Lymph *N*ode involvement, *M*etastasis)
What is the term for severe weight loss in a cancer patient?	Cancer cachexia
What causes cancer cachexia?	Etiology is unclear, perhaps soluble factors produced by the tumor; not from nutritional demands of the tumor

CLINICAL VIGNETTES

A young infant is deficient in NADPH oxygenase. What kind of infections is he more susceptible to?

Bacterial infections because of impaired phagocytosis

A 75-year-old man is noted to have calcified aortic stenosis. What is the mechanism?

The process of dystrophic calcification has taken place on his aged, atherosclerotic aortic valves.

A 5-year-old falls and bumps his knee. Three days later, there is a blue bruise. Why is it blue?

Lysis of erythrocytes causes hemoglobin to break down into other pigments.

A 57-year-old coal miner dies of an emphysematous lung disease. Describe his lungs on autopsy.

Patient has anthracosis (blackened lungs) and a fibroblastic reaction.

A 64-year-old man with renal disease and proteinuria is noted to have bone marrow cells overloaded with protein inclusions. What are they called?

Mott cells or plasma cells with multiple Russell bodies

A 3-year-old child is noted to have the ataxia, psychomotor regression, and dysarthria seen in Neiman-Pick disease type C. What is the mechanism of this disease?

Lysosomal storage disease in which cholesterol is not normally metabolized, so that there are cholesterol accumulations in cells throughout the body.

A 67-year-old smoker has lung cancer metastatic to the pleura. What kind of inflammation might one see in the pleura?

Fibrinous inflammation as a reaction to a fibrinous exudate which can form by stimulation from the cancer cells.

A child is going to receive a living donor liver transplant from his mother. How will the mother's liver regenerate?

Cytokines and polypeptide growth factors induce quiescent liver cells to divide and reconstitute the liver mass.

A 41-year-old woman is diagnosed with cervical carcinoma. Which strains of human papilloma virus are most likely to be involved?

Serotypes 16, 18, 31, 33, and 35

CHAPTER 2

Biochemistry

GENERAL PRINCIPLES

Describe the general steps of protein synthesis:

1. DNA transcribed into mRNA
2. mRNA modified and/or translated into a peptide
3. Protein folding
4. Post-translational modification

What is the significance of the R-group of an amino acid?

Amino acids present in proteins in humans are classified by their R-group, which is the unique functional side-chain moiety. The physical and chemical properties of the R-groups (aliphatic, aromatic, neutral polar, acidic, basic, or sulfur-containing) will influence protein solubility as well as stabilize tertiary protein structure. R-groups also play an important role as buffers by accepting protons under more acidic conditions and donating protons under more basic conditions.

What is an enzyme? What do enzymes do?

An enzyme is a protein that functions to accelerate the rate of a biological reaction by decreasing the activation energy of the reaction. Regulation of enzyme activity allows for adaptation to changing physiologic conditions.

What parameters can influence enzymatic reactions?

Enzyme activity can be affected by changes in temperature, salinity, pH, active site structure, and the presence of competitive and noncompetitive inhibitors.

What are the differences between competitive and noncompetitive enzyme inhibition?

Competitive inhibitors bind reversibly to the active site while noncompetitive inhibitors may bind the active site or distant sites. Competitive inhibition can be overcome by high substrate concentrations whereas noncompetitive inhibition cannot.

What are the general mechanisms of enzyme regulation?

Gene transcription controlling protein synthesis; activation or inactivation by proteolytic enzymes; activation or inactivation by covalent modification (phosphorylation); allosteric regulation by small molecules binding sites distant from the active site; degradation of enzymes by intracellular proteases or in proteasomes

What enzymes participate in DNA replication?

DNA polymerase, DNA ligase, primase

What is the name given to segments of DNA which are spliced out of primary mRNA transcripts?

Introns

Give examples of posttranscriptional RNA modification:

5′ capping, 3′ poly-A tail, splicing

What is a Southern blot?

A technique where electrophoresed *DNA* is transferred to a membrane, which is probed with a "reporter" - labeled DNA sequence. The hybridized membrane is exposed to film to determine the specific size of the targeted DNA (eg, to identify restriction fragment length polymorphisms).

What is a Northern blot?

A technique where electrophoresed *RNA* is transferred to a membrane, which is probed with a "reporter" - labeled DNA sequence. The hybridized membrane is exposed to film to determine if the size of the RNA transcript on the membrane corresponds to the size of a specific known gene transcript in order to measure expression levels of that gene.

What is a Western blot?

A technique where electrophoresed *protein* is transferred to a membrane, which is probed with a "reporter" - labeled antibody. The hybridized membrane is exposed to film to determine if the size of the targeted protein corresponds to the size of a specific known protein in order to measure expression levels of that gene.

What is enzyme-linked immunosorbent assay (ELISA)?

A technique which uses antigen or antibody coupled with a chromogen-tagged enzyme to detect the presence of an antibody or antigen, respectively, in a test sample.

Describe the role of cell membranes in signal transduction:

Cell membranes are the physical barrier that serves to maintain ionic concentration gradients which facilitate nerve conduction as well as facilitated diffusion and active transport of molecules. Cell membranes also contain integral and transmembrane proteins which directly transport signal molecules or which may be involved in second messenger pathways.

What are the intracellular concentrations of Na^+, K^+, and Ca^{2+}?

K^+ is the predominant intracellular ion (140 mEq) while Na^+ (10 mEq) and Ca^{2+} (1-2 mEq) are less concentrated.

What are the extracellular concentrations of Na^+, K^+, and Ca^{2+}?

Na^+ is the predominant extracellular ion (140 mEq) while K^+ (5 mEq) and Ca^{2+} (10^{-4} mEq) are less concentrated.

How are substances transported across biomembranes?

Substances are transported either via diffusion (simple or facilitated) or by active transport (primary or secondary). The important difference between these two processes is that active transport requires energy input by hydrolysis of ATP whereas diffusion requires no energy input.

What is the difference between simple diffusion and facilitated diffusion?

Simple diffusion is driven by the concentration gradient of the molecule that is moving across the membrane. Due to the nature of the lipid bilayer of cell membranes, molecules that are capable of diffusion are small and hydrophobic. Facilitated diffusion is driven by the electrochemical gradient across the membrane.

What is the difference between primary and secondary active transport?

Primary active transport relies on energy released from hydrolysis of ATP by ATPases in cell membranes to move ions and other molecules across cell membranes. Secondary active transport utilizes the electrochemical gradient established by primary active transport to move larger molecules (ie, sugars and amino acids) across cell membranes.

What is the biochemical significance of albumin?

Albumin has several important biochemical roles. It serves as a marker of nutritional depletion, is an osmotic regulator of fluid shifts between intravascular and extravascular spaces, and also functions as a transport protein. Albumin is a small, highly polar molecule, which at physiologic pH has a high capacity for nonspecific binding of ligands (ie, drugs) and for buffering changes in pH by binding protons.

In what clinical situations would a patient's caloric needs be increased?

Extensive burns, pregnancy, increased physical activity level, postsurgery, or posttrauma

What is the purpose of glycolysis?

To anaerobically metabolize glucose to produce ATP as well as to create substrates for other biochemical pathways (ie, pentose phosphate pathway) and, especially in RBCs, to create 2,3-bisphosphoglycerate which regulates the affinity of oxygen for hemoglobin

What is the purpose of the tricarboxylic acid (TCA) cycle?

In cells that have mitochondria, the TCA cycle uses fat, carbohydrate, and protein substrates to produce reduced coenzymes ($FADH_2$ and NADH) which are used in the generation of ATP in the electron transport chain. The TCA cycle does not use oxygen in any of its reactions, but it requires oxygen for reoxidation of reduced coenzymes. The TCA cycle is also involved in the production of substrates for storage molecules.

What is the purpose of the electron transport chain?

To produce ATP via a series of redox reactions using NADH and $FADH_2$ produced in the TCA cycle

What is gluconeogenesis and where does it occur?

Gluconeogenesis is a metabolic pathway that produces glucose from pyruvate. It can occur only in the liver, kidney, and intestinal epithelium.

What is the pentose phosphate shunt and where does it occur?

The pentose phosphate shunt is a metabolic pathway that produces ribose-5-phosphate to be used in nucleotide synthesis and NADPH to be used in fatty acid and steroid biosynthesis. This pathway occurs in the liver, adrenal cortex, and lactating mammary glands.

Which proteins are involved in movement of oxygen within the human body?

Hemoglobin is a protein responsible for oxygen transport and is found exclusively in RBCs. Myoglobin is a protein that stores oxygen in the cytoplasm of skeletal and striated muscle cells and delivers it when needed to mitochondria.

Which are considered to be "normal" variants of hemoglobin?

Adult hemoglobin is mostly HbA $(\alpha_2\beta_2)$ and a small percentage (4%) HbA_2 $(\alpha_2\gamma_2)$. Fetal hemoglobin is a normal hemoglobin during fetal life and comprises <1% of adult hemoglobin.

Give examples of common pathologic hemoglobin variants:

Hemoglobin S, hemoglobin C, and hemoglobin E

What parameters influence the degree of oxygen saturation of hemoglobin?

The oxygen affinity for hemoglobin is regulated by $[H^+]$, $[CO_2]$, $[2,3\text{-BPG}]$, temperature, and metabolic needs of the tissue.

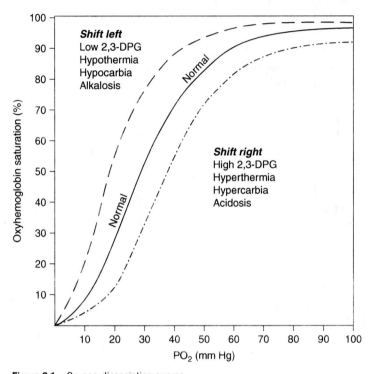

Figure 2.1   Oxygen dissociation curves.

DNA/RNA/PROTEIN PATHOLOGY

What autosomal recessive disorder results in the inability to repair thymidine dimers which form in DNA after exposure to UV light?

Xeroderma pigmentosum

What is the common abnormality in lysosomal storage diseases?

A deficiency in a lysosomal enzyme which leads to accumulation of the enzyme's substrate in various tissues in the body (eg, Gaucher disease "crumpled tissue paper cells")

Which vitamin is required for collagen synthesis?

Vitamin C

What syndrome is the result of defective collagen synthesis causing hyperextensible skin, hypermobile joints, and a tendency to bleed?	Ehlers-Danlos syndrome, also associated with the presence of berry aneurysms
In what syndrome is defective collagen (type I) synthesis associated with blue sclerae and multiple bone fractures due to minimal trauma?	Osteogenesis imperfecta
Which syndrome is associated with long limbs, kyphosis, cardiac abnormalities, and a mutation of the fibrillin gene?	Marfan syndrome

NUTRITIONAL DISORDERS

What is marasmus?	A nutritional deficiency of *both* total calories and protein
What age group is usually affected by marasmus?	Children less than 1 year
What is kwashiorkor?	A nutritional protein deficiency in the setting of adequate total calorie intake
What are the distinguishing features of kwashiorkor?	*M*alabsorption (atrophy of intestinal villi); *E*dema—most important; *A*nemia; *L*iver is fatty; *S*ubcutaneous layer still present *Kwashiorkor lacks **MEALS** with protein
What is the significance of the edema seen in kwashiorkor?	Due to protein deficiency and decreased oncotic pressure
What dermatologic findings are associated with kwashiorkor?	Depigmented bands in hair and skin

VITAMINS AND MINERALS

Which are the fat-soluble vitamins?	Vitamins A, D, E, K *KADE*
Why are fat-soluble vitamins potentially toxic?	Fat-soluble vitamins accumulate in body fat stores. This can lead to toxic blood levels of a substance and with additional redistribution of fat-stored substance into the blood; toxic levels are not easily correctable.

What are the symptoms associated with vitamin A deficiency?

Ocular abnormalities—xerophthalmia, night blindness, and keratomalacia (corneal softening); squamous metaplasia of respiratory tract

Describe the role vitamin A plays in producing vision:

Rhodopsin is a visual pigment found in rod cells of the retinal which contains vitamin A, specifically in the form of 11-*cis*-retinal. With light, 11-*cis*-retinal is converted to all-*trans* retinal which initiates transduction of a nerve impulse in the optic nerve.

Briefly describe the metabolic pathway by which vitamin A is obtained from the diet:

Vitamin A is found in animal products in the form of retinol, retinal, and retinoic acid. The provitamin form, β-carotene, is found in plant products. β-Carotene is metabolized to all-*trans* retinol by β-carotene dioxygenase in the small bowel. Retinol and retinoic acid are stored in the liver as retinol palmitate.

What foods contain high amounts of vitamin A in the form of retinoids?

Liver; egg yolk; butter

What foods contain β-carotene?

Carrots; leafy green vegetables

What are the changes seen in hypervitaminosis A?

Alopecia; liver damage; bone changes

What is the role of vitamin K in clotting cascades?

Vitamin K is necessary for the carboxylation of glutamyl residues in the synthesis of activated clotting factors.

Vitamin K is used for the production of which clotting factors?

Factors II, VII, IX, and X, protein C and protein S

Why are newborn infants susceptible to vitamin K deficiency?

Placental transfer of vitamin K is very limited and the fetal liver does not store significant quantities. Breast milk is a good source of vitamin K. Most infants born in hospitals are given vitamin K at birth as prophylaxis.

How do children and adults get vitamin K?

Dairy products; yellow and green vegetables; synthesized by intestinal flora

What does deficiency of vitamin E cause?   Erythrocyte fragility (hemolysis)

What symptoms are caused by vitamin D deficiency?   Rickets; Osteomalacia; Tetany (hypocalcemia)

*Bones **ROT** without vitamin D

What is an important source of vitamin D?   Milk and dairy products

What occurs with an excess of vitamin D?   Hypercalcemia—vitamin D regulates calcium absorption in the gut and bone reabsorption. Hypercalcemia may result in hypercalciuria and nephrolithiasis.

What are the symptoms of hypercalcemia?   Bone pain; kidney stones; constipation; central nervous system (CNS) symptoms—depression, confusion, stupor

*Stones, bones, groans (abdominal pain), and psychiatric overtones

Which form of vitamin D is the active form?   1,25-Dihydroxycholecalciferol $(1,25\text{-}(OH)_2\ D_3)$

Which form is the storage form of vitamin D?   25-Hydroxycholecalciferol $(25\text{-}OHD_3)$

Which form of vitamin D is consumed in milk? D_2 (ergocalciferol)

Which form of vitamin D is formed by sun exposure on skin? D_3 (cholecalciferol)

How does sarcoidosis affect vitamin D metabolism?   In sarcoidosis, epithelioid macrophages contribute to increased conversion to activated vitamin D leading to hypercalcemia.

Which are the water-soluble vitamins?   B vitamins; vitamin C; folic acid

Which are the B complex vitamins? $B_1\ B_2,\ B_3,\ B_5,\ B_6$

*All Bs except 12

What food sources contain the B complex vitamins?   Leafy green vegetables; whole grain cereals; animal products: meat, fish, and dairy

What is the psychiatric syndrome of B_1 deficiency?

Wernicke-Korsakoff syndrome

What is the usual setting for Wernicke-Korsakoff syndrome?

Alcoholics with malnutrition (lacking B_1)

What are the characteristic findings of a Wernicke triad?

*M*ental confusion; *O*phthalmoplegia/ *N*ystagmus; *A*taxia

*Wernicke patients *MOAN*

What symptom is characteristic of a Korsakoff psychosis?

Confabulation

What degenerative changes are seen in the brains of patients with Wernicke-Korsakoff?

Hemorrhagic lesions of mamillary bodies and paramedian gray matter

What cardiac syndrome is associated with B_1 deficiency?

Wet beriberi

What is wet beriberi?

Fluid retention associated with myocardial dysfunction (high-output cardiac failure)

What type of cardiomyopathy is associated with wet beriberi and thiamine deficiency?

Dilated cardiomyopathy

What is dry beriberi (also due to thiamine [B_1] deficiency)?

Peripheral neuropathy and atrophy of extremities

What biochemical pathways use B_1 as a cofactor?

Oxidative carboxylation for α-keto acids (pyruvate and α-ketoglutarate); transketolase in hexose monophosphate (HMP) shunt

What biochemical pathway uses riboflavin?

Oxidation and reduction using flavin adenine dinucleotide (FAD) and flavin mononucleotide (FMN)

*2*F*s go with ribo*F*lavin (B_2)

What is the triad of dermatitis, dementia, and diarrhea called?

Pellagra (eg, Niacin deficiency)

What are the biochemical pathways that use niacin (B_3)?

Reduction and oxidation reactions with nicotinamide adenine dinucleotide (NAD) and nicotinamide adenine dinucleotide phosphate (NADP)

*N reactions go with Niacin

What diseases can cause B_3 deficiency and symptoms of pellagra?

Hartnup disease because of inadequate tryptophan absorption in the gut and inadequate reabsorption in the renal tubules; carcinoid syndrome because tryptophan is being used by the tumor to synthesize serotonin instead of niacin.

What is the biochemical function of vitamin B_5?

Fatty acid synthesis—part of coenzyme A (CoA)

What antituberculosis medication predisposes to vitamin B_6 deficiency?

Isoniazid (INH)

What biochemical pathways need vitamin B_6?

γ-Aminobutyric acid (GABA) production (neurotransmitter); transamination cofactor; decarboxylation reaction cofactor

What food products contain cobalamin?

Animal products contain cobalamin, but it is exclusively synthesized by bacteria. Cobalamin is not present in plant products.

What is a likely cause of the vitamin B_{12} deficiency in a Japanese immigrant?

Diphyllobothrium latum (fish tapeworm)

What are the causes of B_{12} deficiency?

Vegan diet; *D. latum*; pernicious anemia; Crohn disease (terminal ileum)

What causes cobalamin deficiency in pernicious anemia?

Lack of intrinsic factor

Which test localizes cobalamin (B_{12}) deficiency?

Shilling test

*12 *Cobalt* colored *shillings*

What biochemical pathways require vitamin B_{12}?

Homocysteine methylation to methionine; methylmalonyl-CoA to succinyl-CoA

What neurologic complication may result from B_{12} deficiency?

Abnormal myelin production

Table 2.1 Vitamin Review

Vitamin	Name
Vitamin A	Retinol (think retin A)
Vitamin B_1	Thiamine
Vitamin B_2	*Rib*oflavin (think 2 sides of ribs)
Vitamin B_5	Pantothenate (think pantothenate has five vowels)
Vitamin B_6	Pyridoxine (think pyridoXine and siX)
Vitamin B_{12}	Cobalamin

What vitamin is a required supplement during very early pregnancy to prevent neural tube defects?

Folic acid

What is the most common vitamin deficiency in the United States?

Folic acid deficiency

What does folic acid deficiency cause?

Macrocytic, megaloblastic anemia without neurologic symptoms (as opposed to vitamin B_{12})

What biochemical pathways require folic acid?

Methylation reactions; synthesis of nitrogenous bases (purines and thymine)

What disease is caused by deficiency of vitamin C?

Scurvy (ie, collagen deficiency which results in synthesis of defective connective tissue and can lead to poor bone formation in infants and abnormal bleeding and loss of teeth in adults)

What biochemical pathway requires vitamin C?

Cross-linking collagen
*Vitamin C Cross-links Collagen

What deficiency is caused by eating raw eggs (which contain avidin)?

Biotin deficiency. Avidin binds biotin in the gut and prevents biotin absorption.

What are the symptoms of biotin deficiency?

Dermatitis and gastroenteritis

Which mineral deficiency is associated with Menke disease, an X-linked disease with symptoms of kinky hair and mental retardation?

Copper deficiency

What autosomal recessive (AR) disease is caused by an increase in copper accumulation characterized by decreased ceruloplasmin, hepatolenticular degeneration, asterixis, dementia, Kayser-Fleischer rings on cornea, and choreiform movements?	Wilson disease
What is the treatment for Wilson disease?	Penicillamine
Give examples of essential trace elements:	Iron, zinc, chromium, selenium, magnesium, and copper

POISONING/CHEMICAL INJURY

How does cyanide work?	Prevents oxidative metabolism by inhibiting cytochrome oxidase
What are the antidotes for cyanide poisoning?	Thiosulfate; hydroxocobalamin
What are the pathological findings associated with carbon tetrachloride (CCl_4) exposure?	Centrilobular necrosis and fatty change of the liver
How does CO cause death?	CO binds hemoglobin with a much greater affinity ($20\times$) than oxygen, preventing oxygen transport to tissues, and causing extensive hypoxic injury.
How does methanol cause blindness?	Methanol is metabolized to formic acid and formaldehyde by alcohol dehydrogenase, causing metabolic acidosis and retinal and optic nerve damage.
What is the treatment for methanol poisoning?	Ethanol or dialysis. Ethanol competes for metabolism by alcohol dehydrogenase preventing conversion of methanol (and also ethylene glycol) to formic acid and formaldehyde.
What kidney damage is associated with ethylene glycol?	Acute tubular necrosis
What are the treatments for ethylene glycol toxicity?	Fomepizole, ethanol

What is the antidote for limited ingestion of mercuric chloride?

Raw egg whites—mercuric chloride will bind albumin to form a nearly insoluble precipitate

What red blood cell changes are seen in lead toxicity?

Basophilic stippling

Why does lead toxicity cause a hypochromic, microcytic anemia?

Lead toxicity results in decreased heme synthesis, producing cellular changes similar to those seen in iron-deficiency anemia.

What enzyme does lead inhibit in heme synthesis?

δ-Aminolevulinic acid (ALA) dehydratase

What x-ray findings are consistent with lead toxicity?

Increased radiodensity of long bone epiphyses

What renal syndrome is associated with lead toxicity?

Fanconi syndrome

What is Fanconi syndrome?

Impaired renal reabsorption of amino acids, glucose, and phosphate

What are the antidotes for lead poisoning?

Succimer; penicillamine; calcium ethylenediaminetetraacetic acid (EDTA); dimercaprol

Table 2.2 Antidotes

Overdose	Antidote
Acetaminophen	N-Acetylcysteine
Benzodiazepines	Flumazenil
β-Blockers	Glucagon
Opioids	Naloxone
Tricyclic antidepressants	Sodium bicarbonate
Quinidine	Sodium bicarbonate
Iron	Deferoxamine
Warfarin	Vitamin K

What are the symptoms of cholinesterase inhibitor poisoning with organophosphates?	Salivation; Lacrimation; Urination; Diarrhea; Salivation; Bradycardia; Miosis
	*SLUDS syndrome with BM
What is the antidote for organophosphate poisoning?	Atropine
What are the symptoms of anticholinergic intoxication?	Blurry vision, mydriasis, dry and flushed skin, fever, delirium and hallucinations, decreased bowel sounds or ileus, and urinary retention
	*Blind as a bat, dry as a bone, red as a beet, hot as Hades, and mad as a hatter

ADVERSE EFFECTS OF DRUGS

Which antibiotic is associated with gray baby syndrome and fetal aplastic anemia?	Chloramphenicol
Which class of antihypertensive drugs causes side effects of cough and angioedema?	Angiotensin-converting enzyme (ACE) inhibitors
Which drug can cause side effects of gingival hyperplasia, hirsutism, and folate deficiency?	Phenytoin
Which drug can cause profuse cutaneous flushing (ie, red man syndrome)?	Vancomycin
What lipid-lowering agent is associated with severe flushing?	Niacin
Which drugs have a side effect of diabetes insipidus?	Demeclocycline; lithium; methoxyflurane
Which drugs have lupus-like symptoms?	Hydralazine; INH; Procainamide; Phenytoin
	*It's not HIPP to have lupus-like side effects
Which drugs cause side effects of pulmonary fibrosis?	Busulfan; Bleomycin
	*Bleo makes it hard to blow

Which drugs are associated with photosensitivity reactions?	*S*ulfonamides; *A*miodarone; *T*etracycline *SAT for a photo
Which drug is associated with tendonitis in children?	Fluoroquinolones *Fluoroquinolones hurt attachments to kid's bones
Which drug is associated with hemorrhagic cystitis?	Cyclophosphamide
Which drugs are associated with agranulocytosis?	*C*lozapine; *C*arbamazepine; *C*olchicine *Three *C*s of Agranulo*C*ytosis
Which drugs are associated with gynecomastia?	*S*pironolactone; *D*igitalis; *C*imetidine; *E*strogen; *K*etoconazole **S*ome *D*rugs *C*reate *E*nlarged *K*nockers

BIOCHEMICAL DISEASES

What autosomal recessive disease is characterized by hypoglycemia, jaundice, and cirrhosis with lab values showing an increase in fructose-1-phosphate and a decrease in phosphate values?	Hereditary fructose intolerance
What enzyme is deficient in hereditary fructose intolerance?	Aldolase B
Foods containing what ingredients should be avoided in hereditary fructose intolerance?	Fructose and sucrose
What benign syndrome is characterized by fructose appearing in blood and urine?	Essential fructosuria
What enzyme is abnormal in essential fructosuria?	Fructokinase
What AR disease is characterized by cataracts, mental retardation, hepatosplenomegaly, and accumulation of toxic substances such as galactitol?	Galactosemia

What enzyme is deficient in galactosemia? How is this related to galactitol production?	Galactose-1-phosphate. As a result of this deficiency, galactose-1-phosphate may be metabolized by other enzymes (ie, aldose reductase) into substances, such as galactitol, which become toxic in excessive amounts.
What food contents must be avoided with galactosemia?	Galactose and lactose
What is the main clinical finding associated with deficiencies in any of the glycolytic enzymes?	Hemolytic anemia (because RBCs depend solely on glycolysis for energy)
What enzyme deficiency causes altered mental status and lactic acidosis as well as an increase in pyruvate and alanine levels?	Pyruvate dehydrogenase deficiency
What is the treatment for pyruvate dehydrogenase deficiency?	Increase dietary fat and ketogenic amino acids
Which are the two purely ketogenic amino acids?	1. Leucine 2. Lysine
What inheritance pattern does glucose-6-phosphate deficiency follow?	X-linked recessive
What drugs/foods precipitate hemolytic anemia in glucose-6-phosphate deficient patients?	Primaquine and antimalarials; sulfa drugs; antituberculosis drugs; fava beans
What is the enzyme deficiency in alkaptonuria?	Homogentisic acid oxidase, which is an enzyme in the tyrosine breakdown pathway
What disease results from an inherited defect in the amino acid transporter for cystine, ornithine, arginine, and lysine in the kidney and kidney stones made of cystine?	Cystinuria
Which amino acids does cystinuria affect?	*C*ystine; *O*rnithine; *A*rginine; *L*ysine *COAL*
What disease is caused by disrupted degradation of branched chain amino acids, has decreased amounts of α-keto acid dehydrogenase, and is characterized by mental retardation, CNS abnormalities, and urine that smells like maple syrup?	Maple syrup urine disease

What are the three branched amino acids?	1. Isoleucine 2. Leucine 3. Valine *I Love Vermont maple syrup
What enzyme is deficient in PKU?	Phenylalanine hydroxylase; PKU can also result from reduced amounts of tetrahydrobiopterin, a necessary cofactor for phenylalanine hydroxylase.
What foods must be eliminated from the diet in patients with PKU?	Any foods containing phenylalanine
What amino acid must be added to the diet?	Tyrosine; without the ability to synthesis tyrosine from phenylalanine, tyrosine becomes an essential amino acid.
How are most cases of PKU discovered?	Screening tests done at birth and 2 weeks of age
A deficiency in which enzyme in the purine salvage pathway can cause SCID?	Adenosine deaminase
What is the inheritance pattern in Lesch-Nyhan syndrome?	X-linked recessive
What enzyme is deficient in Lesch-Nyhan syndrome?	Hypoxanthine-guanine phosphoribosyltransferase (HGPRT) in the purine salvage pathway. This leads to increased serum uric acid and clinical features including mental retardation, self-mutilation, aggression, gout, and choreoathetosis.
Which glycogen storage disease is characterized by glucose-6-phosphatase deficiency?	von Gierke disease
Which glycogen storage disease is characterized by deficiency of lysosomal α-1,4-glucosidase?	Pompe disease
Which glycogen storage disease has a deficiency of the debranching enzyme α-1,6-glucosidase?	Cori disease
Which glycogen storage disease is characterized skeletal muscle phosphorylase deficiency?	McArdle disease *McArdle is a myoglobinuria and muscle problem

Which X-linked recessive lysosomal storage disease is characterized by deficiency of α-galactosidase A?	Fabry disease
What two lysosomal storage diseases are X-linked recessive?	1. Hunter syndrome 2. Fabry disease
What X-linked recessive lysosomal storage disease is associated with deficiency of iduronate sulfatase?	Hunter syndrome *A **Hunter** with a gun should not have clouded corneas or severe mental retardation (but a **Hurler** does)
What AR lysosomal storage disease is characterized by a deficiency of α-iduronidase?	Hurler syndrome
What two lysosomal storage diseases result in accumulation of mucopolysaccharides?	1. Hunter syndrome 2. Hurler syndrome
What lysosomal storage disease is characterized by a deficiency of β-glucocerebrosidase?	Gaucher disease *GauCher: problems with GC—Gathered Crinkled cells, GlucoCerebroside increase, and β-GlucoCerebrosidase deficiency
What AR disease is caused by deficiency of hexosaminidase A?	Tay-Sachs disease
What AR disease is caused by a deficiency of sphingomyelinase?	Niemann-Pick disease
What lysosomal storage disease is characterized by a deficiency of galactosylceramide β-galactosidase with an accumulation of galactocerebroside in the brain?	Krabbe disease
What lysosomal storage disease is characterized by deficiency of arylsulfatase A?	Metachromic leukodystrophy

CLINICAL VIGNETTES

A 10-month-old child is found after being abandoned by his parents. On physical examination, the child is grossly underweight and has severe growth retardation. There is obvious loss of muscle and subcutaneous fat. What is the diagnosis?

Marasmus

A 3-year-old child is rescued by child protective services and brought to clinic for evaluation. On physical examination, the child has obvious growth retardation and muscle wasting, but he has preservation of subcutaneous fat. The child also has severe edema of the face, hands, and feet. What is the most likely diagnosis?

Kwashiorkor

A 35-year-old woman presents with night blindness, frequent bone fractures, and increased bleeding when injured. She reports having diarrhea whenever she eats certain grain-containing foods. What is the diagnosis?

Celiac sprue with fat-soluble vitamin deficiency

A 7-year-old white boy presents with frequent respiratory infections, growth retardation, rickets, and fatty stools. His mother remarks that his skin is always salty. What is the most likely diagnosis?

Cystic fibrosis with fat-soluble vitamin deficiency

A 45-year-old woman presents with night blindness, dry eyes, and dry skin. She is a self-proclaimed "picky-eater," eating mostly breads and pasta. She does not eat animal products and dislikes most vegetables. What is the most likely cause of her symptoms?

Vitamin A deficiency

A 3-day-old girl infant presents to the ER with seizures. Her birth history was insignificant except that she was born at home with the help of a midwife. Her parents report no history of trauma, but on computed tomography (CT), there is a large subdural hematoma. What is the likely mechanism of this injury?

Vitamin K deficiency and hemorrhagic disease of the newborn

*K is for Klotting

A 4-year-old child from Asia presents with bending of several bones in the lower extremity. On x-ray, the bones are bowed and malformed with deficient calcification of the osteoid matrix. What is the diagnosis and vitamin deficiency?

Rickets and vitamin D deficiency

A 47-year-old white man presents to the ER after being found under an overpass. He has a history of polysubstance abuse. When questioned, he gives strange answers that seem implausible, and he is easily confused. On physical examination, he appears malnourished, is ataxic, and has nystagmus. What is the vitamin deficiency?

B_1 (thiamine) deficiency

A 12-year-old immigrant from Uganda presents to the clinic with cheilosis, angular stomatitis, glossitis, seborrheic dermatitis, and corneal vascularization. What is the vitamin deficiency?

B$_2$ (riboflavin) deficiency

A 92-year-old white man presents with diarrhea, dementia, and dermatitis of gradual onset. On physical examination, he also has beefy glossitis. What is the most likely vitamin deficiency?

Vitamin B$_3$ (niacin) deficiency
*3 Ds go with B$_3$

An 82-year-old presents with alopecia, gastroenteritis, and a rash. He has low blood pressure and labs show adrenal insufficiency. What is the vitamin deficiency?

Vitamin B$_5$ (pantothenate)

A 69-year-old Hispanic jail inmate presents with new-onset convulsions and hyperirritability. His past medical history is significant for tuberculosis, which is currently being treated. Which vitamin may be deficient?

Vitamin B$_6$ (pyridoxine)

A 34-year-old vegan presents with vision problems and numbness and tingling in his legs. Lab values show a macrocytic and megaloblastic anemia. What is the most likely vitamin deficiency?

Vitamin B$_{12}$ (cobalamin)

A 78-year-old immigrant from a small fishing village in Japan presents with paresthesias in his extremities, vitiligo, and is found to have a macrocytic, megaloblastic anemia. What is the most likely diagnosis?

Vitamin B$_{12}$ deficiency with *D. latum* infection

A 48-year-old immigrant from a poor town in Russia presents with poor wound healing, fragile skin, and easy bruising. On physical examination, he has many bruises, open sores, and swollen gums with many teeth missing. Lab values show anemia. What is the vitamin deficiency?

Vitamin C (ascorbic acid)

A 35-year-old white woman is found dead at her home. She was going through a divorce and her family suspects that her husband has done something that resulted in her death. At autopsy, the pathologist recognizes a distinct scent of bitter almonds and notes no abnormalities except for scattered petechial hemorrhages. What is the most likely cause of death?

Cyanide poisoning

A 78-year-old Chinese man is diagnosed with stomach and esophageal cancer. For most of his life, his diet included smoked fish and cured foods. What chemical carcinogen has he been exposed to?

Nitrosamines

A 62-year-old plant employee presents with liver failure associated with cirrhosis and angiosarcoma of the liver. He claims that exposure to chemicals on the job while making polyvinyl chloride (PVC) piping has caused his illness. What chemical exposure is likely?

Vinyl chloride

A 45-year-old shipbuilder presents with weight loss and difficulty breathing. Chest x-ray shows a mass and a biopsy performed diagnoses mesothelioma. To what was this man exposed?

Asbestos

A 66-year-old man with hepatocellular carcinoma works at a peanut shelling and processing company. What environmental exposure is likely?

Aflatoxin

A family is found dead in their home after a large ice storm and power outage. There was an old gas heater warming the home. At autopsy, the bodies have a cherry-red coloration of the lips, viscera, and muscles. What is the most likely cause of death?

Carbon monoxide (CO) poisoning

A 57-year-old presents to the ER with blindness. He says that he drank a bottle of homemade moonshine last night. What has this man been poisoned with?

Methanol (methyl alcohol)

A 49-year-old leather tanner presents with hematuria. He is diagnosed with transitional cell carcinoma of the urinary bladder. What environmental exposure has been implicated in the formation of bladder cancer?

Aniline dyes

A 2-year-old child is rushed to the ED after drinking some green fluid in the garage while his parents were not looking. His urine shows calcium oxalate crystals. What did the child drink?

Antifreeze containing ethylene glycol

A 67-year-old industrial plant worker presents with a triad of symptoms including chloracne, impotence, and visual disturbance. What chemical exposure is most likely responsible?

Polychlorinated biphenyls (PCBs)

A 57-year-old paper mill worker has been exposed to mercuric chloride, an antifungal agent. What symptoms should be watched for with exposure to mercuric chloride?

Gastrointestinal ulceration; renal damage and calcification

A 3-year-old child is brought to clinic with developmental delays and irritability. The mother mentions that she is renovating their historic home. On physical examination, the child has gray lines on his gums and teeth and a foot drop. Lab values show a hypochromic, microcytic anemia. What is the cause of this child's symptoms?

Lead toxicity from lead paint chips

A 3-year-old presents to the ER with decreased alertness and fluctuating consciousness. The child's mother gave the child aspirin because it had the flu. The child is found to have hypoglycemia and liver biopsy shows fatty microvesicular change. What is the diagnosis?

Reye syndrome (aspirin with viral illness)

A 64-year-old man presents with fever, painful cramping, and profuse diarrhea. He had a wound infection that was successfully treated with oral clindamycin 1 week ago. What is the diagnosis?

Pseudomembranous colitis (*Clostridium difficile*)

A 35-year-old is brought to the ER with severe hypertension and diaphoresis. She said that the symptoms began while she was at a wine and cheese party. She denies all medication except for an antidepressant. Which antidepressant drug class causes these symptoms of tyramine crisis?

Monoamine oxidase inhibitors (MAOI)

A 23-year-old woman undergoing a tonsillectomy has a severe reaction to inhaled anesthetics. The anesthesiologist administered halothane and succinylcholine before the patient's core temperature rose to above 104°F. What drug treats this condition?

Dantrolene (treats malignant hyperthermia)

A 46-year-old African American woman suffers from bloating, cramps, and osmotic diarrhea each time she consumes dairy products. What is the likely cause of her discomfort?

Lactase deficiency

A 56-year-old African American man presents with symptoms of hemolytic anemia. Heinz body precipitate is found within red blood cells. The man is currently taking a sulfonamide antibiotic for an infection. What enzyme is likely to be deficient in this patient?

Glucose-6-phosphate dehydrogenase

A 30-year-old healthy man presents for a regular checkup with complaints of occasional muscle and bone aches. He mentions that occasionally his urine turns black when it is allowed to sit for a few hours. What is the most likely diagnosis?

Alkaptonuria/ochronosis

A 17-month-old child is brought to the clinic for developmental delay. The birth history was uneventful and the child was full-term when he was born at home in the presence of a midwife. On physical examination, the child is fair-skinned and has eczema on his arms. The mother says that he has a strange musty odor. What is the most likely diagnosis?

Phenylketonuria (PKU)

A full-term child is born to African American parents. Upon initial physical examination, it is obvious that the child has a complete lack of pigment in his skin, eyes, and hair. What congenital enzyme deficiency can result in albinism?

Tyrosinase deficiency leading to melanin deficiency

An 8-month-old child presents to the ER with a severe upper respiratory infection. He has required multiple hospitalizations in the past months for various life-threatening infections. Lab values show severe B-cell and T-cell deficiencies. What is the most likely diagnosis?

Severe combined immunodeficiency disease (SCID)

A 4-year-old white boy is brought to clinic by his mother. She is very worried about his developmental delay, as well as other disturbing behaviors including aggression and self-mutilation. He has also had an unusual diagnosis of gout last year. What is the most likely diagnosis?

Lesch-Nyhan syndrome

CHAPTER 3

Genetic Pathology

GENERAL PRINCIPLES

What is the normal human chromosomal complement?	46,XX or 46,XY
What is the normal human haploid number?	23
What is aneuploidy?	Possessing a chromosome number that is not a multiple of the normal haploid number, typically arising from an error in meiosis or mitosis
What are the most common causes of aneuploidy?	Meiotic nondisjunction or failure of chromosomal separation during anaphase of meiosis I (anaphase lag)
What are the most common aneuploidies?	Trisomy and monosomy (Trisomy 21 is the most common chromosomal disorder.)
What is the condition of having one or more additional sets of the haploid number of chromosomes?	Polyploidy (eg, tetraploidy or triploidy)
What is the term for a specific copy of a gene?	Allele
What is the term for loss of part of a chromosome?	Deletion
What is an inversion?	Chromosomal rearrangement resulting from two break points on the same chromosome, with subsequent reversal and reincorporation into the chromosome.

What is the term for two nonhomologous chromosomes exchanging segments?

Translocation

What is a Robertsonian translocation?

An exchange of chromosomal segments between two acrocentric chromosomes, typically resulting in one large and one small chromosome. The small chromosome is often lost.

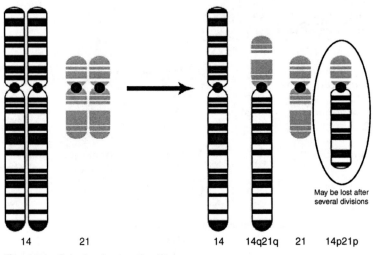

Figure 3.1   Robertsonian translocation.

What type of chromosome has either two short arms or two long arms due to faulty separation of the centromere during meiosis?

Isochromosome

What is the process by which all but one X chromosome in each cell is randomly inactivated early in embryonic development?

Lyonization

What does lyonization produce?

Barr bodies

What is genetic mosaicism?

An individual's cells are a mixture of differing genotypes (eg, some cells are normal while others have trisomy 21, or X0, or show variable lyonization. Lyonization is a normally occurring mosaicism in which approximately half of a woman's cells have maternal X inactivation while the remaining cells have paternal X inactivation.

CHROMOSOMAL ABNORMALITIES

What is the major cause of Down syndrome?	Trisomy 21, usually from maternal meiotic nondisjunction
What are the clinical features of Down syndrome?	Flat nasal bridge, low-set ears, upslanting epicanthal folds, wide-set eyes, simian crease, endocardial cushion cardiac malformations (including ASD, VSD), esophageal atresia, and mental retardation
What is the name given to another characteristic of Down syndrome in which there are small white spots around the border of the iris?	Brushfield spots
Down syndrome patients are at increased risk of developing which conditions later in life?	Early onset Alzheimer disease and both acute lymphoblastic and myeloid leukemias
What is Edwards syndrome and what are the clinical characteristics?	Trisomy 18—newborn with mental retardation, rocker-bottom feet, micrognathia (small lower jaw), prominent occiput, and congenital cardiac malformations
What is Patau syndrome and what are the clinical characteristics?	Trisomy 13—newborn with mental retardation, deafness, microphthalmia, microcephaly, cleft lip and palate, polydactyly, cardiac defects, clenched fists, rocker-bottom feet, and holoprosencephaly
What is the most common cause of a 47,XXY karyotype?	Maternal meiotic nondisjunction
What is the name and clinical phenotype observed in individuals with 47,XXY genotype?	Klinefelter syndrome—tall-statured male with hypogonadism, mild gynecomastia, infertility, and a Barr body seen on buccal smear preparation
Are males with a 47,XYY karyotype easily distinguished from males with a normal 46,XY karyotype?	No, but they are generally tall-with an increased risk of having learning difficulties and/or behavioral problems.
What is the karyotype and common phenotype seen in Turner syndrome?	45,XO—short-statured female, webbed neck, widely spaced nipples, delayed puberty

What cardiovascular anomaly is most often seen with this syndrome?

Coarctation of the aorta

What test could be performed to conclusively diagnose this syndrome?

Karyotype

What is the common phenotype seen in trisomy X (47,XXX)?

Mild mental retardation, menstrual irregularities, and two Barr bodies

What causes a condition characterized by a weak, cat-like cry, severe mental retardation, microcephaly, and congenital heart defects?

Partial deletion of the short arm of chromosome 5 (cri du chat syndrome)

What genetic defect results in DiGeorge syndrome or velocardiofacial syndrome?

Microdeletion of chromosome 22q11

What shared clinical features are associated with microdeletion of chromosome 22q11?

Craniofacial anomalies including cleft palate, congenital heart defects, mental retardation, and increased risk of schizophrenia

What unique features may be used to distinguish DiGeorge syndrome from velocardiofacial syndrome?

Thymic and parathyroid hypoplasia with resultant variable degrees of T-cell immunodeficiency and hypocalcemia

What is genomic imprinting?

An epigenetic process related to differences in DNA methylation of an allele inherited from the mother or the father. DNA methylation results in inactivation of a gene or possibly an entire chromosome.

What two syndromes are associated with genetic imprinting of the long arm of chromosome 15?

1. Prader-Willi
2. Angelman syndrome

Which syndrome is associated with the deletion of a normally active paternal allele of chromosome 15 and what are the clinical features?

Prader-Willi (*P* for paternal)— mental retardation, truncal obesity, hypogonadism, and small hands and feet

Which syndrome is associated with the deletion of a normally active maternal allele of chromosome 15 and what are the clinical features?

Angel*M*an's syndrome (*M* for maternal)— mental retardation, mutism, seizures, ataxia, inappropriate laughter

Table 3.1 Common Chromosome Disorders

Disorder	Inheritance	Abnormality
Down syndrome	Autosomal	Trisomy 21
Edwards syndrome	Autosomal	Trisomy 18
Patau syndrome	Autosomal	Trisomy 13
Klinefelter syndrome	Sex	47,XXY
Turner syndrome	Sex	45,X
Trisomy X	Sex	47,XXX
Supermale	Sex	47,XYY
Cri du chat syndrome	Autosomal	Partial deletion of chromosome 5
DiGeorge or velocardiofacial syndrome	Autosomal	Microdeletion of chromosome 22q11
Prader-Willi syndrome	Autosomal	Deletion of paternal chromosome 15
Angelman syndrome	Autosomal	Deletion of maternal chromosome 15

INHERITANCE PATTERNS

What is the term for having two identical alleles for a given gene?	Homozygous
What is the term for having two different alleles for a given gene?	Heterozygous
What is the term for having only one copy (allele) of a gene?	Hemizygous
What is a point mutation?	Mutation or changing of a single nucleotide
What is a frameshift mutation?	Deletion or insertion of one or more nucleotides that is not a multiple of three, therefore changing the transcriptional reading frame

What is a missense mutation?

Point mutation that causes substitution of one amino acid for another in the protein sequence. It can be conservative (has no effect on protein function) or nonconservative (usually affects protein function deleteriously).

What is a nonsense mutation?

Point mutation that changes the encoded amino acid to a stop codon and causes formation of a truncated version of the protein. It is almost always deleterious.

What is a silent mutation?

Point mutation in which the single base change does not code for a different amino acid, so no disease condition arises

What is a trinucleotide repeat mutation?

Expansion of a repeated sequence of three nucleotides

What is the term describing the tendency for a disorder to increase in severity or appear at an earlier age as it is passed on to the next generation?

Anticipation—often seen with trinucleotide repeat mutations

A disorder in which only one copy of the mutant gene is necessary to cause disease is what type of inheritance?

Autosomal dominant (AD)

A disorder in which two copies of a mutant gene are necessary to cause disease is what type of inheritance?

Autosomal recessive (AR)

What pattern of inheritance causes disorders usually in males and creates heterozygous female carriers due to a mutant gene on the X chromosome?

X-linked recessive

What is co-dominance?

Two alleles share dominance (eg, AB blood group)

What is variable expressivity?

Identical genotypes display a range of phenotypic manifestations and/or severities

What is incomplete penetrance?

Not all individuals with a mutant genotype show the mutant phenotype

What type of inherited genetic disorder is the result of the combined action of the alleles of more than one gene and usually has more complex hereditary patterns?	Polygenic disorder
What are some examples of polygenic disorders?	Obesity, atherosclerosis, alcoholism, autism, schizophrenia, baldness, cleft palate, idiopathic gout, diabetes mellitus, high blood pressure

AUTOSOMAL DOMINANT DISORDERS

What AD connective tissue disease is caused by a mutation in *fibrillin*?	Marfan syndrome
What are the hallmark defects of this disease?	• Skeletal—tall, thin, arachnodactyly • Ocular—ectopia lentis (dislocation of ocular lens) • Cardiovascular—aortic dilation leading to aortic aneurysm or dissection; mitral valve prolapse
A woman with Marfan syndrome and her normal husband wish to have children. What is the probability that their child will have Marfan syndrome?	50%
What is the genetic mutation and the pattern of inheritance for Huntington disease?	AD inheritance of a trinucleotide repeat (CAG) on chromosome 4
What is the physical cause of Huntington disease?	Atrophy of caudate nuclei, putamen, and frontal cortex
What are the resulting symptoms and at what age do they commonly manifest?	Huntington disease typically presents later in life (40-50 years) with involuntary erratic movements (choreiform or extrapyramidal movements) and slow but progressive cognitive decline.
What molecular genetic tool may be used for early diagnosis of this disease?	PCR or DNA sequencing; previously restriction fragment length polymorphism (RFLP) studies were used

What is the explanation for the observation of anticipation, especially associated with paternal transmission?

A progressive expansion of the trinucleotide repeat from generation to generation, which is more likely occur amongst the vast number of sperm produced by the father than the small number of ova produced by the mother.

What AD disease is caused by a mutation of the low-density lipoprotein (LDL) receptor resulting in high serum levels of LDL cholesterol and early onset on atherosclerosis?

Familial hypercholesterolemia

What are the other characteristics of this disease involving deposits of cholesterol in certain areas of the body?

- Xanthomas—deposits in skin and tendons
- Arcus corneae—deposits around periphery of cornea

What AD disorder consists of telangiectases (dilated capillaries) of the skin and mucous membranes with periodic bleeding ranging from epistaxis (nosebleeds) to gastrointestinal hemorrhage?

Hereditary hemorrhagic telangiectasia, otherwise known as Osler-Weber-Rendu syndrome

What AD disorder is characterized by bilateral destruction of renal parenchyma due to multiple expanding cysts, ultimately leading to renal failure?

Autosomal dominant polycystic kidney disease (ADPKD)

In the AD disorder hereditary spherocytosis, what causes the characteristic spheroidal erythrocytes?

Defects of the erythrocyte membrane proteins, most commonly *spectrin*

What test is used to diagnosis hereditary spherocytosis?

Osmotic fragility test

What type of anemia often results from defective erythrocytes?

Hemolytic anemia due to trapping and destruction of the erythrocytes in the spleen

What are the phakomatoses ("neurocutaneous syndromes")?

Neurofibromatosis (NF) 1 and 2, tuberous sclerosis, von Hippel-Lindau disease (VHL), Sturge-Weber syndrome, and ataxia telangiectasia

Which phakomatoses are hereditary and what are the inheritance patterns?

- Autosomal dominant—NF1 and NF2, tuberous sclerosis, VHL
- Autosomal recessive—ataxia telangiectasia
- Nonhereditary/sporadic—Sturge-Weber syndrome

What are the hallmarks of neurofibromatosis 1 (NF1) or von Recklinghausen disease?

Multiple neurofibromas (tumors) anywhere on the body

- Café au lait spots (pigmented skin lesions)
- Lisch nodules—pigmented iris hamartomas
- Skeletal lesions—scoliosis, bone cysts
- Greater risk of developing other tumors—Wilms tumors, pheochromocytoma

What is the hallmark of NF2?

Bilateral acoustic neuromas

What are the clinical features of tuberous sclerosis (incomplete penetrance, variable expressivity)?

Cerebral hamartomas (tubers); renal angiomyolipomas and cysts; hypopigmented skin macules ("ash-leaf spots"); mental retardation; seizures

What are the characteristics of von Hippel-Lindau (VHL) disease?

Capillary hemangioblastoma (or cavernous hemangioma) of cerebellum, retina, or sometimes brain stem and spinal cord; cysts in pancreas, liver, and kidneys; propensity to develop renal cell carcinoma

A mutation in what type of gene is the cause of von Hippel-Lindau disease?

Tumor-suppressor gene (specifically the *VHL* gene)

On which chromosome is this gene located?

Chromosome 3 (short arm)

What AD disease is the most common growth plate disorder and a major cause of dwarfism?

Achondroplasia

What are the hallmarks of achondroplasia?

Skeletal abnormalities; shortened arms and legs, but relatively normal-length trunk; large head with protruding forehead and depression at the root of the nose

What diseases are caused by trinucleotide repeat expansion?

Huntington disease (AD), myotonic dystrophy (AD), Friedreich ataxia (AR), fragile X syndrome (X-linked)

What are the features of myotonic dystrophy?

Muscular dystrophy and myotonia; cataracts; hypogonadism; frontal balding

The finding of bilateral leukocoria (white reflection) when checking for a red reflex on an infant screening exam is concerning for what disease process?

Retinoblastoma

Would this type of retinoblastoma be hereditary (familial) or sporadic?

Hereditary (AD), because it is present bilaterally.

What is the two-hit hypothesis?

The concept that both alleles of a gene must be mutated for a cancer to develop. If the first mutation is inherited (as in hereditary retinoblastoma) the likelihood of developing cancer is increased as only one sporadic mutation is needed to acquire "two-hits."

What gene is mutated in retinoblastoma?

Retinoblastoma 1 (RB1), a tumor-suppressor gene on chromosome 13

Is a child with bilateral retinoblastoma at an increased risk for other cancers later in life?

Yes, because the mutated RB1 gene is present in other tissues, which may subsequently acquire sporadic mutations.

What primarily AD group of disorders is the result of a mutation in type I collagen?

Osteogenesis imperfecta (OI)

What are the hallmarks of this disease?

Brittle bones often resulting in fractures, easy bruising, blue sclera in some types, hearing loss, and dentinogenesis imperfecta in some types

Which type of OI is the result of a null allele, and which types of OI are the results of missense mutations?

• OI type I—null allele
• OI types II, III, IV—missense mutations

AUTOSOMAL RECESSIVE DISORDERS

What pattern of inheritance do most metabolic pathway disorders exhibit?	AR inheritance
A mother with phenylketonuria (PKU), an AR disease, and a normal homozygous father are expecting their first child. What odds can you give them that their child may or may not have PKU?	There is a 0% chance that the child will have PKU since both of the father's alleles are normal, but there is a 100% chance that the child will be a carrier.
What deficiency characterizes the AR diseases Tay-Sachs, Gaucher, Niemann-Pick, and Hurler syndrome?	Single lysosomal enzyme deficiency
What lysosomal enzyme is deficient in Tay-Sachs disease?	Hexosaminidase A (a gangliosidase) is deficient, leading to accumulation of GM_2 ganglioside in the neurons
What are the signs and symptoms of Tay-Sachs disease?	Blindness, increasing central nervous system (CNS) degeneration and dementia, cherry-red spot on the macula, vegetative state before death at about 2-3 years of age
In what ethnic group do carriers for Tay-Sachs disease occur at the frequency of about 1 in 30 individuals?	Ashkenazi Jewish from Eastern Europe
What AR disorder is the most common lysosomal storage disease?	Gaucher disease
What enzyme is deficient in Gaucher disease, and what accumulates as a result?	Glucocerebrosidase is deficient; glucocerebrosides accumulate in phagocytic cells
Which type of Gaucher disease is marked by glucocerebroside accumulation in the CNS, with no detectible amounts of glucocerebroside in the body, hepatosplenomegaly, and death at a very early age?	Type II Gaucher disease
Type I Gaucher disease (adult, nonneuronopathic, chronic) manifests with what symptoms?	Hepatosplenomegaly; skeletal erosions; mild anemia; detectable, but still small, amounts of glucocerebrosidase

What are Gaucher cells?	Distended phagocytic cells with histologic appearance of "crumpled tissue paper" cytoplasm
What is type III (juvenile) Gaucher disease?	Intermediate between types I and II, involves the brain and other organs
What disease is caused by a deficiency of sphingomyelinase and a resulting accumulation of sphingomyelin in phagocytes?	Niemann-Pick disease
What is the histological finding in this disease?	*Foam* cells of the mononuclear phagocytic system
What are the clinical manifestations?	Hepatosplenomegaly; CNS degeneration; cherry-red spot in macula of eye in about 50% of cases; early death
What is the cause of Hurler syndrome?	Deficiency of α-l-iduronidase resulting in accumulation of mucopolysaccharides (dermatan sulfate and heparan sulfate)
How does Hurler syndrome present?	Protuberant abdomen with splenomegaly; large head with course features; corneal clouding
How is Hurler syndrome different from the clinically similar Hunter syndrome?	Hunter syndrome is X-linked recessive, lacks corneal clouding, and is milder. Hurler syndrome is AR.
What are the four common AR glycogen storage diseases?	von Gierke (type I), Pompe (type II), Cori (type III), and McArdle (type V)
How can von Gierke disease be differentiated from Pompe disease?	The two differ in the distribution of glycogen accumulation. • von Gierke disease is secondary to a deficiency of glucose-6-phosphatase and therefore glycogen accumulation predominately in the liver and kidney. • Pompe disease is due to a deficiency of α-1,4-glucosidase, which is present in all tissues, leading to glycogen accumulation in all tissues, including heart, skeletal muscle, and brain.

What signs should one look for when examining a patient if von Gierke disease is suspected?	Massive hepatomegaly causing a prominent abdomen; fat deposits in cheeks and buttocks; convulsions due to hypoglycemia
What is the prognosis for a patient with Pompe disease?	Poor—death due to cardiac failure before age 3
What is the cause of Cori disease?	Deficiency of debranching enzyme amylo-1,6-glucosidase
What are the clinical manifestations of this disease?	Cardiomegaly; hepatomegaly; muscle hypotonia; hypoglycemia
What is the enzyme deficiency and resulting problem in McArdle syndrome?	Deficiency of muscle phosphorylase with subsequent accumulation of glycogen in the muscle, leading to muscle cramps and weakness with exercise
A 4-week-old baby boy is brought to the ER with vomiting and diarrhea. The parents say this happens after breast-feeding, and they also question you about the baby's persistent yellow color. Physical examination reveals cataracts in the eyes and hepatomegaly. What disease should you suspect, and what should a diagnostic test detect?	Galactosemia; lack of galactose-1-phosphate uridyl transferase activity in leukocytes or erythrocytes
What other symptoms will appear if the disease progresses in galactosemia?	Mental retardation; cirrhosis of the liver with resulting hepatic failure; failure to thrive
What causes the cataracts in galactosemia?	Accumulation of galactitol
What simple solution will keep these symptoms from appearing or ameliorate them and reverse the cataracts?	Removal of galactose from the diet
What similar, but less common, AR disorder is characterized only by infantile cataracts?	Galactokinase deficiency galactosemia
What disorder of amino acid metabolism is characterized by pronounced mental deterioration by 6 months of age, hyperphenylalaninemia, seizures, hypopigmentation of the skin, eyes, and hair, and musty body odor?	PKU

What enzyme is deficient?	Phenylalanine hydroxylase is deficient, leading to the inability to convert phenylalanine to tyrosine and resulting in high (toxic) levels of phenylalanine.
What is the treatment and prognosis?	• Treatment—phenylalanine-free diet • Prognosis—good as long as screening for PKU identifies the disease very early and the parents/patient are compliant with a phenylalanine-free diet to prevent progressive mental/neurologic deterioration
What disease is the result of a buildup of homogentisic acid secondary to a deficiency of homogentisic oxidase?	Alkaptonuria
What are the features of this disease?	Severe arthritis; urine discoloration/darkening with exposure to air; ochronosis
What is ochronosis?	A term describing the pigmentation or darkening of fibrous tissue or cartilage
What is the prognosis of alkaptonuria?	Not life threatening, but can be crippling due to the severe ochronotic arthritis
What rare AR disease is characterized by high concentrations of keto acids in the urine?	Maple syrup urine disease
What can be the consequences if this disease goes untreated?	Severe mental retardation and physical disabilities. These can be ameliorated with a protein-modified diet.
What is the most common life-shortening genetic disorder among the white population?	Cystic fibrosis
What is the genetic problem?	Mutation of the cystic fibrosis transmembrane conductance regulator (CFTR) gene, located on chromosome 7, which is inherited in an AR manner

What is the mechanism of disease?	The deficiency of chloride channel proteins resulting in impaired chloride transport. In the lungs, GI tract, and pancreas, chloride secretion is impaired leading to increased sodium and water reabsorption resulting in more viscous secretions. In sweat glands, chloride reabsorption from sweat is impaired, resulting in increased sodium loss.
What are the more common clinical manifestations of this disease?	Chronic pulmonary infections and cough; meconium ileus; fibrotic pancreas and salivary glands; cirrhosis of the liver; obstruction of the; epididymis and vas deferens in males
What organism most commonly causes the pulmonary infections?	*Pseudomonas aeruginosa*
What test is used to diagnosis CF?	Sweat test—reabsorption of chloride is defective leading to an increased concentration of sodium chloride in the sweat ducts. A positive neonatal screening test is not adequate for diagnosis; it must be confirmed with a sweat test.
A mother with sickle cell anemia and a father who knows he is a carrier have a newborn son, so a test is performed to determine if the baby has the disease. What are the chances the child is affected, and what is the diagnostic test?	• 50% chance the child has sickle cell anemia and 50% chance he is a heterozygous carrier • Diagnostic test—peripheral blood smear to identify abnormal (sickle-shaped) erythrocytes
What type of mutation causes the sickle cell form of hemoglobin S (HbS)?	Missense point mutation of the sixth amino acid of the β chain, changing the glutamate to valine
What are the characteristics of sickle cell anemia?	Vaso-occlusive crises; hand-foot syndrome; hemolytic anemia (fatigue, paleness, jaundice); increased risk of infection, especially from the encapsulated organisms (*Haemophilus influenza, Neisseria meningitidis, Streptococcus pneumonia*); delayed growth

X-LINKED

Why do X-linked recessive disorders affect males and females unequally?

Since males are genotypically XY, a single mutant allele will lead to disease phenotype, while females require the typical two mutant alleles (as with AR inheritance) to express disease phenotype.

What is the mechanism of disease in hemophilia A (classic hemophilia)?

A deficiency in coagulation factor VIII

What are the clinical manifestations?

Easy bruising; hemarthroses leading to crippling joint deformities; propensity to massive hemorrhage after trauma or surgery; absence of petechiae

What are the clinical characteristics of Hunter syndrome?

Hepatosplenomegaly, micrognathia, retinal degeneration, mental retardation, diffuse joint stiffness, coarse facies; clinically very similar to Hurler syndrome but less severe

What enzyme is deficient in Hunter syndrome?

L-Iduronosulfate sulfatase enzyme

What accumulates in the tissues in Hunter syndrome?

Dermatan sulfate and heparan sulfate (mucopolysaccharides)

What X-linked recessive disorder usually presents within the first year of life with gross motor developmental delay and hypotonia, with physical examination showing impaired growth and neurologic findings including hyperreflexia, spasticity, and choreoathetosis?

Lesch-Nyhan syndrome

What is the enzymatic deficiency and resulting accumulating substance in Lesch-Nyhan syndrome?

Hypoxanthine-guanine phosphoribosyltransferase (HGPRT), leading to an accumulation of uric acid

What is the prognosis of Lesch-Nyhan syndrome, and what other hallmark characteristics will appear with time?

Prognosis is dependent on severity of HGPRT deficiency, if complete deficiency prognosis is poor with death typically by the first or second decade

- Self-mutilating behavior (eg, biting fingers, lips, etc)
- Mental retardation
- Gouty arthritis
- Aggressive behavior

What metabolic pathway does the enzymatic deficiency in Lesch-Nyhan syndrome affect?

Purine salvage pathway

What are the clinical characteristics of Fabry disease (angiokeratoma corporis diffusum universale)?

Fabry presents in childhood with the following and often results in death by the third to fifth decade:

- Angiokeratomas
- Burning pain the extremities
- Febrile episodes
- Corneal opacities
- Cardiac complications including stroke and renal failure

What enzyme is deficient in Fabry disease?

α-Galactosidase A

What accumulates in the visceral organs and vascular tissues in Fabry disease?

Ceramide trihexosidase

What are the classic features of Duchenne muscular dystrophy (DMD)?

Muscle weakness, proximal > distal; lordosis; pseudohypertrophy of the calf muscles; progressive immobilization and wasting leading to early death typically through respiratory compromise

What diagnostic laboratory parameter should be assessed in DMD?

Serum creatinine kinase levels (will be elevated if DMD present)

What is the prognosis of DMD?

Poor—death results most often from failure of the respiratory muscles, usually by the early twenties

What is the chromosomal defect in Fragile X syndrome?

Expanded trinucleotide repeat sequence of CGG in the 5′-untranslated region of *FMR-1* gene on the X chromosome (X-linked), leading to instability and breakage

What are the clinical features of Fragile X syndrome?

Males with mental retardation, macroorchidism, and large, everted ears

What three qualities make Fragile X different from both classic X-linked dominant or X-linked recessive disorders?

1. Carrier or transmitting state exists in 20% of males with the mutation and can transmit the mutation through their daughters
2. The number of affected (mentally retarded) carrier females is much higher than would be predicted by strictly X-linked recessive inheritance
3. Sherman's paradox—anticipation is observed

Overall, the inheritance most closely resembles X-linked dominant with variable penetrance and anticipation observed.

Table 3.2 Summary of Genetic Disorders

Disorder	Inheritance Pattern	Genetic or Chromosomal Error
Marfan syndrome	AD	*Fibrillin* gene
Huntington disease	AD	Chromosome 4 trinucleotide repeat
Familial hypercholesterolemia	AD	LDL receptor genes
Hereditary hemorrhagic telangiectasia or Osler-Weber-Rendu	AD	*Endoglin, Alk-1*
Adult polycystic kidney disease	AD	*PKD1, PKD2,* and *PKD3* genes
Hereditary spherocytosis	AD	*Spectrin* gene
Type 1 neurofibromatosis or von Recklinghausen disease	AD	*NF1* gene
Tuberous sclerosis	AD	Several loci for *TSC* genes
von Hippel-Lindau disease	AD	*VHL* gene on chromosome 3
Achondroplasia	AD	*FGFR3* gene
Myotonic dystrophy	AD	Chromosome 19 trinucleotide repeat
Retinoblastoma	AD	*RB1* gene
Osteogenesis imperfecta	AD	α_1 and α_2 chains of collagen type I genes
Tay-Sachs disease	AR	Hexosaminidase A gene

Table 3.2 Summary of Genetic Disorders (Continued)

Disorder	Inheritance Pattern	Genetic or Chromosomal Error
Gaucher disease	AR	Glucocerebrosidase gene
Niemann-Pick disease	AR	Sphingomyelinase gene
Hurler disease	AR	α-L-Iduronidase gene
von Gierke disease	AR	Glucose-6-phosphatase gene
Pompe disease	AR	α-1,4-Glucosidase gene
Cori disease	AR	Amylo-1,6-glucosidase gene
McArdle syndrome	AR	Muscle phosphorylase gene
Galactosemia	AR	Galactose-1-phosphate uridyl transferase gene
Galactokinase deficiency galactosemia	AR	Galactokinase gene
Alkaptonuria	AR	Homogentisic oxidase gene
Maple syrup urine disease	AR	Branched-chain keto acid dehydrogenase gene
Cystic fibrosis	AR	CFTR gene on chromosome 7
Sickle cell anemia	AR	Hemoglobin gene
Phenylketonuria	AR	Phenylalanine hydroxylase gene
Hemophilia	X-linked recessive	Coagulation factor VIII gene
Lesch-Nyhan syndrome	X-linked recessive	HGPRT gene
Fabry disease	X-linked recessive	α-Galactosidase A gene
Duchenne muscular dystrophy	X-linked recessive	*Dystrophin* gene
Hunter syndrome	X-linked recessive	L-Iduronosulfate sulfatase gene
Fragile X syndrome	X-linked	Trinucleotide repeat in *FMR-1* gene

Abbreviations: AD, autosomal dominant; AR, autosomal recessive; *Alk*-1, activin receptor-like kinase 1; CFTR, cystic fibrosis transmembrane conductance regulator; FGFR3, fibroblast growth factor receptor 3; FMR-1, fragile mental retardation-1; HGPRT, hypoxanthine-guanine phosphoribosyltransferase; LDL, low-density lipoprotein; NF1, neurofibromatosis 1; PKD, polycystic kidney disease; RBI, retinoblastoma 1; TSC, tuberous sclerosis complex; VHL, von Hippel-Lindau.

CLINICAL VIGNETTES

A newborn baby presents with a flat nasal bridge, low-set eats, simian crease, and ventricular septal defect. What is the most likely diagnosis? What other features may be present that would also support the diagnosis?

Down syndrome

Also look for upslanting epicanthal folds, wide-set eyes, and expect developmental delay/mental retardation

A tall-statured 25-year-old man presents with hypogonadism, slight gynecomastia, and fertility problems. A single Barr body is observed in a buccal smear preparation. What condition is most likely?

Klinefelter syndrome, 47,XXY

A 9-month-old girl presents to the ER with limpness and increasing motor incoordination. Examination reveals a cherry-red spot in the macula of the eyes. What disease should be suspected?

Tay-Sachs disease

A 14-month-old boy presents with a protuberant abdomen and abnormally large head with coarse features. Corneal clouding is observed upon further examination, and palpation of the abdomen in the left upper quadrant reveals an enlarged spleen. What is the most likely diagnosis?

Hurler syndrome

A 16-year-old girl presents with complaints of muscle cramps and fatigue when she exercises for only a short period of time at school. However, resting seems to alleviate these symptoms. Urine analysis reveals the presence of myoglobin. What disease should be suspected?

McArdle syndrome

A short-statured, 17-year-old girl presents with poor breast development and amenorrhea. Widely spaced nipples and a webbed neck are noted on examination. What condition should you suspect?

Turner syndrome, 45,XO

A 9-year-old boy presents with hypogonadism, small hands and feet, truncal obesity, and mental retardation. What are the genetic mutation and diagnosis?

Paternal deletion of the long arm of chromosome 15—Prader-Willi syndrome

A 30-year-old woman presents with the complaint of pain and stiffness in her hip and knee joints. She is also concerned because she noticed for the first time a color change in her urine to black if it was left standing for a few hours. History reveals that no one else in her family has this problem. Physical examination reveals a slightly dark, dusty color of the cartilage of her ears and the sclera of her eyes. What disease should you suspect, and what is causing the symptoms?

Alkaptonuria; buildup of homogentisic acid due to deficiency of homogentisic oxidase

A 2-year-old girl presents with hepatosplenomegaly, micrognathia, and stiffness in her joints. Further examination reveals retinal degeneration, but no corneal clouding. What do you suspect?

Hunter syndrome, a very similar disease to Hurler syndrome except that it is an X-linked recessive disorder

A 20-month-old boy is brought in by his mother because he has not started walking. Physical examination reveals hyperreflexia, choreoathetoid movements, and spasticity. Serum and urine chemistries indicate elevated uric acid levels. What disease is most likely indicated?

Lesch-Nyhan syndrome

A 5-year-old boy presents with "clumsiness," lordosis, and overall muscle weakness. Physical examination reveals apparent hypertrophy of the calf muscles and an irregular heart beat. What disorder is indicated?

Duchenne muscular dystrophy (DMD)

CHAPTER 4

Microbiology in Pathology

BACTERIA

What are the various bacterial morphologies?	Cocci (circular), bacilli (rods), spiral (spirochetes), branching/filamentous
What other feature along with morphology is used to distinguish bacteria?	Gram stain (positive or negative)
What substance in the cell wall is unique to gram-negative bacteria?	Lipopolysaccharide (endotoxin)
What effects does lipopolysaccharide (LPS) have on the infected host?	It causes macrophage activation, complement activation, and Hageman factor activation which, via cytokine release and pathway activation, can cause fever, hypotension, edema, and possibly diffuse intravascular coagulation (DIC).
What substance in the cell wall is unique to gram-positive bacteria?	Teichoic acid
What structure of bacteria facilitates adherence to surfaces (eg, IV lines)?	Glycocalyx
What is the phase of bacterial growth that represents a "no-growth" phase due to depletion of available nutrients?	Stationary phase
What are the encapsulated bacteria?	*Streptococcus pneumoniae, Neisseria meningitidis, Haemophilus influenzae,* and *Klebsiella pneumoniae*

What are the obligate intracellular bacteria?	*Rickettsia* and *Chlamydia*—these organisms cannot synthesize their own ATP
What are the facultative intracellular anaerobes?	*Neisseria, Salmonella, Brucella, Listeria, Legionella, Yersinia, Francisella,* and *Mycobacterium*
What are the obligate anaerobic bacteria?	*Clostridium, Bacteroides,* and *Actinomyces*
What are the spore-forming bacteria?	*Clostridium tetani, Clostridium perfringens,* and *Bacillus anthracis*
What are the most common spirochetes?	*Borrelia, Leptospira,* and *Treponema*
What gram-positive cocci is catalase and coagulase positive?	*Staphylococcus aureus* (occurs in clusters)
What gram-positive cocci occur in chains?	*Streptococcus* (catalase negative)
What are the major groupings of *Streptococcus* species?	Alpha-hemolytic, beta-hemolytic, and nonhemolytic
How are beta-hemolytic *Streptococcus* species further subdivided?	Into groups A, B, C, D, and G according to Lancefield antigens (specific carbohydrates expressed in the bacterial cell wall)
Infection with which bacteria (usually bacteremia) is associated with concurrent colon cancer?	*Streptococcus bovis*
What gram-negative rod can cause malignant otitis externa in diabetics, hot tub folliculitis, and pneumonitis especially in patients with cystic fibrosis?	*Pseudomonas aeruginosa*
What are the gram-negative cocci (diplococci)?	*Neisseria gonorrhoeae* and *N. meningitidis*
Which bacterium has no cell wall and commonly is associated with high IgM titers?	*Mycoplasma pneumoniae*
What stain should be done to detect and help classify most bacteria?	Gram stain

Which bacteria generally do not Gram stain well?	*Treponema, Rickettsia, Mycoplasma, Legionella, Chlamydia,* and *Mycobacterium*
What technique is used to visualize Treponemes?	Darkfield microscopy with florescent antibody staining
What antibody serum test is most specific for syphilis?	Fluorescent Treponemal Antibody–Absorption test (FTA-Abs)
What are the common causes of false positive VDRLs?	Viral infection, drugs, rheumatic fever, SLE, and leprosy
What stain should be done to detect *Mycobacterium*?	Acid-fast stain helps detect "red snappers"
What stain can help detect *Legionella* and fungi like *Pneumocystis jiroveci* (formerly carinii)?	Silver stain
What stain can help detect *Campylobacter* and *Borrelia*?	Giemsa stain
What culture media is needed to isolate *N. gonorrhoeae*?	Thayer-Martin media
What culture media is needed to isolate *H. influenza*?	Chocolate agar
What culture media is required to isolate *Legionella*?	Charcoal yeast with high concentrations of iron and cysteine
What bacteria grow pink colonies on MacConkey agar?	Lactose-fermenting enteric bacteria, including *Escherichia coli, Enterobacter, Serratia,* and *Klebsiella*
What test can be used to distinguish among nonlactose fermenting bacteria?	Oxidase test—*Shigella, Salmonella,* and *Proteus* are oxidase negative, *Pseudomonas* is oxidase positive
Which bacteria produce superantigens?	*Staphylococcus aureus* (TSST-1) and *Streptococcus pyogenes* (Scarlet fever-erythrogenic toxin)
Which bacteria produce A-B toxins?	*Corynebacterium diphtheriae, Vibrio cholerae, E. coli,* and *Bordetella pertussis*
What is the Shiga toxin?	A toxin produced by *Shigella* and *E. coli* O157:H7 that cleaves host cell rRNA
What bacterium is associated with skin infection after animal bites?	*Pasturella multocida*

VIRUSES

In general, what laboratory techniques are used to detect/identify viruses?	PCR, viral culture, antibody tests
What is the genetic ploidy of viruses?	All viruses are haploid (1 copy the complete DNA or RNA genome) except retroviruses which are diploid. This should not be confused with number of strands of DNA or RNA, as some viruses are single stranded while others are double stranded.
Where do DNA viruses undergo replication in host cells?	All DNA viruses undergo replication in the nucleus except for poxviruses where it occurs in the cytoplasm.
Where do RNA viruses undergo replication in host cells?	All RNA viruses undergo replication in the cytoplasm, except influenza virus and retroviruses (both of which replicate in the nucleus).
What is a Tzanck test and what does it detect?	This is a smear of sample taken from an opened vesicle used to detect multinucleated giant cells seen in herpes infections including HSV-1, HSV-2, and VZV (*varicella*).
What virus causes fever, pharyngitis, lymphadenopathy, atypical T cells, and a positive heterophile antibody test?	Ebstein Barr virus (EBV), causing infectious mononucleosis
What virus classically has inclusions that look like "owl's eyes"?	Cytomegalovirus (CMV)
What virus is associated with fever, emesis, jaundice, and Councilman bodies (acidophilic inclusions) in the liver?	Yellow fever virus (Flavivirus)
What viral infection produces paresthesias, headache, fever, central nervous system (CNS) excitability, foaming at the mouth, and paralysis?	Rabies virus
What is the name and location of the inclusion body seen in rabies virus infection?	Negri bodies—eosinophilic, cytoplasmic inclusion in neurons, most commonly in pyramidal cells of the hippocampus

What and why must a confirmatory test be done if an HIV ELISA comes back positive?

ELISA is a screening test, therefore highly sensitive but may result in false-positive test results. HIV Western blot is needed to confirm the diagnosis because it is highly specific; therefore, a positive result on Western blot will confirm the ELISA diagnosis and a negative result on Western blot will identify a false-positive ELISA test.

What neoplasms are associated with HIV infection?

Kaposi sarcoma (HHV-8), primary CNS lymphoma, non-Hodgkin lymphoma, and cervical carcinoma (HPV)

What serologic marker/s would be expected to be positive in an individual vaccinated against Hepatitis B virus?

Hepatitis B surface antibody (HBsAb) only

What serologic marker/s would be expected to be positive in an individual who cleared a previous Hepatitis B infection?

HBsAb and Hepatitis B core antibody (HBcAb)

What serologic marker/s would be expected to be positive in an individual who was a chronic carrier of Hepatitis B virus?

Hepatitis B surface antigen (HBsAg) and HBcAb

FUNGI

What is a dimorphic fungus?

A fungus that can exist in either a mold (hyphal) or yeast form, typically dependent on temperature. Therefore, the fungus will be a mold in the soil and yeast if in the body.

*Mold in cold and yeast in heat

Name two examples of dimorphic fungi:

1. *Histoplasma*
2. *Blastomyces*

What systemic mycosis is endemic to the Mississippi and Ohio River valley and is acquired through contact with bat or bird droppings?

Histoplasmosis

What is the classic histologic description of *blastomyces*?

Yeast with broad-based budding

Give a morphologic description of the fungi responsible for causing pneumonia in a patient who had traveled to the southwestern United States:

Spherule filled with endospores (Coccidioidomycosis)

What fungus commonly causes bilateral pneumonia in immunocompromised patients?

Pneumocystis jiroveci

What population of patients is particularly at risk of acquiring opportunistic infections with *Mucor* spp.?

Diabetics, especially in ketoacidosis (most commonly rhinocerebral abscesses)

What fungus causes meningitis in immunocompromised patients and can be detected using either India ink staining or latex agglutination?

Cryptococcus neoformans

What is the classic appearance of *Cryptococcus*?

Yeast with extremely thick capsular halo and narrow, unequal-based budding

What are the possible presentations/manifestations of *Aspergillus* infection?

Allergic bronchopulmonary aspergillosis; Aspergilloma, aka "fungus ball"; Angioinvasive aspergillosis

What is the morphologic appearance of *Aspergillus*?

Septated hyphae (mold) with 45° angle branching and occasionally a fruiting body will be seen.

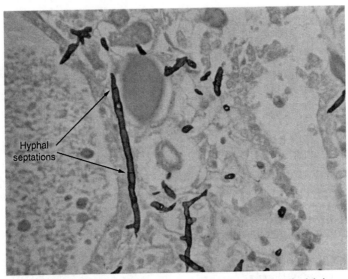

Figure 4.1 Fungal forms are identified in a background of necrotic debris. Fungal hyphae are septated with 45° angle branching, consistent with *Aspergillus fumigatus*. (Reproduced, with permission, from OHSU.)

What is the morphologic difference between *Mucor* and *Aspergillus*?	*Mucor* has wide hyphae and no septae, while *Aspergillus* has 45° branching and septae.
What is the morphologic appearance of *Sporothrix schenckii*?	Cigar-shaped budding yeast forms
What fungus has pseudohyphae, budding yeast, and germ tubes?	*Candida albicans*
What stain can be helpful in detecting fungi?	Silver stain or periodic acid Schiff (PAS) stain
What media is used to culture most fungi?	Sabouraud agar
What fungal organisms are considered dermatophytes?	*Microsporum, Trichophyton,* and *Epidermophyton*
What laboratory technique can be used to diagnose dermatophyte infection?	KOH prep and Wood lamp

PROTOZOA

What is the common presentation of giardiasis?	Bloating, flatulence, diarrhea (often foul smelling), most commonly seen in hikers or campers
What are the forms and appearances of *Giardia lamblia*?	Trophozoite and cyst forms—the trophozoite has the classic "owl-eye" appearance on wet prep but looks like a "folded leaf" on H&E in a small bowel biopsy
What stain is helpful in the detection of the *protozoa Leishmania* and *Plasmodium*?	Giemsa stain
What infection has trophozoite ring forms on blood smear?	Malaria—*Plasmodium*
What are the various species of that cause malaria and which is the most virulent?	*Plasmodium vivax, P. ovale, P. malariae, P. falciparum—P. falciparum* results in the most severe infection
What infection has "maltese cross" (merozoite) forms in addition to trophozoite ring forms on peripheral blood smear?	Babesiosis—because of its similar clinical presentation and ring forms it can be misdiagnosed as malaria.

What stain can help in detecting *Cryptosporidium*?

Acid-fast stain (highlights cysts)

What is the classic computed tomography (CT) or magnetic resonance imaging (MRI) finding associated with cerebral toxoplasmosis?

Multiple ring-enhancing lesions

If amebas are found on microscopic examination of cerebrospinal fluid, infection with which organism should be considered?

Naegleria fowleri

HELMINTHS

What are the three major categories of medically important helminths?

1. Cestodes
2. Nematodes
3. Trematodes

What are the segments of cestodes called?

Each segment of a cestode is a reproductive unit containing eggs and is called a "proglottid." Cestodes are commonly known as tapeworms.

How can the cestodes be distinguished morphologically?

Taenia spp. cannot be distinguished by evaluation of ova. Examination of a gravid proglottid or scolex is necessary to differentiate the members of this group. The ova of the fish tape worm (*Diphyllobothrium latum*) have "knob-like" projections at one end.

What cestode infection, commonly acquired from dogs, causes liver cysts that if ruptured can cause severe anaphylaxis?

Echinococcus granulosus

What trematode infection is associated with increased risk of cholangiocarcinoma?

Clonorchis sinensis

What nematode classically produces ova with mucous plugs at both ends of the egg?

Trichuris trichiura (whipworm)

What are the two species included in the group commonly referred to as hookworms?

1. *Necator americanus*
2. *Ancylostoma duodenale*

CLINICAL VIGNETTES

A 65-year-old woman living at home presents with fever, shortness of breath, and productive cough. Chest x-ray is consistent with right middle lobe pneumonia. Sputum sample is most likely to show what type of organism?

Gram-positive cocci in chains (*Streptococcus pneumoniae*)

A 23-year-old man presents with two-day history of painful, swollen, erythematous knee with no known trauma. Gram stain of the joint aspirate reveals gram-negative diplococci. What is the diagnosis and causative organism?

Septic joint/arthritis—*N. gonorrhea*

A 45-year-old woman with poorly controlled type II diabetes mellitus presents with severe pain of her left ear. The pain is worse with movement or touching of the left tragus. What is the diagnosis and common causative organism?

Otitis externa—*P. aeruginosa* (can progress to malignant otitis in this population)

A 60-year-old man from the central United States presents to the hospital 10 days after returning from a spelunking expedition with fever, nonproductive cough, and shortness of breath. What is the causative organism and what media is needed for culture?

Histoplasma—Sabouraud agar is used for culture. (Culture is the gold standard for diagnosis, however, it has a long intubation time and either identification on sputum sample or antibody tests maybe tried while awaiting the results.)

An HIV positive man presents with headache, neck pain and stiffness, and confusion. A lumbar puncture is performed, what special tests should be performed on the patient's CSF?

India ink staining to look for *Cryptococcus* (think capsule) and cryptococcal antigen

A 50-year-old man with a past medical history significant for a trauma related splenectomy presents with fever and fatigue. He was hiking in hills of Vermont 1 week ago. He is found to have a hematocrit of 32% and a decreased haptoglobin. Peripheral blood smear shows RBS with central pallor and Giemsa stain shows ring and maltese cross forms. What is the diagnosis and what concomitant infection is the patient at risk for?

Babesiosis—up to 20% of patients with *Babesia* infections will also have Lyme disease (*Borrelia burgdorferi*) as both are transmitted by the *Ixodes tick*. This patient is at risk for severe infection given his previous splenectomy.

A 17-year-old young woman presents with a 5-week history of headache, gradual weakness, lethargy, ataxia, and behavior changes. What encephalitis could she have?

HSV-1 encephalitis

A 64-year-old man presents to your clinic with mood changes and deterioration. Concerned, you examine his pupils, and find that they can accommodate but do not react (constrict) to light. What test should you order?

Rapid plasma reagent (RPR) or Venereal Disease Research Laboratories (VDRL) treponemal tests. The patient has Argyll Robertson pupils, which is highly suggestive of tertiary or neurosyphilis.

An 18-year-old girl presents with sore throat, low grade fever, and fatigue. On examination she is found to have nonexudative pharyngitis, anterior and posterior cervical lymphadenopathy, and a mildly enlarged spleen. What is the cause of her illness and what can confirm the diagnosis?

EBV—confirm with Monospot (heterophile antibody test) and peripheral blood smear may show atypical lymphocytes.

A 3-month-old infant is given honey as a cold remedy. The parents bring the infant to the emergency room when the infant becomes quiet and flaccid. What infection should be suspected and what is the mechanism?

Clostridium botulinum—bacterial toxin inhibits release of acetylcholine at neuromuscular junctions

Cigar-shaped budding yeast are seen on microscopic examination of a swab specimen obtained from a patient with multiple open sores on hand and forearm. What leisure activity does this patient likely participate in?

Gardening, likely roses

CHAPTER 5

Hematology and Immunology

HEMATOLOGY

Anatomy/Histology

What cells are derived from pluripotent hematopoietic stem cells (think—what are the components of a CBC with differential)?

- Proerythrocyte → Reticulocyte → *Erythrocytes* (RBCs)
- Lymphoid stem cell → Lymphoblast → *Lymphocytes* (T and B cells*)

  *B cells can go on to become plasma cells
- Myeloid stem cell → Monoblast → *Monocytes*
- Myeloid stem cell → Megakaryoblast → Megakaryocyte → *Platelets*
- Myeloid stem cell → Myeloblast → Promyelocyte → Myelocyte → Metamyelocyte → Band cell → *Neutrophils, Eosinophils, Basophils*

  **Cell types listed in bold are components of a CBC

What are the various types of leukocytes (white blood cells) and what are their unique features?

See Table 5.1 on the following page.

Table 5.1 Types of Leukocytes

Type of Leukocyte	Normal Percentage in Peripheral Blood**	Unique Histologic Features and Type of Granules	Function
Basophils*	<1% WBCs	Dense basophilic (blue) granules that contain, heparin histamine, leukotrienes	Mediate allergies responses
Eosinophils*	1% to 6%	Eosinophilic (red) granules that contain histamine and major basic protein	Provide immune response to helminthic and protozoan infections
Neutrophils*	40% to 75%	Multilobulated nucleus (vs bilobed) and azurophilic granules (lysosomes) that contain lysozyme, myeloperoxidase, and lactoferrin	Acute inflammatory response and phagocytosis
Monocytes	2% to 10%	Large cell with kidney shapes nucleus	Differentiate into macrophages within tissues
Lymphocytes* Includes both T and B cells	20% to 45%	Small, round cell with little cytoplasm surrounding a dense nucleus	*T cells*—mediate cellular immune response; include both cytotoxic (MHC I, CD8) and helper T cells (MHC II, CD4) *B cells*—mediate humoral immune response; can act as antigen presenting cell (APC) and differentiate into plasma cells
Mast cells		Granules which contain histamine, heparin, and chemotactic factors	Bind IgE and mediate allergic reactions, including type I hypersensitivity reactions

Table 5.1 Types of Leukocytes (Continued)

Type of Leukocyte	Normal Percentage in Peripheral Blood	Unique Histologic Features and Type of Granules	Function
Macrophages		Ameboid cell shape with cytoplasmic inclusions of phagocytized materials	Differentiated from monocytes; phagocytic cells in tissues; can function as an APC
Plasma cells		Eccentric nucleus with "clock-face" chromatin and perinuclear clearing ("perinuclear hoff")	Produce antibodies

*These are granulocytes.
**Those in italics are found in a standard WBC differential panel and are those WBCs found in blood (the others are more commonly found in tissue).

Define erythrocytosis:	An increased number of RBCs (eg, as seen in polycythemia vera)
Define leukocytosis:	An increased number of WBCs (eg, as seen in infection or leukemia)
Define anisocytosis:	The presence of an increased amount of RBC size variation
Define poikilocytosis:	The presence of an increased amount of RBC shape variation
Define reticulocytosis:	An increased number of immature RBCs

Pathology—RBCs

What does the *hemoglobin* (Hb) on a CBC measure?	The concentration of hemoglobin in the blood (the normal range for men is 13-15 g/dL and for women is 12-15 g/dL).
What does the hematocrit (Hct) measure?	A percentage of the total volume of erythrocytes relative to the total blood in a sample. Typically, Hct = 3 × Hb. The normal range for men is 40% to 45% and for women is 35% to 45%.

What are the three major categories of anemia?

1. Microcytic (MCV <80)
2. Normocytic (MCV 80-100)
3. Macrocytic (MCV >100)

What does the mean corpuscular volume (MCV) measure?

The average volume of red blood cells (RBCs). Since this is the average measurement it does not identify mixed cell populations, therefore a mixed anemia (microcytic and macrocytic may have a normal MCV).

What are common etiologies of microcytic anemia?

Iron deficiency anemia, thalassemia, lead poisoning, or anemia of chronic disease

*Iron deficiency is by far the most common

What are common etiologies of normocytic anemia?

Anemia of chronic disease hemolytic anemias, acute hemorrhage, aplastic anemias, renal failure

What are common etiologies of macrocytic anemia?

Vitamin B_{12} deficiency or folate deficiency (megaloblastic anemia), alcoholism, chronic liver disease, drugs that block DNA synthesis, significant reticulocytosis

Mechanistically, what causes anemia?

1. Decreased production of RBCs
   a. Deficiency of nutrients (eg, iron) or proteins needed for hematopoiesis
   b. Bone marrow failure
   c. Decreased erythropoietin (typically secondary to renal failure)
2. Increased destruction or loss of RBCs
   a. Hemolysis
   b. Hemorrhage

To evaluate anemia of an unknown origin, what should you remember to order?

Reticulocyte count; this should be elevated with acute blood loss or hemolysis and low (<1%) with decreased RBC production.

What is the most common cause of iron depletion?

Chronic blood loss; seen often in menstruating women. In older patients and men, check stool for microscopic blood (ie, due to colorectal cancer).

What labs would you order to differentiate iron deficiency anemia from anemia of chronic disease?

See Table 5.2 below.

Table 5.2 Lab Values—Iron Deficiency Anemia versus Anemia of Chronic Disease

	Iron Deficiency	Anemia of Chronic Disease
Serum iron	↓	↓
Ferritin*	↓	Varies
% Transferrin saturation	↓↓	↓
TIBC (total iron-binding capacity)	↓	↓

*Remember, ferritin is an acute phase reactant and may be elevated in inflammatory/infectious processes, resulting in misinterpretation.

What causes α-thalassemia?

It is the result of mutations in α-globin genes leading to underproduction or absence of α-globin protein. There are four α-globin genes; severity of disease is a reflection of the number of genes involved.
1. Missing 1 copy of the gene results in a silent carrier state; no anemia is present although patients may have slightly decreased MCV.
2. Missing 2 copies of the gene leads to α-thalassemia trait, which typically manifests as mild microcytic hypochromic anemia and may be clinically mistaken for iron deficiency anemia.

What is hemoglobin H disease ("Hb H")?

The form of α-thalassemia in which patient lacks three α-globin chains, leading to production of β-tetramers. This results in mild to moderate microcytic hypochromic anemia with target cells and Heinz bodies, hepatosplenomegaly, and jaundice.

What is hemoglobin Barts ("Hb Barts")?

All four α-globin genes are missing, leading to complete absence of α-globin chains and production of γ-tetramers and resulting in severe fetal anemia, hydrops fetalis, and often intrauterine fetal demise.
In both Hb H and Hb Barts, the abnormal tetramers have a higher affinity for oxygen than normal hemoglobin resulting in impaired oxygen delivery to tissues.

*Bart = Babies die

What causes β-thalassemia minor and how does it present?

Underproduction of β chain (heterozygote). This is the milder form of β-thalassemia, with mild to moderate anemia.

What causes β-thalassemia major and how does it present?

Absence of β chain. Patients present early in childhood with severe anemia requiring repeated blood transfusions. Often patients have slowed growth and over time can develop sequelae of secondary hemochromatosis, including cardiac failure.

What are the major etiologies of hemolytic anemias?

- Autoimmune (idiopathic, drug related, or underlying disease)
- Nonimmune mediated (microangiopathic, hypersplenism, secondary to cardiac prosthesis, etc)
- RBC membrane defects—both acquired and congenital (hereditary spherocytosis, elliptocytosis, paroxysmal nocturnal hemoglobinuria [PNH], Wilson disease)
- Hemoglobinopathies (sickle cell disease, thalassemia, HbC)
- Enzyme defects (G6PD deficiency most commonly)

Mechanistically, what are the two ways that hemolysis occurs?

1. Intravascular (as the name implies, RBCs destroyed within the blood vessels)—often more severe anemia; labs show hemoglobinemia, hemoglobinuria, and low haptoglobin (eg, microangiopathic, ABO incompatibility)
2. Extravascular (aka within the reticuloendothelial system)—labs show elevated serum bilirubin and lactate dehydrogenase (LDH) (eg, RBC membrane defects)

What are the two categories of autoimmune hemolytic anemias?

1. Warm agglutinin (IgG)—typically more chronic; seen in chronic disease (eg, SLE, CLL) and drugs; primarily extravascular hemolysis
2. Cold agglutinin (IgM)—acute anemia; seen in infections such as mycoplasma and mononucleosis

What are schistocytes and how do they form?

Schistocytes are fragmented RBCs, resulting from mechanical/sheering damage to the RBCs, often seen in DIC or with mechanical heart valves.

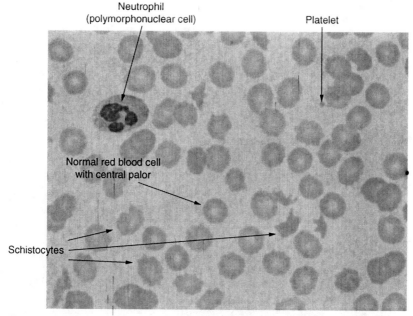

Figure 5.1 Schistocytes and bite cells among otherwise normal red blood cells, a single polymorphonuclear cell, and platelets. (Reproduced, with permission, from OHSU.)

What are spherocytes?

Small round erythrocytes that have lost their central pallor and biconcave shape, formed secondary to a defective cytoskeletal protein. The sphere is the shape with the least surface tension but also the least flexible, resulting in frequent damage to the cell as it passes through the reticuloendothelial system (ie, the spleen).

What cytoskeletal proteins are defective in hereditary spherocytosis?

Spectrin and ankyrin

What test is used to confirm hereditary spherocytosis?

Osmotic fragility test

What is the definitive treatment for hereditary spherocytosis?

Splenectomy. Howell-Jolly bodies (basophilic nuclear remnants) are seen on blood smear after splenectomy.

What specific genetic mutation results in sickle cell anemia?

Single amino acid replacement of glutamine with valine on the hemoglobin β chain. Mutated hemoglobin is referred to as Hb S.

How does the mutation in sickle cell anemia actually lead to anemia?

The mutation in hemoglobin leads to decreased red blood cell deformability/elasticity. As the RBCs traverse the capillaries they do not have the normal elastic properties to distort as they pass through, instead the low oxygen tension promotes "sickling" of the cells. The repeated "sickling" of the cells damages the cell membrane, this damage in addition to the misshapen nature of the cells leads to increased destruction of RBCs in the spleen.

What are some clinical findings associated with sickle cell anemia?

Anemia, cholelithiasis, pain crisis, dactylitis (painful and swollen hands and feet), and autosplenectomy

What are some other hemoglobinopathies?

- Hemoglobin C—similar clinical picture as HbS; most common in West Africa
- Hemoglobin E—range of illness from asymptomatic to severe; most common in Southeast Asia

What two microscopic findings are associated with glucose-6-phosphate dehydrogenase (G6PD) deficiency?

1. *Heinz bodies*—membrane-bound precipitants of denatured hemoglobin secondary to oxidation of iron; can result in bite cells.
2. *Bite cells*—partially devoured RBCs, where macrophages have taken a "bite" out, typically to remove a Heinz body.

How does disseminated intravascular coagulation (DIC) occur?

Coagulation sequence is activated; microthrombi form; platelets, fibrin, and coagulation factors are consumed; and fibrinolytic mechanisms begin

What are the common causes of DIC?

Sepsis, trauma, malignancy (particularly acute promyelocytic leukemia), obstetric complications (eg, preeclampsia), transfusions

What lab findings characterize DIC?

- High—prothrombin time (PT), partial thromboplastin time (PTT), fibrin split products (D-dimer)
- Low—platelet count

What is aplastic anemia?

Failure or destruction of pluripotent bone marrow precursor cells, resulting in pancytopenia

What WBC finding is associated with macrocytic/megaloblastic anemia?

Hypersegmented neutrophils seen in vitamin B_{12}/folate deficiency

Pathology—Coagulation and Platelets

Which coagulation factor is deficient in hemophilia A?

Factor VIII

Which coagulation factor is deficient in hemophilia B?

Factor IX

What is the most common bleeding disorder?

von Willebrand disease

How does a deficiency in von Willebrand factor (vWF) lead to increased bleeding?

Directly results in impaired platelet adhesion and also decreased half-life of factor VIII.

Where is vWF stored?	It is stored within Weibel-Palade bodies within the vascular endothelial cells.
Which lab value measures the activity of the extrinsic pathway of the coagulation cascade?	Prothrombin time (PT): from this measurement a standardized number is calculated and reported as the INR (international normalized ratio).
Which lab value measures the activity of the intrinsic pathway?	Partial thromboplastin time (PTT)
What medication prolongs the PT/INR (with a normal PTT)?	Warfarin—the INR is typically monitored closely in patients on warfarin therapy.
What disease processes prolong the PT/INR?	Liver disease, vitamin K deficiency, DIC (early), Factor VII deficiency, lupus anticoagulant
What medication prolongs the PTT?	Heparin
What disease processes prolong the PTT (with a normal PT)?	Factor deficiencies (VII, IX, XI, XII), clotting factor inhibitors, von Willebrand disease, lupus anticoagulant
What is immune thrombocytic purpura (ITP)?	An autoimmune disorder where autoantibodies form against platelets
What population most often gets ITP?	Young women, 20 to 40 years old
What characterizes ITP?	Prolonged bleeding time with normal PT and PTT. The patient has pinpoint (petechial) hemorrhages, easy bruising, ecchymoses, low platelet count, but an increased number of megakaryocytes in the bone marrow.
What is thrombotic thrombocytopenic purpura (TTP)?	A condition with widespread formation of hyaline thrombi and consumption of platelets that leads to thrombocytopenia and microangiopathic hemolytic anemia
What might you see microscopically in TTP?	Schistocytes (fragmented red blood cells)
What is the pentad of symptoms seen in TTP?	Fever, thrombocytopenia, microangiopathic hemolytic anemia (MAHA), neurological changes, and renal failure

What causes Bernard-Soulier disease?

Mutation in GpIb resulting in a defect in platelet adhesion

What causes Glanzmann thrombasthenia?

Mutation in GpIIb/IIIa, again resulting in defective platelet *aGGregation*

*G for Glanzmann and aGGregation

What is the most common congenital thrombophilia?

Factor V Leiden—a mutation in Factor V (replacement of arginine with glutamine) conferring resistance to degradation by protein C and therefore leading to increased active factor V and a prothrombotic state. Other less common congenital thrombophilias include: prothrombin G20210A mutation, protein C deficiency, protein S deficiency, and antithrombin deficiency.

Give two examples of common acquired thrombophilias/hypercoagulable states:

1. Malignancy
2. Antiphospholipid antibodies (anti-cardiolipin antibodies and lupus anticoagulants)

IMMUNOLOGY

Anatomy/Physiology

What is the reticuloendothelial system and what does it include?

It is part of the immune system, consisting of phagocytes, primarily macrophages and monocytes, located in the reticular connective tissue such as the spleen and lymphoid tissues. It includes the bone marrow, thymus, spleen, lymph nodes, MALT (mucosa-associated lymphoid tissues), Kupffer cells within the liver, and microglia within the CNS.

What are the two histological portions of the spleen?

1. Red pulp—splenic sinuses filled with blood
2. White pulp—lymphoid aggregates

What type of cell is found in the periarterial lymphatic sheath (PALS) of the spleen?

T cells make up the PALS, while B cells make up the follicles within the white pulp.

What is the function of the thymus?	The thymus is a primary lymphoid organ and the site of T-cell differentiation and maturation.
Does a person's thymus grow larger or smaller with age?	The thymus grows larger from birth through onset of puberty; thereafter the thymus grows smaller as it involutes.

Pathology—Immunodeficiencies

What are the four immunodeficiencies that affect B cells and how do they differ in their mechanism?

1. Bruton agammaglobulinemia—X-linked recessive; decrease *production/number* of B cells resulting in low levels of all immunoglobulins; patients have multiple recurrent bacterial infections
2. Severe combined immunodeficiency (SCID)—most commonly X-linked; decreased *production/number* of B and T cells; patients have multiple bacterial, viral, fungal, and protozoal infections
3. Wiskott-Aldrich syndrome—X-linked recessive; decreased *activation* of B cells to encapsulated bacteria ($\downarrow$ IgM); classic triad of symptoms include pyogenic infections, thrombocytopenic purpura, and eczema
4. Selective IgA deficiency—unclear etiology, likely *defect in isotype switching*; patient have recurrent sinus and lung infections, may also have milk allergies and diarrhea; anaphylaxis with transfusion of blood products containing IgA

What is DiGeorge syndrome?

A syndrome associated with deletion of chromosome 22q11.2, leading to failure of the thymus and parathyroid glands to develop and with other congenital abnormalities including cardiac malformations, cleft palate, and abnormal facies.

What infections are patients with DiGeorge syndrome more susceptible?

Viral and fungal infections secondary to T-cell deficiency

| What is the deficit in Chédiak-Higashi syndrome? | This syndrome is the result of a defect in phagocytic cell microtubular function resulting in impaired lysosome degranulation and therefore poor immunity against bacteria. |

Pathology—Immune Responses

What are the classic features of a granuloma?	A collection of epithelioid histiocytes with scattered multinucleated giant cells. The granuloma may or may not contain necrosis.
Give examples of granulomatous diseases:	Tuberculosis, fungal infections, leprosy, cat scratch disease (*Bartonella*), sarcoidosis, Wegner, syphilis, Crohn disease
What HLA allele is associated with ankylosing spondylitis?	B27
What HLA allele is associated with postgonococcal arthritis?	B27
What HLA allele is associated with acute anterior uveitis?	B27
What HLA allele is associated with rheumatoid arthritis?	DR4
What HLA allele is associated with chronic active hepatitis?	DR3
What HLA allele is associated with primary Sjögren syndrome?	DR3
What HLA alleles are associated with type I diabetes mellitus?	DR3 and DR4
Name the four types of hypersensitivity reactions:	1. Type I—immediate hypersensitivity/anaphylactic and atopic reactions 2. Type II—antibody-mediated cytotoxicity 3. Type III—immune-complex disorders 4. Type IV—cell-mediated or delayed-type hypersensitivity

What is the mechanism for type I hypersensitivity reaction?	Exposure to allergen (antigen), antigen then cross-links IgE on presensitized mast cells and basophils resulting in release of vasoactive amines including histamine, followed by allergic end-organ responses
What are the two phases of type I hypersensitivity?	1. Immediate response occurring within 1 hour of exposure 2. Delayed (late) phase response within 3 to 12 hours after exposure
What characterizes the immediate response?	Cross-linked IgE, mast cell activation, histamine release, vasodilation, vascular leakage, and glandular secretions
What characterizes the late response?	New cytokine and leukotriene synthesis, tissue infiltration, tissue destruction, and mucosal epithelial cell damage
How can one identify a type I hypersensitivity reaction?	There must be a specific exposure, short time frame until symptoms occur, specific allergens, and characteristic symptoms.
What is the mechanism for type II reaction (antibody-mediated)?	IgG or IgM are produced and bind to antigen, leading to phagocytosis or lysis by activated complement or Fc receptors
What are some examples of a type II hypersensitivity reaction?	Autoimmune hemolytic anemia, Goodpasture syndrome, and erythroblastosis fetalis (hemolytic disease of the newborn)
Which syndrome creates organ-specific antibodies against the basement membranes of the lung and kidney?	Goodpasture syndrome
What is the mechanism of type III reaction?	Antigen-antibody immune complex deposits, usually in vessel walls, result in acute inflammation (neutrophils) and tissue damage
Give two examples of type III hypersensitivity reactions:	1. Arthus reaction (local) 2. Serum sickness (systemic)
What is the Arthus reaction?	Antibodies complex with various foreign proteins causing a cutaneous vasculitis and localized tissue necrosis

What is the mechanism of type IV reaction?	Activated T lymphocytes activate macrophages and secrete cytokines causing T-cell-mediated cytotoxicity.
What is special about type IV reactions?	This is the only hypersensitivity reaction that does NOT involve antibodies.
What is the classic example of a delayed type IV reaction?	A reactive purified protein derivative (PPD) (tuberculin skin test) will be positive within 48 to 72 hours.
What are some examples of type IV hypersensitivity reactions?	PPD skin test; contact dermatitis; type 1 diabetes mellitus; Guillain-Barré syndrome; multiple sclerosis

ONCOLOGY

What type of leukemia is most common in children?	Acute lymphoblastic leukemia (ALL)
What type of leukemia is most common in young adults, 15 to 40 years old?	Acute myeloblastic leukemia (AML)
What are the characteristic findings of AML on peripheral smear?	Significantly increased circulating myelocytes (blasts) with *Auer rods* present
What are the unique risks, benefits, and the chromosomal abnormality associated with type M3 (promyelocytic) AML?	Increased risk of severe DIC, but responds well to treatment with all-trans retinoic acid (vitamin A), including inducing differentiation of myeloblast. Associated with t(15;17) translocation.
What chronic leukemia is most common in older people, ages >60?	Chronic lymphocytic leukemia (CLL)
What genetic change defines chronic myelogenous leukemia (CML)?	The Philadelphia chromosome, t(9;22) translocation, resulting in the *bcr-abl* fusion gene and protein. Imatinib and other tyrosine kinase inhibitors (anti-*bcr-abl*) provide targeted therapy against the fusion protein.
What genetic alteration is associated with Burkitt lymphoma?	t(8; 14) translocation, involving the c-myc oncogene on chromosome 8 and Ig heavy chain locus on chromosome 14

What is the classic histologic description of Burkitt lymphoma?

Monomorphous sheets of lymphoid cells with high mitotic rate and occasional tingible body-laden macrophage (macrophages containing apoptotic debris) create a "starry sky" appearance.

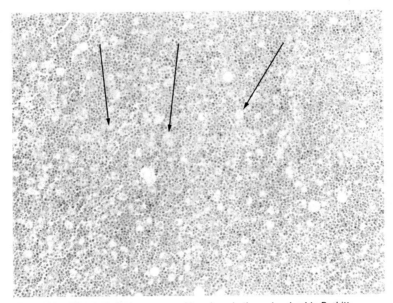

Figure 5.2 "Starry-sky" appearance of lymph node tissue involved in Burkitt lymphoma. The stars in the sky (arrows) are tingible body-laden macrophages, and the dark sky is sheet of malignant lymphocytes. (Reproduced, with permission, from OHSU.)

What genetic alteration is associated with follicular (B cell) lymphoma?

t(14; 18) and expression of bcl-2 involved in apoptosis

Table 5.3 Notable Chromosomal Translocations

Malignancy	Associated Translocation
CML	t(9;22)—*bcr-abl* fusion
AML-M3 (acute promyelocytic leukemia)	t(15;17)
Burkitt lymphoma	t(8;14)—*c*-myc activation
Follicular lymphoma	t(14;18)—*bcl*-2 activation
Mantle cell lymphoma	t(11;14)
Ewing sarcoma	t(11;22)

What is the most common type of Hodgkin lymphoma?

Nodular sclerosing Hodgkin disease

Who usually gets Hodgkin lymphoma?

Bimodal age distribution: 15 to 35 years and >50 years

What is the characteristic cell of Hodgkin disease?

Reed-Sternberg cell

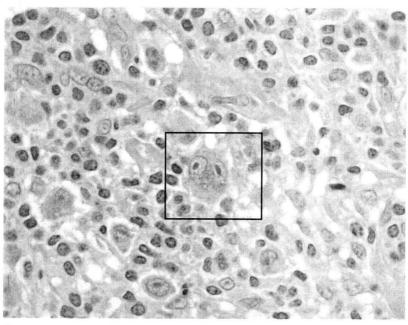

Figure 5.3 Binucleated Reed-Sternberg cell seen in Hodgkin lymphoma. (Reproduced, with permission, from Wettach T, et al: *Road Map Pathology*, New York: McGraw-Hill, 2009; fig 17-3B.)

What virus is clearly oncogenic in Burkitt lymphoma and may also be associated with Hodgkin lymphoma?

Epstein-Barr virus (EBV)

What malignancy is induced by the oncogenic virus HTLV-1?

Adult T-cell leukemia (HTLV-1 = human T-cell leukemia virus 1)

What lymphoma usually occurs in older adults?

Diffuse large cell lymphoma

What aggressive lymphoma usually presents in children?	Lymphoblastic lymphoma (T cells)
A patient is found to have a tumor in her thymus. What is the most likely diagnosis and what underlying disease may she have?	The patient likely has a thymoma, the most common tumor of the thymus, and may have myasthenia gravis (MG). Approximately 30% to 45% of patients with thymomas have MG and ~15% of patients with MG will be found to have thymomas.

TRANSPLANTATION

What is an autograft?	Tissue implanted from self (donor and recipient are the same person)
What is an allograft?	Tissue implanted from genetically different donor of the same species as the recipient
What is a xenograft?	Tissue implanted from a donor of a different species (eg, porcine heart valves in humans)
What is a syngeneic graft?	Transplant between genetically identical individuals (eg, bone marrow transplant between identical twins)
What antigen labeling system is most important for predicting transplant rejection?	HLA system (especially Class I, DR/DQ)
Name the four types of transplant rejections:	1. Hyperacute (minutes to hours) 2. Acute humoral (within first few months) 3. Acute cellular (within first few months) 4. Chronic (months to years and episodic)
What is the mechanism for hyperacute rejection?	Humoral—there is a preformed cytotoxic antibody to the donor antigen, usually at the level of the vascular endothelium
What histological changes characterize hyperacute transplant rejection?	Fibrinoid necrosis and thrombosis

What is the mechanism of acute vascular rejection?

Humoral—antibodies to the donor antigen develop over time

What histologic changes characterize acute humoral/vascular rejection?

Arteritis, necrosis, thrombosis, and neutrophilic infiltration

What is the mechanism of acute cellular rejection?

Cell-mediated—the recipient's $CD4^+$ and $CD8^+$ lymphocytes attack donor cells

What histologic changes characterize acute cellular rejection?

Lymphocytes/mononuclear cell infiltration; interstitial and tubular inflammation

What causes chronic rejection?

Any disturbance in the ability of the host and graft to tolerate one another

What histologic changes characterize chronic rejection?

Vascular changes, especially intimal hyperplasia and fibrosis

Describe GVHD:

The donor's lymphocytes in the graft immunologically attack the recipient's cells (outside of the graft) because the graft lymphocytes recognize the recipient's cells as "non-self."

What characterizes GVHD clinically?

Skin rash, jaundice, and diarrhea

What can be done to attempt to prevent GVHD?

Irradiated the donor cells to eliminate leukocytes

If a person is deficient in polymorphonuclear neutrophils (PMNs), what types of infections are they most susceptible to?

Infections caused by *Staphylococcus, Aspergillus, Candida,* and gram-negative bacteria

Deficiency in T cells makes you susceptible to what types of infections?

Mycobacteria, fungi, parasites, viruses

Deficiency in antibodies makes you susceptible to what types of infections?

Encapsulated organisms and viruses

Deficiencies in complement make you susceptible to what types of infections?

Neisseria, especially *Meningococcus*

TRANSFUSION MEDICINE

In ABO blood groups, what is Landsteiner rule?

If you lack the RBC antigen, you make the antibody to it (type A antigen blood has anti-B antibodies).

Which blood type is the universal recipient?

Type AB, because they have formed neither anti-A or anti-B antibodies in their plasma.

What does Rh⁺ indicate?

The presence of the D antigen on the person's RBCs.

What is Rh immune globulin?

Immunoglobin G (IgG) anti-D antibodies in a purified preparation; given to Rh? mothers in pregnancy to prevent hemolytic disease of the newborn

What does the direct antiglobulin test (DAT or direct Coombs) detect?

The DAT detects the presence of antibodies coating the patient's RBC surface in vivo.

What does the indirect antiglobulin test (IAT or indirect Coombs) detect?

The IAT detects RBC antibodies in the patient's serum (in vitro binding of IgG).

Describe the process for performing both the DAT and IAT:

- DAT—The patient's RBCs are washed (removing the patient's plasma) and then incubated with Coombs reagent (anti-human globulin). If agglutination of the RBCs occurs the test is positive, indicating that antibodies on the surface of the patient's RBCs were present and bound the Coombs reagent in order to agglutinate.
- IAT—The patient's serum is extracted (RBCs removed) and incubated with standard RBCs that have known antigenicity. Then the Coombs reagent is added. If agglutination occurs the test is positive, indicating presence of antibodies in the patient's serum binding to an antigen on the standard RBCs and then binding Coombs reagent in order to agglutinate.

In addition to the Rh system, what are some other clinically significant RBC antigens?

Kidd (causes severe acute hemolytic transfusion reactions), Duffy, and Kell

What tests are performed on donated blood to screen for human immunodeficiency virus (HIV) contamination?

Standard tests for anti-HIV-1 and HIV-2 antibodies. HIV-1 p24 antigen (by ELISA) and HIV nucleic acid testing are also used specifically to detect very early infection.

What is used as an anticoagulant in blood components?

Citrate

How does the anticoagulant work?

It binds calcium ions, making them unavailable to be used as cofactors in the coagulation cascade.

What are the available blood components for transfusion?

Red blood cells (RBCs); fresh frozen plasma (FFP); platelets (PLT); cryoprecipitate (cryo from FFP)

How many units of whole blood does the average adult have in his/her body?

8 to 10 units

On average, giving 1 unit of packed RBCs should raise the hemoglobin level by how much?

1 g/dL

What type of RBCs should be given to patients who have had previous problems with febrile reactions to blood products, or who will be chronically transfused?

Leukocyte-reduced RBCs since they decrease the risk of human leukocyte antigen (HLA) autoimmunization and the risk of transfusion reactions

What should be used as an intravascular volume expander?

Albumin, crystalloid, or colloid; *not* FFP

When might you give a patient platelets?

Prophylactic use for extremely low platelet counts (<10,000/μL); prior to surgery for low platelet counts (typically <50,000/μL); to aid coagulation in actively bleeding patients

What is the usual dose of platelets?

1 unit in adults, or 10 mL/kg in pediatrics

What are *apheresis platelets*?

Platelets collected from a single donor during an apheresis procedure

What does cryoprecipitate contain?

Factor VIII, factor XIII, fibrinogen, and von Willebrand factor

What is the most common metabolic side effect of massive blood transfusion?	Alkalosis due to the citrate anticoagulant converting to bicarbonate in the liver
What correlates to the severity of a febrile nonhemolytic transfusion reaction?	The number of leukocytes present in the blood component
What is a risk of FFP transfusion?	Allergic/anaphylactic reactions
What causes these allergic reactions?	The patient has IgE antibodies against plasma proteins in the transfused blood
What type of patients will have anaphylactic reactions?	Patients who are IgA deficient and have preformed IgA antibodies
What can be done to prevent anaphylactic reactions in these individuals?	Use washed RBCs and platelets or use plasma from other IgA-deficient patients
What causes TRALI (transfusion-related acute lung injury)?	The donor's antileukocyte antibodies react with the recipient's leukocytes.
What characterizes TRALI clinically?	Pulmonary edema, fever, tachypnea, cyanosis
What infection are blood-transfusion recipients at greatest risk for?	Bacterial contamination (*not* HIV or hepatitis)

CLINICAL VIGNETTES

A patient reports severe nausea and dizziness within an hour of eating shrimp. What type of hypersensitivity reaction is this?

Type I hypersensitivity

A 4-year-old child has allergic rhinitis, eczema (atopic dermatitis), and asthma. What is the hypersensitivity type?

Type I hypersensitivity

A woman is Rh⁻ and pregnant with her second Rh⁺ child. If she does not receive anti-Rh immunoglobulin during either pregnancy, what will likely happen?

Erythroblastosis fetalis, or hemolytic disease of the newborn, will result since the mother will likely have anti-Rh antibodies in her bloodstream, from the first pregnancy, that will cause hemolysis of the second fetus's RBCs.

A newborn baby shows signs of anemia and jaundice within the first 24 hours of life. What might he have?

Hemolytic disease of the newborn (due to Rh factor incompatibility or ABO blood group incompatibility between mother and infant)

A woman starts to feel exhausted and light-headed a week after beginning a course of penicillin. What is this?

Autoimmune hemolytic anemia, which is a type II hypersensitivity reaction to a drug (the body forms antibodies to the drug, the antibody binds the drug on the RBCs, resulting in hemolysis)

A patient develops an itchy, raised, red rash 2 to 3 days after using a new brand of laundry detergent. What is this?

Contact dermatitis, which is a type IV hypersensitivity reaction

A patient begins receiving a blood transfusion. He develops fever, chills, hypotension, and DIC. What happened?

Acute hemolytic transfusion reaction. The patient received RBCs with an antigen to which he had previously formed alloantibodies, such as ABO antigens or Kidd antigen.

A child receives a bone marrow transplant from his healthy brother. Several months later he develops a rash, jaundice, and diarrhea. What is this reaction?

Graft-versus-host disease (GVHD)

An alcoholic man presents with anemia. Would you expect his mean corpuscular volume (MCV) to be high or low? What is he probably deficient in?

Expect him to have megaloblastic anemia with a high MCV, either as a direct result from the chronic alcohol use or secondary to concomitant vitamin B_{12} and/or folate deficiency.

A 53-year-old man has been feeling tired recently. His hemoglobin level is 8.0. What should you be sure to order?

Check for occult blood in the stool and order a colonoscopy to evaluate for possible colorectal cancer.

An elderly woman has lung cancer. What might characterize her anemia of chronic disease?

Decreased RBC life span, microcytosis, impaired iron metabolism, and possible refractoriness or lack of response to erythropoietin

A 7-year-old girl has an elevated white blood cell (WBC) count, easy bruising, and fatigue. What should she be evaluated for?

Acute lymphoblastic leukemia—the most common type of cancer in children under age 15

A 17-year-old girl notices a swollen lymph node in her neck and biopsy shows Reed-Sternberg cells. What disease is likely?

Hodgkin disease

CHAPTER 6

Cardiovascular Pathology

EMBRYOLOGY

What is the ductus arteriosus?	It connects the pulmonary artery to the proximal aorta, effectively by passing the lungs during fetal development.
What happens if the ductus doesn't close after birth?	If it remains patent after birth, the neonate becomes hypoxic (patent ductus arteriosus, PDA).
The sinus venosus gives rise to which parts of the cardiovascular system?	A portion of the wall of the right atrium and the coronary sinus
The bulbus cordis gives rise to which parts of the cardiovascular system?	The proximal aorta and the pulmonary arteries
What is the function of the ductus venosus?	To provide a direct passageway for nutrient-rich blood from the placenta to pass through the developing liver to supply the developing heart
What happens to the ductus venosus at birth?	It becomes obliterated and fibrosed, forming the ligamentum venosum.

ANATOMY

Define the anatomic components of the cardiovascular system:	Heart, macrovasculature (aorta, arteries, large arterioles, veins), microvasculature (small arterioles, postcapillary venules, capillaries), and lymphatics

Name the four heart valves in the direction of blood flow:

1. Tricuspid valve
2. Pulmonary valve
3. Mitral valve
4. Aortic valve

What structure provides the base of attachment for the cardiac valves?

The so-called "fibrous skeleton" of the heart, which is composed of dense connective tissue and has three main components: the septum membranaceum, the trigona fibrosa, and the annuli fibrosi. The base of each cardiac valve is attached to the annuli fibrosi.

What is the anatomic location of the carotid bodies and what is their function?

The carotid bodies are located near the bifurcation of the common carotid artery (bilaterally), and they function as chemoreceptors monitoring levels of carbon dioxide and oxygen in the blood.

What is the anatomic location of the carotid sinus and what is their function?

The carotid sinuses are dilatated segments of the internal carotid artery (bilaterally), and they contain baroreceptors which detect changes in blood pressure and transmit this information to the central nervous system.

At what anatomic location does lymphatic fluid reenter the bloodstream?

Either via the thoracic duct at the confluence of the left internal jugular and left subclavian veins or via the right lymphatic duct at the confluence of the right internal jugular and right subclavian veins.

Which two organs do not have lymphatic drainage?

1. Central nervous system
2. The bone marrow

HISTOLOGY

Name the three microscopically identifiable "coats" of blood vessel walls:

1. Tunica (L. "coat") intima
2. Tunica media
3. Tunica adventitia

Which additional named structures of blood vessel walls are identifiable in arteries?

Internal elastic lamina (separates the tunica intima from the tunica media) and the external elastic lamina (separates the tunica media from the tunica adventitia)

What is the cellular composition of the tunica intima?

A single layer of endothelial cells supported by a subendothelial layer of loose connective tissue with scattered smooth muscle cells.

Of what are the internal and external elastic lamina composed? What are the functions of these structures?

Elastin. Gaps in the internal elastic lamina (aka fenestrae) allow nutritive substances from the blood to diffuse to cells located deeper in the vessel wall. The elastic properties of both the internal and external lamina serve to modulate the degree of pressure variation in vessels during systole and diastole.

What is the cellular and extracellular composition of the tunica media?

Concentric layers of smooth muscle cells admixed with variable amounts of elastic fibers, type III collagen, proteoglycans, and glycoproteins produced by the smooth muscle cells

What is unique about the tunica media of the carotid sinus?

It is thinner than the tunica media in other vessels which allows baroreceptors in this segment of the internal carotid artery to detect changes in blood pressure and transmit this information to the central nervous system.

What is the composition of the tunica adventitia?

Type I collagen and elastic fibers

What are vasa vasorum?

Arteries, capillaries, and venules in the tunica adventitia and outer tunica media of larger vessels that provide nutrients to these outer layers

Describe the innervation of blood vessels:

In vessels containing smooth muscle cells, sympathetic nerve fibers discharge norepinephrine to cause vasoconstriction. Vessels that supply blood to skeletal muscles also have cholinergic innervation to cause vasodilation. Density of innervations is higher in arteries than in veins.

Which histologic layer of the wall of the heart is homologous with the tunica intima of blood vessels?

Endocardium

Where do branches of the Purkinje system terminate within the heart?

In the subendocardial layer, which also contains veins and other nerve branches

What cells compose the myocardium and to what fibrous structure are they associated?	The myocardium is composed of cardiac muscle cells (aka cardiomyocytes). These cells are arranged in layers which form a complex spiral around the chambers of the heart. Many cardiomyocytes are anchored to the fibrous cardiac skeleton.

PHYSIOLOGY

What is cardiac output (CO)?	The volume of blood pumped by the heart per unit time. CO (mL/minute) = stroke volume (mL/beat) × heart rate (beats/minute)
What is ejection fraction (EF)?	Of the volume of blood present in the left ventricle at the end of diastole (EDV), EF is the percentage of that volume that is pumped per beat. Normal EF ≥ 55%. EF = (SV/EDV) × 100
Changes in which variables will affect cardiac output?	Stroke volume and heart rate
Changes in which variables will affect stroke volume?	Preload, afterload, and contractility
At which phase of the myocardial action potential does calcium enter the cardiomyocytes?	Phase 2 (plateau)—calcium enters via voltage-gated calcium channels
What is the consequence of calcium influx on cardiomyocyte contraction?	Calcium influx triggers additional calcium release from the sarcoplasmic reticulum. Calcium binds troponin C inducing a conformational change in troponin I and movement of the troponin-tropomyosin complex out of the actin filament active site. When this active site is bound by myosin, cross-bridges form and contraction can occur.
What is the function of the three cardiac troponins?	1. Troponin C binds calcium and is bound to both troponin T and troponin I 2. Troponin T is bound to tropomyosin 3. Troponin I is bound to actin and holds the troponin-tropomyosin complex in place

How is the smooth muscle contraction apparatus different from the cardiac muscle contraction apparatus?

Smooth muscle contraction is dependent on calcium binding calmodulin to activate myosin light chain kinase and phosphorylate myosin leading to cross-bridge formation and contraction. Smooth muscle contraction does not involve troponins.

Which phase of the pacemaker action potential undergoes diastolic depolarization?

Phase 4—the membrane potential will spontaneously depolarize as sodium conductance is increased, this accounts for the automaticity of the sinoatrial (SA) and atrioventricular (AV) nodes and subsequently for heart rate

PATHOLOGY

General Principles

What is the leading cause of death in the United States?

Heart disease

What entities are included in the category "heart disease"?

Coronary artery disease (CAD), cardiomyopathy, ischemic heart disease, hypertension, valvular disease, heart failure, and inflammatory heart disease

What other now common chronic condition increases a patient's risk of experiencing a cardiovascular event?

Diabetes mellitus

What modifiable risk factors can increase a patient's risk of experiencing a cardiovascular event?

Smoking, sedentary lifestyle, obesity, and hyperlipidemia

What is hyperlipidemia?

A state of having elevated quantities of lipid substances—cholesterol and triglycerides, in the blood

What is a clinical sign associated with hyperlipidemia?

Xanthomas—yellow to white waxy deposits commonly involving skin of the eyelids or Achilles tendon

How do xanthomas appear microscopically?

Diffuse dermatitis consisting of foamy histiocytes (lipophages)

Which laboratory tests may be used to assess for myocardial infarction?	Troponin and/or CK-MB are used to assess for cardiac infarction. Historically, myoglobin, LDH, AST levels were also used.
When do cardiac troponin levels increase after a myocardial infarction and how long will the levels remain elevated?	Levels will rise approximately 3 to 6 hours after infarction and may remain elevated for as long as 14 days after the event. (Note—there is a latent period, therefore if a patient presents with very acute infarction, the troponin level may initially *not* be elevated.)
Which laboratory test is used in diagnosis and management of congestive heart failure?	B-type natriuretic peptide (BNP)

Table 6.1 ECG Findings and Electrolyte Abnormalities

ECG Finding	Electrolyte Abnormality
Peaked T waves	Hyperkalemia
Prolonged QT	Hypocalcemia
Flattened T waves	Hypokalemia
Prominent V waves	Hypokalemia
Wide QRS	Hyperkalemia

Vascular

What are the risk factors for hypertension?	Smoking; Obesity; Diabetes; African American race/Age *SODA*
What is the most common identifiable etiology of hypertension (HTN)?	Renal disease, which accounts for less than 10% of all cases of HTN; the remaining 90% of cases are termed "essential (primary) hypertension" and the underlying cause is not well-characterized.
What are the complications of uncontrolled HTN over time?	Aortic dissection; coronary heart disease; congestive heart failure (CHF); renal failure; stroke
What part of the brain parenchyma does uncontrolled hypertension affect first?	Basal ganglia and internal capsule

What is the difference between hypertensive *urgency* and *emergency*?

Urgency is only high blood pressure (>200/>120), whereas *emergency* is high blood pressure and *end-organ damage*.

What is atherosclerosis?

A process of thickening of the wall of any sized artery as a result of deposition of fatty materials (eg, cholesterol) and subsequent chronic inflammatory response

What are the risk factors associated with atherosclerosis?

Smoking; hypertension; hyperlipidemia; diabetes mellitus

What is the earliest histologic and/or gross finding associated with atherosclerosis?

Fatty streaks in a vessel walls

What do fatty streaks progress into?

Plaques—a nodular accumulation of fatty materials and macrophages which may be associated with cholesterol crystals and calcification

What is the most common arterial location of atherosclerosis?

Abdominal aorta

What is arteriosclerosis? Arteriolosclerosis?

- Arteriosclerosis is a term used to describe "hardening" of medium to large arteries.
- Arteriolosclerosis is a term used to describe "hardening" of small arteries.

  *Note neither of these terms is specific for changes to artery walls due to atherosclerosis.

Define stable angina:

A clinical term used to describe chest pain that develops with exertion or stress and is relieved with rest

Define acute coronary syndrome (ACS):

A term used to describe a clinical presentation which may represent manifestations of one of several underlying pathologic processes. Generally, patients present with chest pain starting a rest or with minimal exertion that is not relieved with rest or nitroglycerine. ACS may represent unstable angina, ST-elevation myocardial infarction (STEMI), or non-ST-elevation MI (NSTEMI).

What is the difference between unstable angina and STEMI/NSTEMI?

In unstable angina, heart muscle is not damaged. In STEMI and NSTEMI, heart muscle undergoes ischemic damage and becomes infarcted.

What is the cause of stable angina?

Stable angina is a clinical scenario that can be caused by decreased blood flow to myocardium (eg, due to narrowing of vessel lumen by atherosclerosis), resistance of vasculature to blood flow, and decreased oxygen-carrying capacity of the blood.

Which drug relieves the chest pain associated with stable angina?

Usually nitroglycerin or vasodilators (ie, calcium channel blockers). If there is decreased oxygen-carrying capacity in the blood, the patient may need blood transfusion or other therapies.

What is the cause of unstable angina?

Atherosclerotic plaque disruption with subsequent platelet plug formation, possibly leading to thrombosis of a coronary vessel

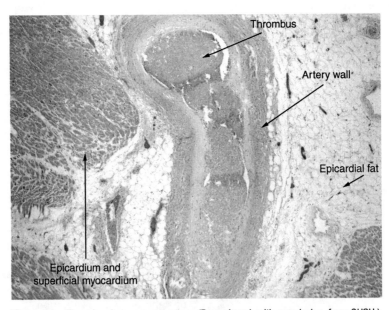

Figure 6.1 Thrombus in a coronary artery. (Reproduced, with permission, from OHSU.)

What is the cause of Prinzmetal angina?	Vasospasm that causes a clinically significant narrowing of the coronary vessels; the etiology of vasospasm is not known.
Which artery is the most commonly affected during acute MI?	Left anterior descending (LAD) *Older LADs usually have MIs
How is an MI diagnosed?	Clinical history and depending on timing of presentation, cardiac enzymes, and abnormal ECG findings
What are the two patterns of MI?	1. Transmural 2. Subendocardial
What areas of the heart are affected with transmural infarctions?	Blood flow to the entire ventricular wall is compromised. Ultimately, necrosis extends from epicardium to endocardium.
What are the typical findings on ECG with transmural infarction?	ST segment elevation or Q waves
What areas of the heart are affected with subendocardial infarctions?	Only the inner one-third of usually the left ventricle wall
What are the ECG findings in acute subendocardial infarcts?	Nonspecific ischemic changes, ST depression
What are the earliest histologic changes associated with infarction?	Early features of coagulative necrosis with blurring of nuclear and cell borders
In general, what are the gross and microscopic changes observable in MI at autopsy?	In general, observable changes will vary depending on amount of elapsed time between infarction and autopsy. Gross changes can include: pallor or hyperemia, necrotic areas, early scar formation, and old scars from previous MI. Microscopic changes can include: blurring of cardiomyocyte nuclei and striations, neutrophils, macrophages, fibrosis, and scar formation.
During healing and repair, what type of necrosis does infracted myocardium undergo?	Coagulative necrosis
When are the first microscopic changes of coagulative necrosis in MI observable?	After 12 hours

What are the first cells to appear in the damaged tissue about 12 hours post-MI?

Neutrophils

*Neutrophils go to a *New* site of injury at *Noon* (8-12 hours after injury)

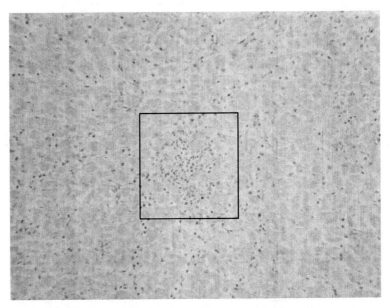

Figure 6.2   Collection of infiltrating neutrophils in myocardium seen during early response to infarction. (Reproduced, with permission, from OHSU.)

What is the most common cause of death within the first 24 to 48 hours post-MI?

Arrhythmia

By the third day, what gross evidence is there that tissue has been damaged by MI?

Area of infarct is pale and beginning to turn yellow with surrounding hyperemia

What cells begin to migrate to the damaged tissue between days 3 and 5 post-MI?

Macrophages

What is the most common cause of death between days 3 and 7 post-MI?

Ventricular wall rupture leading to cardiac tamponade

By 10 days post-MI, what gross changes to the myocardium are obvious?

Yellow necrotic tissue replaced with new gray-white vascular connective tissue

What microscopic changes are seen at 10 days post-MI?

Granulation tissue is forming, macrophages are the predominate cell type

By the fifth week post-MI, what macroscopic and microscopic changes are evident?

Fibrosis of infracted area with scar formation

Which complication of MI causes a friction rub and is likely to occur between 4 days and 3 weeks after the MI?

Fibrinous pericarditis

If after MI, damaged myocardium does not regain full mobility, what complication are patients at higher risk to experience?

Thromboembolic events due to blood stasis near the areas of impaired myocardial mobility

What tests are needed to diagnose pulmonary thromboembolus?

CT-Angiogram (CTA) or less often, ventilation/perfusion (V/Q) scan

From where can pulmonary thromboembolisms arise?

Deep lower extremity leg veins are the most common site (95%), but can also arise in upper extremity veins and within the chambers of the heart (ie, under conditions of dysfunctional pumping) or on damaged valve leaflets. Less commonly, emboli can arise from hepatic or mesenteric sites or from arterial sites if a left-to-right shunt is present.

Are emboli always blood clots?

No. Embolus is a generic term used to describe a mass of substance that originated elsewhere and moved to its current position via the bloodstream. Emboli can be fat, air, thrombus, bacteria (septic emboli), amniotic fluid, or tumor cells.

Which type of clot has lines of Zahn?

Thromboembolus or premortem clot

Which type of clot lacks lines of Zahn, is homogeneous in color, and is easily removed from vessels?

Postmortem clot

What is the triad of preeclampsia?

A pregnant woman presenting with hypertension, edema, and proteinuria

What is eclampsia?

Seizures, plus the triad of preeclampsia

What is the treatment for eclampsia?	Magnesium sulfate and delivery of the baby
What dangerous syndrome associated with preeclampsia is characterized by hemolysis, elevated liver function tests (LFTs), and low platelets?	HELLP syndrome

Inflammatory/Autoimmune

Which acute necrotizing vasculitis in children may be complicated by the development of coronary aneurysms?	Kawasaki disease
Which medium-to-large vessel vasculitis primarily affects young Asian females and may be referred to as "pulseless disease"?	Takayasu arteritis—upper extremity pulses may be weak due to thickening of the aortic arch and/or proximal great vessels
Temporal arteritis (giant cell arteritis) primarily presents in elderly females and often affects branches of which artery?	The carotid artery and in turn the temporal artery and the vascular supply to the eye; therefore temporal arteritis has diagnostic urgency to prevent blindness.
What is Dressler syndrome?	An autoimmune form of fibrinous pericarditis which affects patients several weeks to months post-MI. The exact etiology is unknown, but the autoimmune reaction is believed to be directed toward myocardial antigens. This syndrome may also affect heart surgery patients.
What is the treatment for Dressler syndrome?	Steroids and nonsteroidal anti-inflammatory drugs (NSAIDs)
What are the two major categories of pericarditis?	1. Acute pericarditis 2. Chronic pericarditis
What is constrictive pericarditis?	Chronic pericarditis may result in "constrictive pericarditis" if the pericardium becomes thickened, fibrotic, and subsequently noncompliant. In this case, the pericardium may prevent the heart from expanding appropriately to fill with blood during diastole.

How are forms of acute pericarditis classified?	By the associated type of pericardial effusion: serous, fibrinous, hemorrhagic, purulent, or caseous
What x-ray finding is helpful in diagnosing constrictive pericarditis?	Calcified pericardium
What physical finding of constrictive pericarditis is found on auscultation?	Pericardial knock—the sound produced during rapid ventricular filling
Chest pain and an echocardiogram revealing a "water bottle"-shaped heart would be associated with what diagnosis?	Pericardial effusion
What diseases are associated with hemorrhagic pericardial effusions?	TB and malignancy
Which type of effusion is most common?	Serous
What are some common causes of pericarditis and pericardial effusion?	Infection; renal failure; connective tissue disease

Anatomic

What is cardiomyopathy?	Cardiomyopathy is a general term used to reflect a change in heart muscle structure or functional ability. There are many causes of cardiomyopathy, including acquired and inherited forms, all of which generally manifest clinically and pathologically as one of the three major types of cardiomyopathy.
What are the major types of cardiomyopathy?	Dilated; hypertrophic; restrictive
Which cardiomyopathy is associated with alcoholic abuse and beriberi (thiamine deficiency)?	Dilated
Which cardiomyopathy is the most common?	Dilated
What therapeutic drug is associated with dilated cardiomyopathy?	Doxorubicin

What cardiac abnormality is seen at autopsy in hypertrophic cardiomyopathy?

Myocardial hypertrophy (particularly of the ventricular septum)

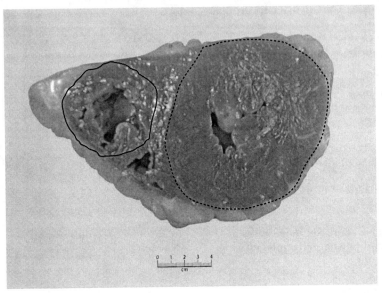

Figure 6.3   Heart—superior view, anatomic position. Right ventricle (solid black) and left ventricle (dashed black). Normal left ventricular myocardial thickness is less than 1.2 cm, this left ventricle measures up to 3.0 cm in maximal thickness. (Reproduced, with permission, from OHSU.)

Mechanistically, what is the major difference between dilated and hypertrophic cardiomyopathy?

Dilated cardiomyopathy will result in systolic dysfunction because the heart becomes so massively enlarged that it cannot pump adequately. In contrast, hypertrophic cardiomyopathy will result in diastolic dysfunction because there is so much extra myocardium that the chambers cannot fill with an adequate quantity of blood.

What is the characteristic shape of the left ventricle (LV) in hypertrophic cardiomyopathy?

Banana shaped

What inheritance pattern is seen in familial hypertrophic cardiomyopathy?

Autosomal dominant

What type of cardiomyopathy may result from systemic processes such as amyloidosis and hemochromatosis?

Restrictive/obliterative cardiomyopathy

Which form of restrictive cardiomyopathy is associated with eosinophilia?

Loeffler obliterative cardiomyopathy

What are the clinical findings in restrictive cardiomyopathy?

Loud S3; normal chest x-ray

Degenerative

What is heart failure? What are the causes of heart failure?

A situation in which the cardiac output is insufficient for the body's needs. Possible causes of decreased pump function include: myocardial infarction, hypertension, valvular disease, and cardiomyopathy. Less commonly, heart failure can occur when the body's needs are increased as in severe anemia, gram-negative sepsis, and thyrotoxicosis.

What are the two major clinical patterns of heart failure?

1. Left heart failure—dyspnea, orthopnea, evidence of decreased systemic perfusion (ie, altered mental status, cool extremities), tachypnea, and crackles on lung examination
2. Right heart failure—edema, nocturia, ascites, hepatomegaly, elevated jugular venous pressure (JVP)

What is the characteristic macroscopic liver finding associated with right ventricular failure?

Nutmeg liver resulting from the appearance of the dilated central veins in contrast to the adjacent pale hepatic parenchyma

What histologic finding might support the diagnosis of antemortem pulmonary congestion?

Hemosiderin-laden macrophages in pulmonary airspaces ("heart failure cells")

What is cardiogenic shock?

A state of inadequate circulation due to failure of the heart to pump a sufficient volume of blood to meet the body's demand.

What is the most common valvular lesion?	Mitral valve prolapse
What disease is associated with floppy valves and a midsystolic click?	Mitral valve prolapse
What is the cause of mitral valve prolapse?	Myxomatous degeneration of the zona fibrosa
Rheumatic fever predominately affects which cardiac valves?	Left-sided high-pressure valves (ie, mitral and aortic) are affected more frequently than right-sided low-pressure valves (ie, tricuspid and pulmonic).
What conditions predispose a patient to developing aortic stenosis?	Congenital bicuspid valve and rheumatic fever

Table 6.2 Murmurs

Murmur Review	
IV drug users	TR
Opening snap	MS (think "OSMS" or Opening Snap MS)
Radiates to axilla	MR (think MR. X has a stinky Axilla)
Pulsatile liver	TR
Syncope	AS (think syncope causes you to fall on your ASs)
Machine-like murmur	PDA (think PDA [as in make out] in the Machine shop)

Traumatic/Emergency

What disease is associated with the development of an abdominal aortic aneurysm (AAA)?	Atherosclerosis
What is the potential life-threatening event that can occur with AAA?	Rupture. Depending on the site of rupture, blood will fill the retroperitoneum or abdominal cavity. The mortality of ruptured AAA is estimated to be 75% to 90%.

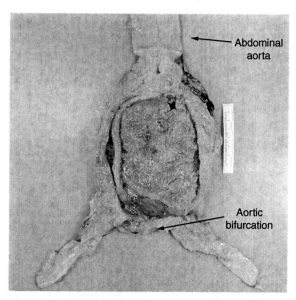

Figure 6.4   Ruptured abdominal aortic aneurysm (AAA). The aorta and iliac vessels have been opened posteriorly, revealing a large mass of acellular debris. (Reproduced, with permission, from OHSU.)

What is the gold standard for diagnosis of traumatic rupture of the aorta?	Aortogram or computed tomography (CT) angiogram
What is the treatment for aortic dissection?	Control hypertension (descending aortic dissection); immediate surgical intervention (ascending aortic dissection)
What is the difference between dissection and aneurysm?	Dissection results when a tear in the tunica intima allows blood to penetrate into and divide the tunica media. Aneurysm is a general term for vascular wall dilation and occurs when the vessel wall is weakened (eg, atherosclerosis).
What genetic disease is associated with aortic dissection in young, particularly male, patients?	Marfan syndrome
What is the cause of aortic dissection in Marfan syndrome?	Cystic medial degeneration of the wall of the aorta (highlighted by loss of elastin)

What are the common causes of cardiac tamponade?

Trauma, iatrogenic trauma, pericarditis, myocardial rupture, hypothyroidism

What collection of signs and symptoms would suggest that a patient is presenting with cardiac tamponade?

Finding a Beck triad (low arterial blood pressure, jugular venous distension, and distant, muffled heart sounds) and/or pulsus paradoxus on physical examination

What is pulsus paradoxus?

Decreased systemic pressure with inspiration (>10 mm Hg)

What is the treatment for cardiac tamponade?

Immediate pericardial window

What is the difference between tension and nontension pneumothorax?

In tension pneumothorax, the volume of air in the pleural cavity increases with each breath, secondary to a tissue flap that essentially creates a one-way valve. Due to the resulting pressure gradient and shifting of mediastinal structures, this can result in compromise of intrathoracic vessels. In nontension pneumothorax the volume of gas remains constant during breathing and there is little to no effect on mediastinal structures.

What signs and symptoms would suggest that a patient is presenting with tension pneumothorax?

Tachycardia, hypotension, decreased heart sounds, distended neck veins, and absent breath sounds on the side of the pneumothorax

What radiologic evidence would support a diagnosis of tension pneumothorax?

Deviation of the trachea to the side of the chest opposite the pneumothorax due to unilateral increased intrathoracic pressure

What is the emergent treatment for tension pneumothorax?

Needle thoracostomy followed by chest tube insertion

How can patients develop a pneumothorax?

They can develop spontaneously (rupture of apical blebs) or after penetrating chest wounds. They are also associated with lung infections, parenchymal lung disease, and lung cancers.

Infectious

What are the clinical characteristics of bacterial endocarditis?	Fever; Anemia; Murmur; Emboli; Osler nodules; Nail hemorrhages; Roth spots; Janeway lesions *FAME ON RJ*
What are the Osler nodes of bacterial endocarditis?	Tender-raised lesions on toes and fingers
What are Roth spots of bacterial endocarditis?	White retinal spots surrounded with hemorrhage
What are the small red lesions on palms and soles of patients with bacterial endocarditis?	Janeway lesions
What is the etiology of Osler nodes, Roth spots, and Janeway lesions?	All are caused in some way by immune complex deposition. In the case of Roth spots and Janeway lesions, the immune complex deposition occurs in vessels leading to small vessel vasculitis.
Which valve is most commonly involved in bacterial endocarditis?	Mitral valve
Which valve is associated with bacterial endocarditis in intravenous (IV) drug users?	Tricuspid valve
Which microorganism is associated with acute bacterial endocarditis producing large vegetations rapidly on previously normal valves?	*Staphylococcus aureus*
Which streptococcus species is associated with smaller vegetations on diseased valves causing subacute bacterial endocarditis?	*Streptococcus viridans*
What is the etiology and organism involved in rheumatic fever?	Immunologically mediated inflammatory response to group A beta-hemolytic streptococcus infection, usually pharyngitis or tonsillitis
What is the Aschoff body of rheumatic fever?	Focal interstitial myocardial inflammation with multinucleated giant cells

What is the usual time span between the tonsillitis infection and the onset of rheumatic fever?	1 to 4 weeks
Do blood cultures show septicemia with streptococcus during rheumatic fever?	No
What is the mechanism of rheumatic fever?	Cross-reactivity between tissues and antistreptolysin antibodies
What is the lab test that helps diagnose rheumatic fever?	Elevated antistreptolysin O (ASO) antibody titers
What is the rash that has central clearing in rheumatic fever?	Erythema marginatum
What is the chronic consequence of fibrotic healing of valves after rheumatic fever?	Chronic rheumatic heart disease
Which valve abnormality is most commonly involved with rheumatic heart disease?	Mitral stenosis (MS)
Infection of the aorta with which organism is associated with aneurysm of the aortic root and aortic arch?	*Treponema pallidum* (tertiary syphilis)—due to disruption of the vasa vasorum
What is the characteristic appearance of the aorta in tertiary syphilis?	The tissue is "wrinkly" and has a tree bark-like appearance.
What are the infectious causes of dilated cardiomyopathy?	Coxsackie virus and Chagas disease (*Trypanosoma cruzii*)
What cardiac abnormalities are associated with chronic infection with *Trypanosoma cruzi*?	Cardiomyopathy, the pathogenesis of which is not well understood

Congenital

Which disease is associated with notched ribs, cystic hygroma of neck, and coarctation of the aorta?	Turner syndrome
What are the cyanotic congenital heart diseases?	*T*etralogy of Fallot; *T*ransposition of the great vessels; *T*ricuspid atresia; *T*runcus arteriosus; *T*otal anomalous venous return; hypoplastic left heart
	*Ts and hypoplastic heart are cyanotic

Which birth defect is associated with cyanosis, death soon after birth, and maternal diabetes?	Transposition of the great vessels
What shape is the heart in transposition of the great vessels?	Egg shaped *Transport the egg
Which congenital heart disease is associated with ventricular septal defect (VSD), pulmonary stenosis, right ventricular hypertrophy, and overriding aorta?	Tetralogy of Fallot
What is the shape of the heart in tetralogy of Fallot?	Boot shaped
What congenital cyanotic heart disease is characterized by wide pulse pressure, single loud S2, and holosystolic murmur of VSD?	Truncus arteriosus
Which cyanotic congenital heart disease is associated with right ventricular heave, wide fixed S2 split, and a snowman-shaped heart?	Total anomalous venous return

Neoplastic

What is the most common type of tumor involving the heart?	Metastatic tumor (most are not primary)
What is the most common primary cardiac tumor in children?	Rhabdomyomas
What disease is characterized by cardiac rhabdomyomas, cortical hamartomas, seizure, mental retardation, and ash-leaf spots of the skin?	Tuberous sclerosis
What is the most common primary cardiac tumor seen in adults?	Myxoma
Where is the most common site of myxoma tumors?	Left atrium
How do myxomas appear microscopically?	Polygonal, hyperchromatic "myxoma cells" with eosinophilic cytoplasm are present in an abundant myxoid background

CLINICAL VIGNETTES

A 67-year-old white man presents with syncope, chest pain, and dyspnea. Physical examination reveals narrow pulse pressure and a murmur that radiates to the carotids. What is the diagnosis?

Aortic stenosis (AS)

A 62-year-old white woman presents to the clinic with occasional chest pain. On physical examination, she has a diastolic blowing murmur, widened pulse pressure, displaced point of maximal impulse (PMI), and left ventricular dilation. What is the most likely diagnosis?

Aortic regurgitation (AR)

A 45-year-old Hispanic woman with a history of rheumatic fever presents with hemoptysis and ruddy cheeks. On physical examination, she has an opening snap and a diastolic rumble, as well as occasional periods of atrial fibrillation on ECG. What is the most likely diagnosis?

Mitral stenosis (MS)

A 54-year-old man has an apical holosystolic murmur that radiates to the axilla, an S3, and a soft S1, as well as left ventricular dysfunction. What is the most likely diagnosis?

Mitral regurgitation (MR)

A 25-year-old IV drug addict presents with chest pain. On examination, he has a harsh holosystolic murmur, increased jugular venous pressure, and a pulsatile liver. What is the most likely diagnosis?

Tricuspid regurgitation (TR)

A 25-year-old healthy woman presents to clinic for a well-woman examination. On physical examination, she has a midsystolic click. What is the most likely diagnosis?

Mitral valve prolapse (MVP)

A 6-month-old is found to have a harsh machine-like murmur during a routine examination. He lives at a high altitude and was exposed to rubella during the first trimester. What is the diagnosis?

Patent ductus arteriosus (PDA)

A 72-year-old white man suffers from chest pain that is usually brought on by exertion. Resting always relieves the symptoms. What is the most likely diagnosis?

Stable angina

A 56-year-old white man complains of increasing chest pain that is not relieved by rest or nitroglycerin. What is the most likely diagnosis?

Unstable angina

A 25-year-old Asian woman presents to the clinic with complaints of intermittent chest pain that is not associated with exercise or stress. Often the chest pain will occur when she is sitting or resting. What is the most likely diagnosis?

Prinzmetal angina

A 62-year-old African American man presents to the ER with severe chest pain which is radiating to his jaw. The pain started an hour ago and is not relieved by nitroglycerin. On physical examination, the patient appears to be in acute distress, looking diaphoretic and pale. The patient has an impending feeling of doom. Electrocardiogram (ECG) is abnormal. What is the most likely diagnosis?

Myocardial infarction (MI)

A 62-year-old white man presents to the ER with fever, pericarditis, and pleural effusion. Six weeks ago he was hospitalized with a massive MI. His labs reveal an elevated erythrocyte sedimentation rate (ESR). What is the most likely diagnosis?

Dressler syndrome

A 79-year-old diabetic presents with altered mental status and dyspnea. Physical examination reveals blood pressure of 98/50. ECG shows a ventricular arrhythmia and chest x-ray shows pulmonary edema. What is the most likely diagnosis?

Silent MI in elderly or diabetic patient

A 17-year-old star athlete collapses on the basketball court and is found to be pulseless. Despite cardiopulmonary resuscitation (CPR), the boy expires. What type of cardiomyopathy is suspected?

Hypertrophic cardiomyopathy

A 45-year-old white man with human immunodeficiency virus (HIV) and tuberculosis (TB) presents with chest pain and cough. Physical examination reveals a friction rub, and ECG shows diffuse ST elevation. What is the most likely diagnosis?

Acute pericarditis

A 28-year-old white man is brought to the ER by ambulance after a motor vehicle accident (MVA). On physical examination, the patient is tachycardic, but heart sounds are distant and quiet. The patient is hypotensive, has distended neck veins, an inward carotid impulse, and pulsus paradoxus, but breath sounds are normal. What is the most likely diagnosis?

Cardiac tamponade (Beck triad)

A 26-year-old white man is brought to the ER after sustaining injuries during a car accident. On physical examination, he is tachycardic with decreased heart sounds, hypotensive, with distended neck veins, and has absent breath sounds on one side. On x-ray, the trachea is deviated to the opposite side. What is the most likely diagnosis?

Tension pneumothorax

A 26-year-old man is brought to the ER after a fall from several stories. Radiologic testing reveals widened mediastinum with loss of the aortic knob. What is the most likely diagnosis?

Traumatic rupture of the aorta

A 35-year-old woman presents with shortness of breath and chest pain. She just arrived from Australia the day before. On physical examination, she is tachycardic and tachypneic with a fixed split S2 and loud P2. What is the most likely diagnosis?

Pulmonary embolus (PE)

A 28-year-old arrives at the ER after being thrown from a vehicle during an MVA. He has multiple broken bones including his left and right femurs. He has no chest or head injuries but begins complaining of shortness of breath and dies suddenly. What is the most likely diagnosis?

Fat emboli associated with long bone fracture

A 65-year-old African American man with a past medical history of hypertension presents to the ER with tearing chest pain that is radiating to the back. His blood pressure is 220/110, and he is diaphoretic. What is the most likely diagnosis?

Aortic dissection

A 69-year-old white man presents to the ER with hypotension and back pain. On examination, he has a pulsatile epigastric mass. What is the most likely diagnosis?

Abdominal aortic aneurysm (AAA)

An 18-year-old presents to clinic with fever and tender lesions on her finger and toe pads. On physical examination, a new murmur is detected, as well as retinal hemorrhages and splinter hemorrhages on nail beds. What is the most likely diagnosis?

Bacterial endocarditis

A 59-year-old African American man presents to the ER with severe headache and blood pressure of 200/110. On physical examination, he has papilledema and fundal hemorrhages. What is the diagnosis?

Hypertensive emergency/malignant hypertension

A 23-year-old woman presents to the clinic with chronic hypertension since her teens. She is thin and a nonsmoker. On physical examination, she has a bruit over her left kidney. What is the most likely cause of her hypertension?

Renal artery stenosis from fibromuscular dysplasia

A 24-year-old G1P1 presents with severe headache and swelling of the lower extremities. On physical examination, she is found to have hypertension and edema of hands, feet, and face. Urinalysis (UA) shows proteinuria. What is the diagnosis?

Preeclampsia

A 14-year-old girl presents with arthritis in multiple joints, fever, a new cardiac murmur, rash with central clearing, and subcutaneous nodules. What is the most likely diagnosis?

Rheumatic fever

An 83-year-old man presents to the clinic with complaints of dyspnea on exertion and orthopnea. Physical examination reveals hypotension and tachycardia with a loud S3. Further investigation reveals pulmonary edema with increased pulmonary venous pressure. What is the most likely diagnosis?

CHF, left sided

A 78-year-old man presents with edema in the lower extremity. Physical examination reveals hepatomegaly, ascites, and distended neck veins. What is the most likely diagnosis?

CHF, right sided

A 1-year-old child is brought to the pediatrician by her mother with complaints of several episodes of turning blue during playing. The child squats down when she turns blue and then a few seconds later she resumes playing. What congenital heart disease can cause this symptom?

Tetralogy of Fallot (Tet spells)

CHAPTER 7

Respiratory Pathology

ANATOMY

What is the primary respiratory muscle?

The diaphragm

What are the accessory muscles of respiration?

Intercostals, sternocleidomastoid, scalene, and abdominal muscles

What nerves innervate these muscles for effective ventilation?

Phrenic, intercostals, cranial, and cervical nerves

When are accessory muscles of respiration recruited for ventilation?

When there is a need to increase intrathoracic pressure to force exhalation, like in obstructive lung disease

HISTOLOGY

What types of cells line alveoli?

- Type I pneumocytes—predominant cell type that facilitate rapid diffusion of gases
- Type II pneumocytes—secrete surfactant (dipalmitoyl phosphatidylcholine)

What is unique about type II pneumocytes?

They are capable of regeneration and repair, and are precursors to type I pneumocytes.

What type of cell is a histiocyte?

A type of macrophage

What characteristic inclusion bodies can be found on electron microscopy in the cytoplasm of Langerhans histiocytes?

Birbeck granules (resemble tennis rackets)

PHYSIOLOGY

What is surfactant?

Dipalmitoyl phosphatidylcholine—a complex lipoprotein that coats the surface of alveoli, decreasing surface tension, and preventing collapse at low lung volumes

What increases production of surfactant?

Thyroxine and cortisol

What is residual volume (RV)?

The amount of air in the lungs after maximal expiration

What is expiratory reserve volume (ERV)?

The amount of air that can still be breathed out after normal expiration

What is alveolar volume (V_A) and dead space volume (V_D)?

- V_A—the portion of an inhaled breath that fills the respiratory zone
- V_D—the portion of an inhaled breath that remains in the conducting airways

What is tidal volume (TV or V_T)?

The sum of alveolar and dead space ventilation with quiet breathing

What is inspiratory reserve volume (IRV)?

The amount of air in excess of tidal volume that moves into the lungs on maximal inspiration

What is vital capacity?

The sum of tidal volume, inspiratory reserve volume, and expiratory reserve volume. Alternatively, it is the total volume of air that can be inhaled starting from the point of maximal expiration. Vital capacity is equal to total lung capacity minus residual volume.

What is the functional residual capacity (FRC)?

The resting lung volume at the end of passive expiration which is determined by the opposing elastic forces of the chest wall (outward) and the lungs (inward).

How do you calculate the FRC?

FRC = RV + ERV

What is the total lung capacity (TLC)?

The total amount of air that the lungs can contain (IRV + TV + ERV + RV)

What fraction of the TLC is the normal FRC?

Less than 50%

What is inspiratory capacity (IC)?

The volume of gas that can be taken into the lungs on a full inspiration starting from the functional residual capacity (IC = IRV + TV)

What is compliance?

The change in lung volume produced by a given change in intrapleural pressure (C = ΔV/ΔP)

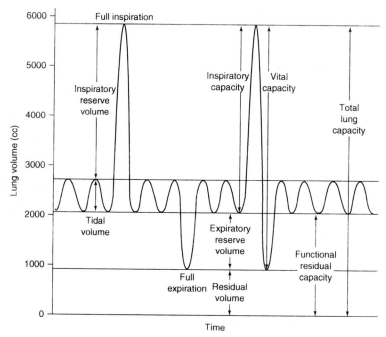

Figure 7.1 Lung volumes.

What conditions decrease compliance?

Restrictive lung diseases like pulmonary fibrosis or pulmonary edema which limit lung volume expansion

Give an example of a disease with increased lung compliance:

Emphysema increases compliance due to the loss of elastic recoil.

Describe the distribution of ventilation in the lungs:

Distribution is unequal, with greater ventilation at the apex and less at the base when in the upright position.

Describe the distribution of perfusion in the lungs:	Distribution is unequal, with greater perfusion at the base and less at the apex when in the upright position.
What kind of resistance circuit is the pulmonary circulation?	Low resistance
What determines blood flow in the normal lung?	The relationship between alveolar and pulmonary vascular pressure
What optimizes gas exchange?	The matching of ventilation and perfusion (V/Q)
What is the strongest factor affecting ventilation?	The maintenance of normal blood pH which is accomplished through the elimination or retention of CO_2
What are the two types of respiratory sensors and where are they located?	1. Chemoreceptors—found in the medulla and aortic and carotid bodies 2. Mechanoreceptors (including stretch and irritant receptors)—found in the chest wall and airways
Chemoreceptors maintain normal blood pH by responding to changes sensed by central and peripheral receptors. What are these changes?	Central chemoreceptors monitor CSF and respond rapidly to changes in hydrogen ion concentration and pCO_2. Peripheral chemoreceptors respond to changes in the partial pressure of arterial oxygen and exert regulatory effect by altering the respiratory rate.
How do chemoreceptors help maintain normal blood pH?	They modulate the rate and depth of breathing in response to how much the receptors are stimulated.
What is the difference between hypoxia and hypoxemia?	Hypoxia is a situation in which tissues are deprived of oxygen needs. Hypoxemia refers to decreased partial pressure of oxygen in the blood.
What happens to hemoglobin during normal conditions at 150 mm Hg PaO_2?	Hemoglobin is completely saturated with four molecules of oxygen. Further increases in PaO_2 have little effect on the oxygen content of blood.

PATHOLOGY

General Principles

What happens when alveolar pressure is greater than arterial pressure?

Perfusion is reduced or completely obstructed.

What two conditions can result in alveolar pressure being greater than arterial pressure?

1. Shock—pulmonary artery pressure falls below alveolar pressure due to severe blood loss
2. Positive pressure ventilation— alveolar pressure rises above the pulmonary artery pressure

What occurs in states of increased oxygen demand?

CO_2 rises and pulmonary vascular resistance falls secondary to the recruitment of unperfused vessels in order to meet oxygen demand.

What happens to blood vessels in localized alveolar hypoxia?

There is local constriction of arterioles supplying the hypoxic area, also known as hypoxic pulmonary vasoconstriction.

How does hypoxic pulmonary vasoconstriction work?

Constriction of blood vessels decreases blood flow to areas of low ventilation and helps maintain ventilation-perfusion matching by directing blood to areas of higher ventilation.

What parameters influence the degree of oxygen saturation of hemoglobin?

The oxygen affinity for hemoglobin is regulated by $[H^+]$, $[CO_2]$, $[2,3\text{-BPG}]$, temperature, and metabolic needs of the tissue. In peripheral tissues where there are conditions of increased acidity, increased $[CO_2]$, and increased $[2,3\text{-BPG}]$, oxygen has a lower affinity for hemoglobin (right shift on the curve means that it takes higher pO_2 to saturate a given percentage of binding sites on hemoglobin). In the lungs where there are conditions of less acidity, decreased $[CO_2]$, and decreased $[2,3\text{-BPG}]$, oxygen has a higher affinity for hemoglobin. This serves to facilitate oxygen unloading in peripheral tissues and oxygen binding in the lungs.

How does carbon monoxide (CO) affect the oxyhemoglobin dissociation curve?

CO binds to hemoglobin with 240 times the affinity of oxygen; consequently, it decreases the O_2 content in blood by decreasing the amount of oxygen bound to hemoglobin. Thus for essentially any pO_2, oxygen saturation of hemoglobin will be reduced if carbon monoxide is present.

What are the factors that affect pulmonary gas exchange?

Mismatching of ventilation with perfusion caused by hypoventilation, decreased FiO_2, shunting, and diffusion impairment

Define shunting:

Deoxygenated blood passes through the pulmonary vasculature without being ventilated.

What are the nonpulmonary causes of hypoxemia?

Inadequate cardiac output, low hemoglobin concentration, and low hemoglobin-O_2 saturation

How does aging affect normal lung function?

Both the total alveolar surface area and the elastic recoil of the lungs decrease

What is dyspnea?

Shortness of breath

What is orthopnea?

Dyspnea occurring when the patient is in the supine position as a result of a decrease in vital capacity caused by abdominal contents exerting force against the diaphragm

What is paroxysmal nocturnal dyspnea?

Dyspnea occurring several hours after lying down and is often associated with congestive heart failure. It is caused by an increase in venous return to the heart resulting in mild pulmonary edema.

What is atelectasis?

Alveolar collapse caused by bronchial obstruction or external compression of the lung parenchyma by tumors, pleural fluid, or air within the pleural cavity.

What is pulmonary alveolar proteinosis?

An uncommon condition characterized by the accumulation of amorphous, periodic acid-Schiff (PAS)-positive material in the alveolar air spaces.

What is a transudative pleural effusion?

Extravasated pleural fluid that occurs secondary to increased capillary pressure or low levels of serum protein

What is an exudative pleural effusion?

A collection of pleural fluid rich in protein and cellular elements that is caused by the altered permeability of vessel walls usually due to inflammation or malignancy

How do you differentiate between transudates and exudates in pleural fluid analysis?

By comparing protein and lactate dehydrogenase levels in the pleural fluid to the serum (Light criteria)

What are the Light criteria and how many must be met to diagnose an exudative pleural effusion?

At least one of the following criteria must be met:
1. Pleural fluid protein >2.9 g/dL (29 g/L)
2 Pleural fluid cholesterol >45 mg/dL (1.16 mmol/L)
3. Pleural fluid LDH >60% of upper limit for serum

What are the principal causes of pleural exudates?

1. Microbial infection
2. Cancer including bronchogenic carcinoma, metastatic neoplasms, and mesothelioma
3. Pulmonary infarction
4. Viral pleuritis

Congenital

What are the most important factors for the survival of premature infants?

Adequate vascularization and surfactant in the lungs; surfactant generally begins to be produced at 32 weeks gestation.

What is pulmonary agenesis?

The complete absence of lungs, bronchi, and vasculature caused by failure of bronchial buds to develop

What is pulmonary hypoplasia?

Poorly developed bronchial tree with abnormal histology found in association with congenital diaphragmatic hernias and bilateral renal agenesis

Describe the association between pulmonary hypoplasia and congenital diaphragmatic hernia:

Herniation of abdominal contents into the thorax compresses the developing lung causing it to become hypoplastic.

What causes infant respiratory distress syndrome (hyaline membrane disease)?

Lack of or inadequate surfactant production plus structural immaturity

How do you measure lung maturity in a premature infant?

By measuring the lecithin-to-sphingomyelin ratio in the amniotic fluid. If the ratio is less than 2:1, the fetal lungs may be surfactant deficient.

What conditions are associated with infant respiratory distress syndrome (hyaline membrane disease)?

Prematurity, maternal diabetes mellitus, and birth by caesarean section

What is Kartagener syndrome?

An autosomal recessive disorder that results in structurally abnormal cilia leading to impaired mucociliary clearance in the airways and reduced sperm motility in the gonads

What cardiac anomaly is associated with Kartagener syndrome?

Situs inversus

What is Langerhans cell histiocytosis (histiocytosis X)?

A disease of the immune system in children that causes proliferation of histiocytes and may result in interstitial lung disease, painful bone swelling, and diabetes insipidus. The finding of diabetes insipidus, exophthalmos, and lytic bone lesions is also called Hand-Schüller-Christian triad. Langerhans cell histiocytosis (LCH) exists on a spectrum from unifocal disease (previously known as eosinophilic granuloma) to multifocal unisystem LCH (Hand-Schüller-Christian) to multifocal multisystem LCH (also called Letterer-Siwe disease).

Anatomic

What is a pneumothorax?

A collection of air or gas in the pleural cavity as a result of disease or injury

What is a hemothorax?

A collection of whole blood in the pleural cavity caused by the rupture of blood vessels resulting from trauma or inflammation

What are the causes of massive hemoptysis (greater than 500 cc of blood)?	Lung cancer, lung cavities containing mycetomas, cavitary tuberculosis, pulmonary hemorrhage syndromes, atrioventricular (AV) malformations, and bronchiectasis
How can you differentiate between a hemothorax and a bloody pleural effusion?	Blood clots are usually present in a hemothorax
What is a chylothorax?	A pleural collection of a milky lymphatic fluid containing microglobules of lipid
Why is a chylothorax always significant?	It implies obstruction of the major lymph ducts usually by an intrathoracic cancer.

Inflammatory/Autoimmune

What are the three most common causes of chronic cough?	1. Asthma 2. Postnasal drip 3. Gastroesophageal reflux disease (GERD)
What are the two major categories of diffuse pulmonary lung disease?	1. Obstructive 2. Restrictive lung disease
What is the key feature in obstructive lung disease?	Increase in resistance of airflow out of the lungs due to the partial or complete obstruction of the airways resulting in lung volumes greater than normal (air trapping)
What is the key feature in restrictive lung disease?	Reduced expansion of lung parenchyma accompanied by a decrease in TLC resulting in smaller than normal lung volumes
How do lung volumes differ in obstructive and restrictive lung disorders?	Obstructive lung disease is characterized by a marked decreased in the 1 second forced expiratory volume (FEV_1) and a normal or increased forced vital capacity (FVC) resulting in a decreased FEV_1/FVC ratio. In restrictive lung disease, the FEV_1 and FVC are both decreased proportionately, resulting in a normal FEV_1/FVC ratio.

Give examples of obstructive pulmonary diseases:	Asthma, emphysema, chronic bronchitis, bronchiectasis, cystic fibrosis, bronchiolitis, tumors, and aspiration of foreign objects
Give examples of restrictive pulmonary diseases:	Adult respiratory distress syndrome (ARDS), pneumoconiosis, sarcoidosis, idiopathic pulmonary fibrosis, and chest wall/skeletal abnormalities
How are chronic restrictive pulmonary diseases categorized?	They are divided by lung response which includes alveolitis, interstitial inflammation, and diffuse fibrosis with or without granuloma formation.
What is asthma?	A condition characterized by episodic, reversible bronchospasm resulting from an exaggerated bronchoconstrictor response to a variety of stimuli
What are the clinical manifestations of asthma?	Bronchoconstriction, airway inflammation, edema, and mucus secretion
What is status asthmaticus?	Severe paroxysm that does not respond to therapy and would persist in the absence of intervention resulting in hypercapnia, acidosis, and severe hypoxia
What is emphysema?	A condition characterized by the permanent enlargement of the airspaces distal to the terminal bronchioles accompanied by destruction of alveolar walls
What are the three types of emphysema?	1. Centrilobular 2. Panacinar 3. Paraseptal
What is the distinctive feature of centrilobular emphysema?	Distal alveoli are spared while the central or proximal parts of the acini formed by respiratory bronchioles are affected.
Where in the lungs are lesions of centrilobular emphysema more common and severe?	Upper lung lobes
What is panacinar emphysema?	Emphysema that results in uniformly enlarged acini from the level of the respiratory bronchiole to the terminal blind alveoli.

Where in the lungs are lesions of panacinar emphysema more common and severe?	Lower lung lobes
What is panacinar emphysema associated with?	Loss of elasticity and α_1-antitrypsin deficiency
What is distinctive about paraseptal emphysema?	The proximal portion of the acinus is normal, while the distal part is predominantly involved.
Where in the lungs are lesions of paraseptal emphysema more common and severe?	Emphysema is more striking adjacent to the pleura, along the lobular connective tissue septa, and at the margins of the lobules.
What is the proposed mechanism to explain alveolar wall destruction and airspace enlargement in emphysema?	Excess protease or elastase activity unopposed by appropriate antiprotease regulation
What is α_1-antitrypsin?	A glycoprotein which is a major inhibitor of serine protease activity, particularly elastase, which is secreted by neutrophils during inflammation
How does smoking contribute to emphysema?	Smoking favors the recruitment of leukocytes and the release of elastase.
What is the classic clinical presentation of emphysema?	Patients are usually dyspneic and have a barrel chest. Their breathing is marked by prolonged expiration, hyperventilation, and relatively normal gas values (*pink puffers*).
What is the classic clinical presentation of chronic bronchitis?	Patients are usually obese, have less prominent dyspnea, and have a decreased respiratory drive. They retain CO_2 and tend to be hypoxic and cyanotic (*blue bloaters*).
What are the complications of chronic obstructive pulmonary disease (COPD)?	Chronic hypoxemia can lead to pulmonary vascular spasm, pulmonary hypertension, and cor pulmonale.
Define chronic bronchitis:	A persistent cough resulting in sputum production for more than 3 months for at least two consecutive years
What contributes to airflow obstruction in chronic bronchitis?	Inflammation, fibrosis with resultant narrowing of the bronchioles, and coexistent emphysema

What is the distinctive feature of chronic bronchitis?

Hypersecretion of mucus

What is chronic bronchiolitis?

Small airway disease characterized by goblet cell metaplasia, inflammation, fibrosis, and smooth muscle hyperplasia

What is bronchiectasis?

The permanent dilation of bronchi and bronchioles due to the destruction of muscle and elastic tissue secondary to infection or obstruction caused by a variety of conditions

Patients with bronchiectasis classically complain of what symptom complex?

Cough with copious amounts of purulent, sometimes fetid, sputum

What are the conditions that commonly predispose to bronchiectasis?

1. Bronchial obstruction caused by tumors, foreign bodies, and mucus impaction
2. Congenital or hereditary conditions like cystic fibrosis, immunodeficiency states, and Kartagener syndrome
3. Necrotizing or suppurative pneumonia

What is usually cultured from the sputum of patients with bronchiectasis?

Mixed flora including staphylococci, streptococci, pneumococci, enteric organisms, anaerobic and microaerophilic bacteria, *Haemophilus influenzae*, and *Pseudomonas aeruginosa*.

What causes restrictive lung disease?

Abnormalities of the chest wall due to bony deformities or neuromuscular dysfunction; interstitial lung disease—characterized by accumulation of substances within the pulmonary interstitium

What are the key changes that occur in restrictive lung disease?

Interstitial fibrosis produces a *stiff lung* with reduced lung compliance necessitating increased respiratory effort.

What are the complications of restrictive lung disease?

Respiratory failure, pulmonary hypertension, and cor pulmonale

What are the prototypic acute restrictive (interstitial) lung disorders?

Acute respiratory distress syndrome (ARDS) and infant respiratory distress syndrome (hyaline membrane disease)

What is acute respiratory distress syndrome (ARDS)?

A syndrome featuring acute respiratory compromise in the absence of left-sided heart failure resulting from diffuse alveolar damage and an increase in capillary permeability causing leakage of protein-rich fluid into the alveoli. This syndrome can be the result of many different etiologies.

What is the mechanism of injury in ARDS?

Necrosis of endothelial and epithelial cells secondary to the release of toxic mediators by neutrophils, the formation of oxygen-derived free radicals, and the activation of the coagulation cascade

What is the classic radiographic finding in ARDS?

Diffuse ground-glass opacification in the lungs

What is the characteristic pathologic finding in ARDS?

Intra-alveolar hyaline membranes composed of fibrin and cellular debris

What is idiopathic pulmonary fibrosis (IPF)?

An interstitial lung disease of unknown etiology that is characterized by chronic inflammation and fibrosis of the alveolar wall

Describe the sequence of events in IPF:

It begins with alveolitis, progresses to fibrosis, and results in a lung filled with cystic spaces (*honeycomb* lung)

What is observed clinically in a patient with IPF?

Patients exhibit respiratory difficulty and eventually become hypoxemic and cyanotic. Cor pulmonale and cardiac failure may result.

What is hypersensitivity pneumonitis (extrinsic allergic alveolitis)?

An immunologically mediated inflammatory lung disease that results in alveolitis. It is often an occupational disease that results from heightened sensitivity to inhaled antigens.

How does hypersensitivity pneumonitis usually present?

The acute reaction presents with fever, cough, dyspnea, and constitutional complaints 4 to 8 hours after exposure. The chronic form of the disease has an insidious onset of cough, dyspnea, malaise, and weight loss.

How does hypersensitivity pneumonitis differ from bronchial asthma?

In bronchial asthma, the bronchi are the focus of injury; whereas in hypersensitivity pneumonitis, damage occurs at the level of the alveoli and results in a restrictive picture.

What are diffuse pulmonary hemorrhage syndromes?

Pulmonary interstitial and vascular disorders that present with hemorrhage. They include Goodpasture syndrome, idiopathic pulmonary hemosiderosis, and vasculitis-associated hemorrhage.

What is sarcoidosis?

A type IV hypersensitivity reaction to an unknown antigen that results in a multisystem disease characterized by noncaseating granulomas in multiple tissues and organs.

Sarcoidosis tends to affect what race and age group?

People of African descent during the teenage or young adult years

What is the most common abnormality seen on routine x-ray in a patient with sarcoidosis?

Bilateral hilar lymphadenopathy

What are the characteristic laboratory findings in sarcoidosis?

Hypercalcemia/hypercalciuria, hypergammaglobulinemia, and increased activity of serum angiotensin-converting enzyme (ACE)

What are the common pathologic changes that occur in sarcoidosis?

Interstitial lung disease; enlarged hilar lymph nodes; anterior uveitis; splenomegaly/hepatomegaly; erythema nodosum of the skin; polyarthritis

What is Mikulicz syndrome?

Bilateral eye and salivary gland involvement in sarcoidosis, tuberculosis, or leukemia

What sort of immunologic response is seen in patients with sarcoidosis?

Patients manifest cutaneous allergy to common skin test antigens like *Candida,* mumps, and purified protein derivative (PPD). They also have a polyclonal hyperglobulinemia.

What is the clinical course of sarcoidosis?

It is largely unpredictable and characterized by either progressive chronicity or periods of activity interspersed with remissions.

How is sarcoidosis diagnosed?	It requires lung or lymph node biopsy demonstrating noncaseating granulomas.
What is Goodpasture syndrome?	A hemorrhagic pneumonitis and glomerulonephritis caused by antibodies to antigens common to glomerular and pulmonary basement membranes
What is idiopathic pulmonary hemosiderosis?	A disease that resembles the pulmonary component of Goodpasture syndrome without the renal component

Environmental/Toxins

What are pneumoconioses?	Environmental lung diseases caused by the inhalation of inorganic particles that result in interstitial lung damage
What is anthracosis?	An environmental disease caused by the inhalation of carbon dust. It is usually endemic in urban areas and causes no harm.
What is coal workers' pneumoconiosis?	An occupational disease caused by the inhalation of coal dust, which contains both carbon and silica
What is silicosis?	A chronic occupational lung disease caused by the exposure to free silica dust
Who typically gets silicosis?	Miners, glass manufacturers, and stonecutters
A retired miner is suspected of having silicosis. The patient must be advised that he may have an increased susceptibility to what other disease?	Tuberculosis
What is *farmer's lung*?	A type of hypersensitivity pneumonitis caused by the inhalation of spores of thermophilic actinomycetes from moldy hay
What is asbestosis?	An environmental disease caused by the inhalation of asbestos fibers that result in diffuse pulmonary interstitial fibrosis

Patients in what occupations have an increased risk of developing asbestosis?	Shipbuilders and plumbers
What is the mechanism of injury in asbestosis?	Injury is initiated by the uptake of asbestos fibers by alveolar macrophages. A fibroblastic response follows and leads to diffuse interstitial fibrosis, particularly in the lower lobes.
What are ferruginous bodies?	Asbestos fibers coated with iron and calcium and found inside macrophages
Ferruginous bodies stain positive with what dye?	Prussian blue
Patients with asbestosis tend to have a predisposition to what type of cancers?	Bronchogenic carcinoma and malignant mesothelioma

Vascular

Where do most pulmonary emboli arise?	More than 95% of PEs arise within the large deep veins of the lower legs, typically the popliteal vein, femoral vein, and iliac vein.
What is Virchow triad?	Risk factors that predispose to vascular thrombosis. It includes (1) endothelial dysfunction, (2) stasis or turbulent flow of blood, and (3) changes in the constituents of blood (hypercoagulability).
What conditions are associated with a hypercoagulable state?	Prolonged bed rest/immobilization, severe trauma, congestive heart failure, high estrogen states, and disseminated cancer
What are the consequences of embolic pulmonary arterial occlusion?	There is an increase in pulmonary artery pressure due to restriction of flow and ischemia of the downstream pulmonary parenchyma. Acute, dramatic elevation of pulmonary artery pressure will cause pulmonary hypertension and possibly life-threatening right-heart failure.

Patients who have experienced a pulmonary embolus are at increased risk of developing additional emboli. What is considered appropriate preventative treatment?

Early ambulation for postoperative or postpartum patients; use of elastic stockings; isometric exercises for bedridden patients; anticoagulation therapy for high-risk patients

What is primary pulmonary hypertension?

Primary pulmonary hypertension can be diagnosed when mean pulmonary pressure reaches one-fourth of systemic pressure, in the absence of any identifiable explanation.

What are the causes of secondary pulmonary hypertension?

1. Cardiac disease—left-to-right shunts, mechanical obstructions on the left side of the heart
2. Inflammatory disease—scleroderma and other vasculitides
3. Lung disease—COPD, recurrent pulmonary emboli, chronic interstitial lung disease, and sleep apnea

What is pulmonary edema?

The abnormal accumulation of extravascular fluid within the lung parenchyma and airspaces

What causes pulmonary edema?

High pulmonary capillary and venous hydrostatic pressure (cardiogenic pulmonary edema) or increased capillary permeability (noncardiogenic pulmonary edema)

Give examples of cardiogenic causes of pulmonary edema:

Left ventricular failure or mitral stenosis

Give examples of noncardiogenic causes of pulmonary edema:

Inflammatory alveolar reactions, pneumonia, shock, sepsis, pancreatitis, uremia, or drug overdose

Give examples of vasculitis-associated hemorrhage syndromes:

Systemic lupus erythematosus, Wegener granulomatosis, and microscopic polyangiitis

What histopathologic characteristic do the vasculitis-associated hemorrhage syndromes have in common?

Necrotizing inflammation of the pulmonary capillaries

| What antibodies are associated with Wegener granulomatosis? | Circulating antineutrophil cytoplasmic antibodies (c-ANCAs) with a cytoplasmic staining pattern |

Infection

What is pneumonia?	A respiratory disease characterized by inflammation of the lung parenchyma (excluding the bronchi) caused by viruses, bacteria, fungi, or irritants
What are the general clinical signs and symptoms of pneumonia?	Fever, chills, muscle stiffness, pleuritic chest pain, cough, blood-tinged or rusty sputum, shortness of breath, rapid heart rate, and difficulty breathing
What are ways to diagnose pneumonia?	Chest x-ray; Gram stain and culture (bacterial); bronchoalveolar lavage (*Pneumocystis carinii* pneumonia [PCP]); serodiagnosis (*Mycoplasma*)
What laboratory finding is classically associated with bacterial pneumonia?	A neutrophilic leukocytosis with an increase in band neutrophils (left shift)
What are the four most common bacteria causing sinus and respiratory infections?	1. *Streptococcus pneumoniae* 2. *Haemophilus influenzae* 3. *Staphylococcus aureus* 4. *Mycoplasma pneumoniae*
What are the common morphologic patterns of pneumonia?	Lobar pneumonia, bronchopneumonia, and interstitial pneumonia

Table 7.1 Patterns of Pneumonia

Morphologic Pattern	Typical Organism	Key Characteristics
Lobar	*Streptococcus pneumoniae*	Intra-alveolar exudates; forms consolidations
Bronchopneumonia	*Staphylococcus aureus, Haemophilus influenzae, Klebsiella pneumoniae, Streptococcus pyogenes*	Inflammatory infiltrates; patchy distribution involving one or more lobes
Interstitial pneumonia (atypical)	*Mycoplasma pneumoniae* Viruses (various)	Diffuse, patchy inflammation localized to the interstitial areas of the alveolar walls

What are the four stages of lobar pneumonia?

1. Congestion
2. Red hepatization
3. Gray hepatization
4. Resolution

What are the potential complications of bacterial pneumonias?

Abscess formation; empyema formation; organization of normal lung tissue into fibrous tissue; bacterial dissemination—meningitis, arthritis, or infective endocarditis

Which pneumonias are the most common in childhood?

Viral pneumonias

What are the commonly implicated viruses?

Influenza, parainfluenza, respiratory syncytial virus (RSV), rhinovirus, and adenovirus

What is Q-fever?

The most common rickettsial pneumonia

What organism causes Q-fever?

Coxiella burnetii

Who typically gets Q-fever?

People working with infected cattle or sheep, people who consume unpasteurized milk from infected animals

What are the features of *atypical pneumonia*?

Acts like a cold; patients may never be febrile; caused often by *Mycoplasma* and viruses; chest x-ray often appears worse than the patient appears (*walking pneumonia*)

What is ornithosis?

An atypical pneumonia that results from inhalation of the dried excrement of birds infected with *Chlamydia psittaci*

What is *Pneumocystis carinii* pneumonia?

The most common opportunistic infection in patients with acquired immunodeficiency syndrome (AIDS) and others with impaired immunity

What sort of lung damage is seen in patients with *Pneumocystis* infection?

Diffuse, interstitial pneumonitis

What is the best way to diagnose *Pneumocystis carinii* **pneumonia?**	Bronchoalveolar lavage, bronchial washing, or sputum

Table 7.2 Features of Selected Pneumonias

Organism	Characteristics	Complications
Streptococcus pneumoniae	Common in elderly or debilitated patients; most common community-acquired	Empyema formation
Staphylococcus aureus	Common in patients with COPD; often a complication of viral disease or a result of blood-borne infection in IVDU	Abscess, formation endocarditis
Streptococcus pyogenes	Often a complication of influenza or measles	Lung abscess
Klebsiella pneumoniae	Common in alcoholic and diabetic patients; also seen in elderly and hospitalized patients	Abscess formation, fibrosis bronchiectasis
Haemophilus influenzae	Common in infants/children and debilitated adults with COPD	Epiglottitis and meningitis in infants/children
Legionella pneumophila	Common in elderly and patients with cardiac, renal, immunologic, or hematologic diseases; associated with inhalation of aerosol from contaminated stored water	GI complications
Pseudomonas aeruginosa	Common in hospitalized and neutropenic patients, patients with cystic fibrosis, burn victims, and patients requiring mechanical ventilation	Abscess formation
Moraxella catarrhalis	Common in adults with COPD; similar to pneumonia caused by *H. influenzae*	

Table 7.2 Features of Selected Pneumonias (Continued)

Organism	Characteristics	Complications
Aspiration bronchopneumonia (anaerobic and microaerophilic bacteria)	Common in markedly debilitated and unconscious patients	Partial chemical pneumonitis from swallowed gastric contents, abscess formation
Mycoplasma pneumoniae	Common in children and young adults; associated with nonspecific cold agglutinins reactive to red cells	Mild and self-limiting; alveolar hyaline membranes

Abbreviations: GI, gastrointestinal; IVDU, intravenous drug use.

What is a lung abscess?	Necrosis of the pulmonary tissue and formation of cavities containing necrotic debris or fluid caused by microbial infection
What are the organisms that frequently cause lung abscesses?	*Staphylococcus, Pseudomonas, Klebsiella, Proteus,* and anaerobic organisms
Who is at risk of developing a lung abscess?	Patients predisposed to aspiration due to loss of consciousness from alcohol/drug overdose, neurologic disorders, or general anesthesia
What are the clinical and radiologic signs of a lung abscess?	Fever, foul-smelling purulent sputum, prominent cough, and x-ray evidence of a fluid-filled cavity
What is the treatment for a lung abscess?	Antibiotic therapy with surgical drainage, if necessary
What is tuberculosis?	A communicable, chronic granulomatous disease caused by *Mycobacterium tuberculosis*

How is tuberculosis spread from person to person?

Inhalation of droplets containing the organism

What is primary tuberculosis?

The form of the disease that develops in a previously unexposed, unsensitized person. It is characterized by the formation of a Ghon complex.

What is a Ghon complex?

The combination of a parenchymal lesion (granuloma) and hilar lymph node involvement

What characterizes the granuloma of tuberculosis?

Central caseous necrosis ("caseating granuloma")

What mycobacterial infection is often seen in AIDS patients with a normal chest x-ray?

Mycobacterium avium-intracellulare

What is secondary tuberculosis?

The pattern of disease that arises in a previously sensitized host either from reactivation of dormant primary lesions or exogenous reinfection

Where do the lesions of secondary tuberculosis localize?

Apical or posterior segments of the upper lobes

What are the clinical signs and symptoms of secondary tuberculosis?

Progressive disability, fever, hemoptysis, pleural effusion, and generalized wasting

What characterizes secondary tuberculosis?

Cavitary lesions

What are the complications of secondary tuberculosis?

Progressive pulmonary tuberculosis from expansion of areas of caseation; lymphatic and hematogenous spread resulting in miliary tuberculosis; extrapulmonary tuberculosis from hematogenous seeding like tuberculous meningitis and Pott disease

What is Pott disease?

Extrapulmonary tuberculosis involving the spine (tuberculous arthritis of the intervertebral joints)

What is intestinal tuberculosis?

Tuberculosis caused by the ingestion of infected milk or the swallowing of coughed-up infectious sputum

Define scrofula:

Tuberculous involvement of the oropharyngeal lymphoid tissue with spread to the lymph nodes in the neck

What is the immune mechanism in the pathogenesis of tuberculosis?

Delayed hypersensitivity reaction

How is tuberculosis diagnosed?

Sputum smear stain for acid-fast bacilli and sputum culture

Is *Mycobacterium tuberculosis* visible on gram-stained slides?

No; *M. tuberculosis* has a waxy coating composed of mycolic acid which is impervious to gram-staining techniques.

What do the bacilli look like on an acid-fast smear?

The bacilli stain red and are nicknamed "red snappers."

Which dimorphic fungi can cause pulmonary disease even in healthy hosts?

Histoplasma capsulatum, Coccidioides immitis, and *Blastomyces dermatitidis*

Which fungi are considered opportunistic infectious agents?

Nonseptate hyphal fungi belonging to the order *Mucorales* and the mold-like fungi belonging to the order *Aspergillus*

How does a fungal infection of the lungs typically manifest?

Cavitary, fluid-filled masses

A researcher studying cacti in the Sonoran desert comes to the clinic complaining of shortness of breath, cough, fever, and unintended weight loss. What is the likely diagnosis?

Coccidioidomycosis

An accurate travel history is important when working-up a patient with an infectious lung disorder. List the endemic lung diseases and the location where each occurs:

- Histoplasmosis—Ohio and Mississippi River valleys
- Coccidioidomycosis—San Joaquin valley and the southwest United States
- Blastomycosis—Ohio and Mississippi River valleys and around the Great Lakes
- Tuberculosis—developing countries

Which fungal infection is characterized by pseudohyphae and budding yeasts in the immunocompromised?

Candidiasis

How does *Candida albicans* infection typically present in immunocompetent hosts?

Superficial infection on the mucosal surfaces of the oral cavity (thrush) or vagina

In the immunocompromised host, candidiasis can become invasive and produce blood-borne dissemination. What are the complications that occur with systemic spread?

Pulmonary, renal, and hepatic abscesses and vegetative endocarditis

How is diagnosis of *Cryptococcus neoformans* frequently made?

Diagnosis is made by visualizing the organism by fungal silver stains or specifically highlighting the capsule by India ink. Detection of the cryptococcal antigen can be made using a latex agglutination test.

What is the most common invasive fungal infection in AIDS patients?

Cryptococcus neoformans

What does *Cryptococcus* look like histologically?

Round, budding yeasts with halo (from the thick capsule)

Invasive forms of aspergillosis and mucormycosis cause what kind of damage?

Vascular necrosis and infarction of blood vessels

What fungus causes *fungus* balls in the lung?

Aspergillosis

Which fungus has a high mortality in immunocompromised patients but is infrequently observed to infect healthy individuals?

Mucor

What is the difference between *Mucor* and *Aspergillus*?

Mucor has wide hyphae and no septae, while *Aspergillus* has 45° branching and septae

What are the two fungus-like bacteria?

1. *Actinomyces israelii*
2. *Nocardia asteroids*

How are infections by *Actinomyces* and *Nocardia* detected?

- Actinomycosis—identification of sulfur granules within the inflammatory exudates
- Nocardiosis—identification of characteristic acid-fast forms in the smears of exudates

What is a complication of a pulmonary infection caused by *Actinomyces* or *Nocardia*?

Abscess formation

What viral pneumonia shows cellular enlargement with nuclear and cytoplasmic basophilic inclusions histologically?

Cytomegalovirus (CMV) pneumonia

What are the two types of inclusions seen in herpes simplex virus (HSV) pneumonia?

1. Eosinophilic ground glass in nucleus
2. Cowdry type A inclusions—central eosinophilic body with surrounding halo

Who gets Varicella zoster pneumonia?

15% of those with chicken pox, usually adults

What does Varicella zoster pneumonia look like on histology?

Inclusions look like those of HSV

Varicella zoster pneumonia kills what type of patients?

Mortality is highest in pregnant patients and the immunocompromised

Describe the histologic appearance of measles pneumonia:

Multinucleated (Warthin-Finkeldey) cells with eosinophilic intranuclear and intracytoplasmic inclusions

What nuclear features are associated with adenovirus pneumonia?

Basophilic "smudges" that fill the nucleus; eosinophilic body with a surrounding halo

What is the histologic difference between influenza pneumonia and parainfluenza pneumonia?

Intracytoplasmic inclusions are present in parainfluenza pneumonia but are absent in influenza pneumonia.

What does respiratory syncytial virus (RSV) bronchiolitis look like?

Small, eosinophilic inclusions surrounded by a clear halo

Neoplasm

What is the most common cancer in the lungs?

Metastatic cancer from extrathoracic organs

What is the most common benign neoplasm in the lungs?

Hamartoma

What is a hamartoma?

A benign tumor-like nodule composed of an overgrowth of otherwise normal mature cells and tissues

What are the histologic categories of lung carcinoma?

1. Nonsmall cell lung carcinoma—includes squamous cell carcinoma, adenocarcinoma (including bronchioalveolar), large cell carcinoma, and carcinoid tumors
2. Small cell lung carcinoma

What is bronchial carcinoid?

A neoplasm derived from neuroendocrine cells present in the pulmonary parenchyma. It spreads by direct extension into the surrounding tissues. Histologically, they look like their intestinal counterparts, but rarely produce carcinoid syndrome.

What is carcinoid syndrome?

A syndrome of facial flushing, wheezing, and diarrhea caused by the release of serotonin from carcinoid tumors

Where do the majority of lung cancers arise?

In the lining epithelium of major bronchi, usually close to the hilus of the lung

What are the common presenting signs and symptoms of lung cancer?

Cough, hemoptysis, bronchial obstruction, and wheezing

Which lung cancers have the strongest association with smoking?

Squamous cell carcinoma and small cell carcinoma

Lung cancers typically metastasize to what organs?

Liver, adrenals, brain, and bones

What are the key features of squamous cell carcinomas?

1. More common in men than women
2. Arise centrally in major bronchi and eventually spread to hilar nodes
3. Are slow to disseminate and late to metastasize
4. Large lesions can undergo central necrosis with cavitation
5. Well-differentiated tumors show keratin pearl formation
6. May be marked by inappropriate parathyroid hormone-like activity with resultant hypercalcemia

What are the key features of adenocarcinomas?

1. More common in women and nonsmokers
2. Usually peripherally located
3. Slow-growing tumors but tend to metastasize early
4. Bronchioalveolar carcinomas tend to present as either a solitary peripheral nodule or as pneumonia-like consolidations on chest x-ray.

What are the key features of large cell carcinomas?

1. Tumors lack differentiation, they are "undifferentiated high-grade carcinomas"
2. Show no evidence of keratinization or gland formation
3. Tendency to spread to distant sites early
4. Peripherally located

What are the key features of small cell lung carcinomas?

1. More common in men than women
2. Strongly associated with smoking
3. Centrally located
4. Composed of small, dark, round-to-oval, lymphocyte-like cells with scant cytoplasm and hyperchromatic nuclei ("oat" cell appearance)
5. Rapidly growing lesions that tend to infiltrate widely and metastasize early
6. Considered the most aggressive and least likely to be cured by surgery
7. Derived from epithelial cells of the lung that have neurosecretory granules
8. Capable of secreting a host of polypeptide hormones like adrenocorticotropic hormone (ACTH), calcitonin, and gastrin-releasing peptide causing paraneoplastic syndrome

What are the typical complications of lung cancer?

Superior vena cava syndrome, Pancoast tumor, Horner syndrome, Endocrine (paraneoplastic), Recurrent laryngeal symptoms (hoarseness), and Effusions

SPHERE of complications

What are paraneoplastic syndromes?

Clinical syndromes that result from the synthesis of bioactive substances produced by a tumor. Symptoms may be endocrine, neuromuscular, musculoskeletal, cardiovascular, cutaneous, hematologic, gastrointestinal, renal, or miscellaneous in nature.

Define superior vena cava syndrome:

Compression of the superior vena cava by a mass that blocks venous return to the heart

What causes superior vena cava syndrome?

More than 95% of all cases are associated with cancers involving the upper chest (lung cancers and lymphoma)

What is the clinical presentation of superior vena cava syndrome?

Coughing, difficulty breathing, and swelling of the face, neck, and upper arms

What is a Pancoast tumor?

A nonsmall cell lung cancer that originates in the upper portion of the lung and extends to other nearby tissues such as the ribs and vertebrae causing Horner syndrome

What is Horner syndrome?

Ptosis, miosis, and anhidrosis resulting from the interruption of the cervical sympathetic plexus by an apical lung tumor

What is malignant mesothelioma?

A rare cancer of mesothelial cells usually arising in the parietal or visceral pleura

What occupational exposure is associated with malignant mesothelioma?

Exposure to asbestos

There is strong epidemiologic evidence linking Epstein-Barr virus to what type of respiratory cancer?

Nasopharyngeal carcinoma

Nasopharyngeal carcinomas occur in high frequency in which patient subgroup?

Asian patients

Most laryngeal cancers present as what type of lesions?

Typical squamous cell lesions

What is the most common presenting feature of vocal cord nodules, papillomas, and squamous cell carcinomas of the larynx?   Hoarseness

CLINICAL VIGNETTES

Hours after birth, a 29-week-old premie is noted to have severe retractions with labored breathing. The baby soon tires and expires. Postmortem histologic examination reveals collapsed alveoli lined with eosinophilic material. What is the likely diagnosis?

Respiratory distress syndrome (hyaline membrane disease)

A 7-year-old boy presents with his parents who note that he quickly becomes short of breath when playing outside, especially in the spring and fall. The boy will occasionally wheeze when he becomes short of breath. With rest, his symptoms go away. What does this presentation suggest?

Asthma, possibly triggered by exertion or allergens

A 65-year-old patient comes in with dyspnea on exertion that is episodic in nature. What does this presentation usually suggest?

Parenchymal lung disease or cardiac dysfunction

A patient comes in with dyspnea that is seasonal and sometimes triggered by environmental exposure. What does this presentation suggest?

Asthma or hypersensitivity pneumonitis

A 35-year-old man complains of chest pain for the last 4 days. He states that his pain is worsened by deep inspiration and describes it as a sharp, stabbing pain. He tells you that he's recovering from a recent cold. What is the likely diagnosis?

Pleuritic chest pain secondary to viral infection

A 45-year-old woman complains of intermittent substernal chest pain, worse after eating spicy meals, and a long-standing history of nocturnal cough. What is the likely diagnosis?

Gastroesophageal reflux disease (GERD)

CHAPTER 8

Gastrointestinal Pathology

EMBRYOLOGY

From which embryologic tissue are most gastrointestinal organs derived?

Endoderm

During which weeks of embryologic development does most visceral organ development occur?

Organogenesis occurs between weeks 3 and 8.

Through what structure does blood flowing to fetus through the umbilical vein arrive in the inferior vena cava?

The ductus venosus

Which adult structure does the umbilical vein ultimately give rise to?

The falciform ligament which contains the ligamentum teres

Which four structures give rise to the diaphragm?

1. Septum transversum
2. Dorsal mesentery of the esophagus
3. Pleuroperitoneal folds
4. Body wall

What adult structures does the ventral pancreatic bud ultimately give rise to?

Main pancreatic duct, uncinate process, and head of the pancreas

What adult structures does the dorsal pancreatic bud ultimately give rise to?

Accessory pancreatic duct and body, isthmus, and tail of the pancreas

Into which three sections is the primitive gut divided?

1. Foregut (pharynx to duodenum)
2. Midgut (duodenum to transverse colon)
3. Hindgut (distal transverse colon to rectum)

ANATOMY

In which way is the division of the primitive gut anatomically relevant?	The division corresponds to anatomic regions of shared blood supply. The foregut is supplied by the celiac trunk, the midgut is supplied by the superior mesenteric artery, and the hindgut is supplied by the inferior mesenteric artery.
Which other gastrointestinal organs are supplied by the celiac trunk?	Liver, gallbladder, and pancreas
What are the three main branches of the celiac trunk?	1. Common hepatic artery 2. Splenic artery 3. Left gastric artery
What are the different anatomic regions of the stomach?	Cardia, fundus, body, antrum, and pylorus
Which gastrointestinal organs are located in the retroperitoneum?	Second, third, and fourth portions of the duodenum, descending colon, ascending colon, and most of the pancreas (except the tail)
Which three ligaments are connected to the liver?	1. Falciform 2. Hepatoduodenal 3. Gastrohepatic ligaments
What structures are contained in the hepatoduodenal ligament?	The hepatic artery, portal vein, and common bile duct
What structures are contained in the gastrohepatic ligament?	The gastric arteries
What is the difference in vascularization above and below the pectinate line?	Above the pectinate line is supplied by the superior rectal artery and drained by the superior rectal vein which drains to the portal vein. Below the pectinate line is supplied by the inferior rectal artery and drained by the inferior rectal vein which drains to the IVC.
Name three major salivary glands associated with the oral cavity:	1. Parotid 2. Submandibular 3. Sublingual

What is an annular pancreas?

A congenital defect in which an abnormal ring or collar of pancreatic tissue encircles the duodenum, causing nausea, vomiting, feeling of fullness, and feeding intolerance in the newborn

HISTOLOGY

What kind of epithelium lines the oral cavity?

Nonkeratinized stratified squamous epithelium

What kind of epithelium lines the esophagus?

Nonkeratinized stratified squamous epithelium

What are the three layers of esophageal mucosa?

1. Epithelium
2. Lamina propria
3. Muscularis mucosa

Describe the muscles of the esophagus:

The upper third of the esophagus contains skeletal muscle, the middle third has both skeletal and smooth muscle, and the lower third consists entirely of smooth muscle.

What type of epithelium lines the stomach?

Simple columnar epithelium

What cell types are found within gastric glands and what do they produce?

- Parietal cells—produce HCl and intrinsic factor
- Mucosal neck cells and lining cells—produce protective mucus
- Neuroendocrine system cells—produce various hormones
- Regenerative cells
- Chief cells—produce precursor enzymes

How is the gastric mucosal barrier maintained?

Through constant mucus and bicarbonate secretion, mucosal blood flow, and prostaglandin synthesis

Name the layers of the wall of the intestine:

From internal to external: mucosa (epithelium, lamina propria, muscularis mucosa), submucosa, muscularis externa, and serosa/adventitia

Where is the submucosal plexus located?

Between the submucosa and the inner layer of the muscularis

What do neurons in the submucosal plexus predominately regulate?

Local secretions, blood flow, and absorption

Where is the myenteric plexus located?

Between the inner (circular) and outer (longitudinal) layers of the muscularis

What do neurons in the myenteric plexus predominately regulate?

Gut motility

What type of epithelium lines the small intestine?

Simple columnar epithelium

What is the major function of the small intestine?

Absorption and enzymatic digestion of amino acids, monosaccharides, and lipids

What determines the absorptive capacity of the small intestine?

Available surface area (mucosal folds, villi, and microvilli)

What type of epithelium lines the large intestine?

The colon is lined by simple columnar epithelium. The anus is lined by simple columnar epithelium to the rectum, then simple cuboidal epithelium to the anal valves, and finally, stratified squamous epithelium beyond the anal valves.

Where are Brunner glands located and what is their function?

In the submucosa of the duodenum—they produce alkaline secretions to neutralize acidic stomach contents

What are the functions of the liver?

Synthesis of serum proteins; processing of dietary amino acids, carbohydrates, lipids, and vitamins; detoxification of pollutants; secretion of endogenous waste products into bile

What laboratory values are used to evaluate hepatocyte function and biliary excretion?

- Hepatocyte function—AST, ALT, lactate dehydrogenase (LDH), serum albumin, prothrombin time (PT), and serum ammonia
- Biliary excretion—serum bilirubin, urine bilirubin, serum alkaline phosphatase, serum γ-glutamyl transpeptidase, and serum 5-nucleotidase

MOUTH AND ESOPHAGUS

Congenital

What is cleft lip?

A failure of fusion of the maxillary and medial nasal processes during embryologic development resulting in a gap in the upper lip while the palate remains intact

What is cleft palate?

A failure of fusion of the lateral palatine processes, the nasal septum, and/or the median palatine processes. The resulting gap leaves the nasal cavity in communication with the oral cavity.

What are the most common congenital anomalies of the esophagus?

Esophageal atresia and tracheoesophageal fistula (TEF)

Define atresia:

The absence of a luminal opening

What is the most frequent type of TEF?

A distal TEF with proximal esophageal atresia

Anatomic

What is achalasia?

The incomplete relaxation of the lower esophageal sphincter with consequent dilatation of the proximal esophagus due to the loss of the myenteric plexus

What is typical of achalasia on barium esophagogram?

"Bird beak" appearance with distal esophageal stenosis and proximal dilation, may see air–fluid (or contrast) line in upper esophagus

What disease causes secondary achalasia and frequently occurs in South America?

Chagas disease

What are the clinical signs and symptoms of achalasia?

Progressive dysphagia, nocturnal regurgitation, aspiration pneumonia, weight loss, cough, and airway obstruction

What malignancy is associated with achalasia? — Esophageal carcinoma

What is diffuse esophageal spasm (DES)? — An esophageal motor disorder due to a functional imbalance between excitatory and inhibitory postganglionic neurons

What is typical of DES on barium esophagogram? — A "cork screw" pattern

What are the clinical signs and symptoms of DES? — Dysphagia and diffuse chest pain

What is the difference between a Mallory-Weiss tear and Boerhaave tear? — A Mallory-Weiss tear is a partial-thickness tear usually at the gastroesophageal junction. Boerhaave tear is a full-thickness perforation in the distal third of the esophagus. Both are associated with recent vomiting.

What factors contribute to esophageal tears or perforation? — Forceful vomiting, gastroesophageal reflux disease (GERD), and procedures such as endoscopy, dilation/intubation of the esophagus, and placement of a nasogastric tube

What are varices? — Tortuous, dilated veins—frequently involving the esophageal, rectal, and epigastric vessels

What condition is associated with esophageal varices? — Portal hypertension

What are the clinical signs and symptoms of esophageal varices? — Patients are usually asymptomatic, but if varices rupture, they can present with hematemesis or lower gastrointestinal (GI) bleed.

Infectious

What are common, painful, recurrent ulcerations of the oral mucosa known as? — Cold sores (aphthous ulcers)

What is the causative agent of cold sores? — Herpes simplex virus (HSV) (usually type 1)

How is HSV transmitted?

HSV transmission requires intimate contact with a person actively shedding the virus
- Type 1 (oral)—transmission via direct contact with lesions through kissing or sharing utensils
- Type 2 (genital)—transmitted sexually or perinatally from infected mother to baby

How does herpes gingivostomatitis manifest in young children (primary infection)?

Fever, sore throat, erythema, and pharyngeal edema, usually followed by ulcerative lesions on the oral and pharyngeal mucosa

What are the diagnostic tools used in HSV detection?

Tzanck test of the vesicular fluid, polymerase chain reaction (PCR), and viral culture

What are the classic microscopic changes seen in herpes infection?

Infected cells clump together to form multinucleated giant cells with eosinophilic, intranuclear viral inclusions

How does *Candida albicans* infection of the mouth or esophagus appear clinically?

Patients present with whitish plaques of curd-like material which can be scrapped off of the mucosal surface.

Who is likely to get oral candidiasis?

Patients undergoing chemotherapy, those with diabetes, chronic debilitating diseases, acquired immunodeficiency syndrome (AIDS) or other types of immunodeficiency, patients on antibiotics, and infants.

What is sialadenitis?

Inflammation of the major salivary glands

What causes sialadenitis?

Etiology can be viral, bacterial, traumatic, or autoimmune.

What are the most common bacterial causes of sialadenitis?

Staphylococcus aureus and *Streptococcus viridans*

What is a common viral cause of sialadenitis?

Mumps

What are some infectious causes of esophagitis in immunosuppressed patients?

Herpes simplex virus (HSV), cytomegalovirus (CMV), and *Candida albicans*

Trauma

What is leukoplakia?	An irregular, whitish patch/plaque caused by epidermal thickening or hyperkeratosis and is believed to be a defense or reparative response to insult. Whereas candidiasis lesion can be scrapped off with mechanical forces, leukoplakia cannot.
What are the most common sites of leukoplakia on the oral cavity?	The vermilion border of the lower lip, the buccal mucosa, and the hard/soft palate
What are the common causes of leukoplakia?	Trauma; tobacco use; alcohol use; infection (Epstein-Barr virus [EBV], syphilis); chemical irritation
What percentage of oral leukoplakia is premalignant (dysplastic)?	5% to 25%
Define a mucocele:	A common lesion of the salivary glands that develops from the accumulation of saliva secondary to blockage and/or rupture of salivary gland ducts
What is the most common cause of mucocele formation?	Trauma

Neoplasm

What is erythroplasia?	A clinical term used to describe lesions of the mucous membranes which are red and nonulcerated
What percentage of erythroplasia undergoes malignant transformation?	More than 50%
The majority of oral cavity malignancies are what type of cancer?	Squamous cell carcinoma
What is the most common age group affected?	Patients older than 40 years

What are the risk factors for oral cancer?

Tobacco use, human papillomavirus (HPV) infection, leukoplakia, erythroplasia, alcohol abuse, and chronic irritation

What are the most common locations of squamous cell carcinoma in the oral cavity?

Ventral surface of the tongue, lower lips, floor of the mouth, gingiva, and soft palate

What is the most frequent site of salivary gland tumors?

Parotid gland (65%-80%)

What is the percentage of parotid gland tumors that are benign?

70% to 80%

What is the most common salivary gland tumor?

Pleomorphic adenoma (also known as "mixed tumor")

What are the key characteristics of pleomorphic adenomas?

They are benign, painless, slow-growing, and have a tendency to recur. Pleomorphic adenomas have been reported to undergo malignant transformation.

What are two other common salivary gland tumors?

1. Warthin tumor
2. Mucoepidermoid carcinoma

What are the key features of a Warthin tumor?

Second most common salivary gland tumor; benign; male > female; smokers > nonsmokers; affects mainly the parotid glands; gross appearance—often multicystic containing "crankcase oil"-like fluid

What is the classic microscopic finding of a Warthin tumor?

Double layer of neoplastic epithelial cells on a reactive lymphoid stroma

What is a key epidemiologic feature of mucoepidermoid carcinomas?

They are the most common type of salivary gland malignancy in children.

What is the classic microscopic finding of mucoepidermoid carcinomas?

Variable mixture of squamous and mucin-producing cells in a cystic or sheet-like pattern

What is the most common malignancy of the esophagus worldwide?

Squamous cell carcinoma

What are the common risk factors for squamous cell carcinoma of the esophagus?	• Alcohol consumption* • Tobacco use* • Long-standing esophagitis • Achalasia • Vitamins A, C, thiamine, or pyridoxine deficiency • High content of nitrites/nitrosamine in diet • Fungal contamination of food • Familial *These are the biggest risk factors and the combination exponentially increases the risk of carcinoma. (This is an example of synergism.)

Inflammatory/Autoimmune

What systemic inflammatory conditions are associated with aphthous ulcerations in the mouth?	Inflammatory bowel disease and Behçet disease
What is an autoimmune cause of sialadenitis?	Sjögren syndrome (bilateral)
What is the clinical presentation of Sjögren syndrome?	Dry mouth (xerostomia), dry eyes (keratoconjunctivitis sicca), an associated second connective tissue disease, and parotid gland enlargement
Sjögren syndrome is associated with what type of malignancy?	Lymphoma
What are the key characteristics of Plummer-Vinson syndrome?	Iron deficiency anemia, glossitis, and esophageal webs
What are esophageal webs?	Thin membranes of normal esophageal tissue (including mucosa and submucosa) appearing in the middle to lower third of the esophagus causing pain and dysphagia (solids > liquids)
What are patients with Plummer-Vinson syndrome at increased risk of?	Squamous cell carcinoma of the pharynx/esophagus
What is esophagitis?	Inflammation of esophageal mucosa
What conditions lead to esophagitis?	GERD, Barrett esophagus, infections, and chemical irritation

What is GERD?	Gastroesophageal reflux disease in which stomach acid refluxes into the esophagus
What are common causes of GERD?	Inappropriate relaxation of the lower esophageal sphincter, a sliding hernia, inadequate esophageal clearance, and delayed gastric emptying
What substances decrease the tone of the lower esophageal sphincter?	Coffee, cigarettes, alcohol, progesterone (pregnancy), chocolate, and calcium channel blockers
What are the classic symptoms of GERD?	Heartburn (often related to eating or lying supine), a sour taste in the mouth, and abdominal or chest pain
What are the complications of GERD?	Esophageal strictures, ulcers, hemorrhage, Barrett esophagus, and esophageal adenocarcinoma
What is Barrett esophagus?	A complication of long-standing GERD that results in intestinal metaplasia in which stratified squamous epithelium above the gastroesophageal junction is replaced with intestinal-type columnar epithelium including goblet cells.
What are the complications of Barrett esophagus?	Adenocarcinoma, stricture, and ulceration

STOMACH

Congenital

Define congenital pyloric stenosis:	Muscular hypertrophy of the pyloric smooth muscle wall causing obstruction
What are the key clinical features of pyloric stenosis?	Palpable mass ("olive") in the epigastric region; persistent, nonbilious projectile vomiting in young infants; male > female
What do the common imaging studies show in patients with pyloric stenosis?	• X-ray—dilated stomach bubble • Ultrasound—elongated pyloric channel (>14 mm) and thickened pyloric wall (>4 mm)

Infectious

What is *H. pylori*?	A spiral, microaerophilic, gram-negative bacterium that infects the mucosal layer of the GI tract and produces urease and cytotoxins
How is *H. pylori* transmitted?	Not well-defined, but may be transmitted via fecal-oral route
What malignancies are associated with chronic *H. pylori* infection?	Adenocarcinoma and lymphoma of the stomach
How is *H. pylori* diagnosed?	Biopsy, serological testing for *H. pylori* antibody, or urease breath test
What percentage of people infected with *H. pylori* develop peptic ulcers?	10% to 20%

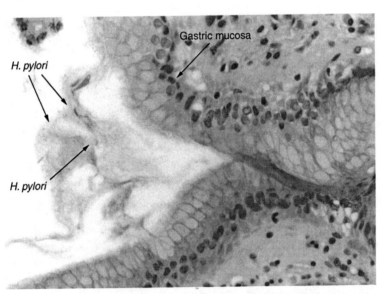

Figure 8.1 Mucosa of gastric fundus. Comma and rod-shaped *H. pylori* are present in fundic gland secretions. (Reproduced, with permission, from OHSU.)

Neoplasm

What are common examples of benign gastric neoplasms?

Leiomyomas; hyperplastic polyps; fundic gland polyps; adenomas

What are the most common malignant tumors of the stomach?

Gastric carcinoma (90%-95%), GI lymphoma, and carcinoid tumors

What are the risk factors for developing gastric carcinoma?

Chronic gastritis; dietary nitrates/smoked food/pickled vegetables; decreased intake of fresh fruits/vegetables; *H. pylori* infection; history of adenomatous polyps

What is *linitis plastica* (leather bottle stomach)?

Diffuse gastric cancer that results in a thickened, rigid stomach caused by the extensive infiltration of neoplastic cells in the gastric wall

What is the name for a firm, palpable left supraclavicular lymph nodes that represents metastatic carcinoma, typically from a primary carcinoma in the thoracic or abdomen?

Virchow node

What is a Krukenberg tumor?

Metastasis of gastric adenocarcinoma to the ovaries. Histologically, these tumors often have signet-ring cell features.

What are the clinical signs and symptoms of gastric carcinoma?

Weight loss, abdominal pain, dysphagia, anorexia, nausea, and vomiting

Inflammatory/Autoimmune

What is chronic gastritis?

Mucosal inflammation with lymphocytic and plasma cell infiltrates leading to gastric gland loss, mucosal atrophy, and intestinal metaplasia

What are the two types of chronic gastritis?

1. Type A or autoimmune chronic gastritis—caused by antibodies to parietal cells
2. Type B or infectious chronic gastritis—caused by *H. pylori*

To which part of the stomach does autoimmune chronic gastritis localize?

The body of the stomach

To which part of the stomach does infectious chronic gastritis localize?

The antrum of the stomach

What is acute gastritis?

Mucosal inflammation with edema and a predominately neutrophil inflammatory infiltrate

What are common causes of gastritis?

Heavy use of nonsteroidal anti-inflammatory drugs (NSAIDs); alcohol consumption and smoking; treatment with chemotherapy; uremia; systemic infection; severe stress (trauma, burn, surgery); ischemia and shock; suicidal ingestion of acids and alkali; mechanical trauma

What is the clinical presentation of gastritis?

Usually asymptomatic, but can cause nausea, vomiting, abdominal pain, hematemesis, and melena

What are peptic ulcers?

Chronic, usually solitary, punched-out erosions of the mucosa occurring mainly in the duodenum or stomach, but can be found in any portion of GI tract exposed to gastric acid and pepsin

What is the classical presentation of PUD?

Localized chronic, intermittent, epigastric burning/aching/gnawing pain accompanied by nausea, vomiting, bloating, and belching

What clinical feature may help distinguish gastric ulcers from duodenal ulcers?

Abdominal pain will be greater with meals if the patient has a gastric ulcer and will decrease with meals if the patient has a duodenal ulcer

What are the complications of PUD?

Hemorrhage, perforation, and gastric outlet obstruction

What conditions are associated with PUD?

H. pylori infection, use of NSAID and/or high-dose corticosteroids, Zollinger-Ellison syndrome, central nervous system (CNS) injuries, sepsis, and extensive burns

How is PUD treated?

- Triple therapy for *H. pylori* infection—amoxicillin/tetracycline, metronidazole, and bismuth
- Proton pump inhibitors, antacids, and H_2 blockers
- Lifestyle changes—decrease tobacco and alcohol consumption

Table 8.1 Classical Differences between Duodenal and Gastric Ulcers

PUD	Pathology	Etiology	*H. pylori*	% of PUD	Eating	Associated ABO
Gastric	Decreased protection against acid	Use of NSAIDs and *H. pylori*	~70%	25%	Worsens pain	A
Duodenal	Increased acid production	Same as above	~100%	75%	Improves pain	O

Abbreviations: NSAIDs, nonsteroidal anti-inflammatory drugs; PUD, peptic ulcer disease.

What is achlorhydria?

The absence of hydrochloric acid (HCl) secretion

How does pernicious anemia cause achlorhydria?

Autoimmune inflammatory cells destroy acid-secreting parietal cells.

What vitamin deficiency is seen in patients with pernicious anemia?

Vitamin B_{12} deficiency

Why is there vitamin B_{12} deficiency with pernicious anemia?

Destruction of the parietal cells results in loss of intrinsic factor needed for B_{12} absorption

What is a hiatal hernia?

A condition in which a portion of the stomach herniates through the esophageal hiatus of the diaphragm

What are the two major types of hiatal hernia?	1. Sliding—the anatomic location of the gastroesophageal junction is displaced cranially and a portion of the proximal stomach is drawn into the mediastinum 2. Paraesophageal—the GE junction is in its normal anatomic position and part of the cardia of the stomach moves into the thorax adjacent to the esophagus *Both can occur simultaneously

HEPATOBILIARY

Congenital

What is Gilbert syndrome?	A benign liver disorder that results in an unconjugated hyperbilirubinemia due to a partial deficiency in the enzymes used to metabolize bilirubin
What is the defective enzyme in Gilbert syndrome?	Glucuronosyltransferase
What is Crigler-Najjar syndrome?	A rare inherited disorder characterized by the absence of bilirubin conjugating enzyme in the liver

Table 8.2 Types of Bilirubinemia

Bilirubinemia	Characteristics	Congenital Causes	Other Causes	Excretion in the Urine?
Conjugated or direct	Water soluble, loosely bound to albumin	Dubin-Johnson and Rotor syndromes	Hepatocellular damage, gallstones, pancreatic cancer, biliary cirrhosis/atresia	Yes
Unconjugated or indirect	Insoluble, tightly bound to albumin	Gilbert and Crigler-Najjar syndromes	Hemolytic anemia, physiologic disease of the newborn, hepatocellular disease	No

Describe the two types of Crigler-Najjar syndrome:

1. Type 1—autosomal recessive, complete absence of conjugating enzyme, elevated levels of unconjugated bilirubin, kernicterus, and death within the first 18 months of life
2. Type 2—less severe, nonfatal form of disease with partial defect in conjugating enzyme

What is Dubin-Johnson syndrome?

An autosomal recessive disorder that results from a defect in the glucuronide transport proteins which carry bilirubin from the liver into the biliary system

What are the key clinical features of Dubin-Johnson syndrome?

Conjugated hyperbilirubinemia, hepatomegaly, and dark pigmentation of the liver

What is Rotor syndrome?

A variant of Dubin-Johnson syndrome characterized by chronic, conjugated hyperbilirubinemia and defective excretion of organic anions into bile. It requires no treatment and has excellent prognosis.

What is a key difference between Dubin-Johnson syndrome and Rotor syndrome?

The liver is darkly pigmented in Dubin-Johnson syndrome and is not pigmented in Rotor syndrome.

What is Wilson disease?

An autosomal recessive disease that results in the accumulation of copper in many organs, mainly the liver, brain, and eyes

What are the clinical characteristics of Wilson disease?

Liver cirrhosis, basal ganglia degeneration (parkinsonian symptoms), psychosis, dementia, and corneal (Descemet membrane) deposits (Kayser-Fleischer rings)

What are the diagnostic lab abnormalities in Wilson disease?

Low levels of serum ceruloplasmin and increased urinary excretion of copper

How do you treat Wilson disease?

Penicillamine, zinc (blocks absorption of copper in the GI tract), and restriction of foods high in copper

What is hemochromatosis?

A condition in which a defect of iron absorption results in excessive iron (hemosiderin) deposition with tissue damage in many organs, primarily the liver, pancreas, and myocardium

What are the clinical characteristics of hemochromatosis?

It is characterized by the triad of hepatomegaly, skin pigmentation, and diabetes mellitus (*"bronze diabetes"*).

What are the types of hemochromatosis?

- Primary disease or hereditary hemochromatosis—autosomal recessive disorder caused by a mutation in the HFE gene
- Secondary disease—associated with chronic blood transfusion therapy, ineffective erythropoiesis, or increased oral intake of iron

What are the diagnostic lab abnormalities in hemochromatosis?

Increased levels of serum iron, transferrin iron saturation, and serum ferritin

What is the treatment of hemochromatosis?

Repeated phlebotomy and deferoxamine

What are patients with hemochromatosis at greater risk of developing?

Congestive heart failure (secondary to myocardial iron deposition) and hepatocellular carcinoma

Anatomic

What is Budd-Chiari syndrome?

A disease characterized by the occlusion (eg, thrombosis) of the hepatic veins, usually accompanied by ascites, hepatomegaly, jaundice, and pain in the abdomen

What is Budd-Chiari often associated with?

Polycythemia vera, hepatocellular carcinoma, and other abdominal neoplasms

What is cholelithiasis?

The presence of stones (cholesterol, pigment, or mixed-type) in the gallbladder

What are the risk factors for cholesterol gallstone formation?

Female sex; obesity; premenopausal; age 40 or slightly older; rapid weight loss; prolonged total parenteral nutrition

*Four Fs: "female, fat, forty, fertile"

How are pigmented stones formed?

Excess insoluble unconjugated bilirubin precipitates around a nidus, forming a stone

What are pigmented stones often associated with?

Hemolytic anemia and bacterial infection

What are the clinical manifestations of gallstones?

Gallstones are usually asymptomatic, but they can cause colicky right upper quadrant pain, nausea, and vomiting, especially after eating.

What are the common complications of gallstones?

Biliary colic; cholecystitis; common bile duct obstruction; ascending cholangitis; acute pancreatitis ("gallstone pancreatitis"); gallstone ileus; mucocele; malignancy

What is a common lab finding in cholelithiasis?

High levels of alkaline phosphatase, indicating an obstructive process

Infectious

What serum marker indicates acute hepatitis B infection?

Anti-HBc IgM (antihepatitis B core immunoglobin M)

What serum antigen indicates active hepatitis B infection or carrier state?

Hepatitis B surface antigen (HBsAg)

What are the screening and confirmatory tests for chronic hepatitis B infection?

- Screening—HBsAg in serum
- Confirmatory—hepatitis B virus, DNA, hepatitis B envelope antigen (HBeAg), or hepatitis B core antigen (HBc Ag) in liver

What serum marker indicates hepatitis B immunity?

Anti-HBsAg (antihepatitis B surface antigen)

Table 8.3 Hepatitis Viruses

Type	Virus	Route	Incubation	Chronicity	Antibody	Medicines
A	Picornaviridae (RNA)	Fecal-oral	15-45 days	None	Anti-HAV	
B	Hepadnaviridae (DNA)	Sex IVDU Transfusion Vertical	30-150 days	2%-7%	Anti-HBs Anti-HBc Anti-HBE	IF-alpha
C	Flaviviridae (RNA)	Sex IVDU Transfusion	15-120 days	70%-85%	Anti-HCV	IF-α ribavirin
D	RNA virus	Sex IVDU Transfusion Vertical	30-150 days	2%-7%	Anti-HDV	IF-α
E	RNA virus-like caliciviruses	Fecal-oral	30-60 days	None	Anti-HEV	

Abbreviations: Anti-HAV, antihepatitis A virus; Anti-HBc, antihepatitis B core; Anti-HBe, antihepatitis B envelope; Anti-HBs, antihepatitis B surface; Anti-HCV, antihepatitis C virus; DNA, deoxyribonucleic acid; GI, gastrointestinal; HDV, hepatitis D virus; HEV, hepatitis E virus; IVDU, intravenous drug use; RNA, ribonucleic acid.

For which of the hepatitis viruses are vaccines currently available?

Hepatitis A and hepatitis B

What are the screening and confirmatory tests for chronic hepatitis C infection?

- Screening—anti-HCV (antihepatitis C virus)
- Confirmatory—HCV, RNA, PCR

What three viruses are associated with an increased risk of hepatocellular carcinoma?

1. Hepatitis C
2. Hepatitis B
3. Hepatitis D

What viral hepatitis is associated with a high rate of acute liver failure in pregnant women?

Hepatitis E

If you are suspicious that a patient has hepatitis A, what are the likely laboratory findings?

Anti-HAV IgM (antihepatitis A virus immunoglobin M) and increased levels of alanine transaminase (ALT), aspartate transaminase (AST), bilirubin, and γ-glutamyltransferase (GGT)

Environmental/Toxins

What is the most common cause of liver disease in the United States?

Alcohol abuse

What are the different stages of alcoholic liver disease?

- Fatty liver—often reversible
- Alcoholic hepatitis—characterized by swollen and necrotic hepatocytes, neutrophil infiltration, Mallory bodies, and fibrosis
- Cirrhosis—irreversible complication

What are the causes of hepatic necrosis?

- Drugs or toxins—acetaminophen, halothane, rifampin, isoniazid, monoamine oxidase (MAO) inhibitors, carbon tetrachloride, and *Amanita phalloides* poisoning
- Fulminant viral hepatitis

What are the clinical signs and symptoms of hepatic failure?

Jaundice, hypoalbuminemia, hyperammonemia, fetor hepaticus (musty body odor), impaired estrogen metabolism leading to hypogonadism and gynecomastia, palmar erythema, spider angioma, and coagulopathy due to impaired synthesis of blood-clotting factors II, VII, IX, and X

What are the clinical features of end-stage liver disease?	Hepatic encephalopathy, asterixis, hyperreflexia, and hepatorenal syndrome

Degenerative

What is cirrhosis?	End-stage liver disease with a loss of normal hepatic architecture
What are the key histologic features of cirrhosis?	Disruption of the architecture of the entire liver with the presence of parenchymal nodules of proliferating hepatocytes that are surrounded by fibrotic tissue
What are the two common causes of cirrhosis?	1. Alcohol abuse 2. Viral hepatitis (usually chronic hepatitis C)
What are the complications of cirrhosis?	• Portal hypertension—with subsequent sequelae (varices, ascites, etc) • Hepatocellular carcinoma • Hepatic encephalopathy • Coagulopathy • Pruritus, jaundice • Other organ involvement—hepatorenal syndrome, hepatopulmonary syndrome
What is portal hypertension?	A vascular disorder of the liver characterized by increased resistance to portal blood flow at the level of the sinusoids with the development of venous collaterals and ascites
How is portal hypertension classified?	By the site of portal venous obstruction: • Prehepatic—caused by portal and splenic vein obstruction secondary to thrombosis • Intrahepatic—caused by vascular obstruction secondary to cirrhosis, metastatic tumor, or schistosomiasis • Posthepatic—caused by venous congestion secondary to constrictive pericarditis, tricuspid insufficiency, congestive heart failure (CHF), or hepatic vein occlusion (Budd-Chiari syndrome)

What is portosystemic shunting?

Abnormal vascular connections between the hepatic portal vein and the systemic circulation

What are the clinical consequences of portosystemic shunting?

Esophagogastric varices, periumbilical collaterals (caput medusa), splenomegaly, and hemorrhoids

What kind of liver damage is associated with chronic right-sided heart failure?

Centrilobular fibrosis (also known as cardiac sclerosis)

What is the appearance of the cut surface of the liver in a patient with chronic heart failure often referred to as?

Nutmeg liver, with areas of red centrilobular congestion alternating with adjacent pale portal areas

What is kernicterus?

The accumulation of unconjugated bilirubin in the brain leading to neurological damage

Kernicterus can be a complication of what disease in the newborn?

Erythroblastosis fetalis (also known as hemolytic disease of the newborn)

What is Reye syndrome?

An acute, noninflammatory encephalopathy with hepatic failure that occurs primarily in children who have taken aspirin during a viral infection

What is fatty liver of pregnancy?

A rare, but serious, condition of pregnancy in which there is an excessive accumulation of fat in hepatocytes causing microvesicular changes

What is the prognosis of fatty liver of pregnancy?

Prognosis is usually good, but disease can progress to hepatic failure, coma, and death.

What is the treatment for fatty liver of pregnancy?

Treatment requires delivery to minimize the risks to the mother and baby. The mother may require intensive care for several days after delivery. In most cases, liver function returns to normal within a few weeks.

Inflammatory/Autoimmune

What is autoimmune hepatitis?

A spectrum of disease in which the body's immune system attack hepatocytes causing inflammation and hepatic dysfunction

What markers are increased in autoimmune hepatitis?

Serum titers of antinuclear, anti-smooth muscle, and anti-liver/kidney microsomal antibodies

What is primary biliary cirrhosis?

A disease characterized by the inflammatory destruction of small bile ducts within the liver that typically affects middle-aged women

What causes primary biliary cirrhosis?

Etiology is unknown, although the presence of antimitochondrial and antinuclear autoantibodies in some patients suggests a possible autoimmune cause

What is secondary biliary cirrhosis?

Biliary injury and fibrosis due to extrahepatic biliary obstruction

What are the typical signs and symptoms of biliary cirrhosis?

Jaundice, pruritus, fatigue, symptoms related to chronic portal hypertension, and hypercholesterolemia (xanthoma/xanthelasma)

What is cholecystitis?

Acute inflammation of the gallbladder usually due to a gallstone obstructing the cystic duct (cholelithiasis)

What is a Murphy sign?

A classical physical finding in acute cholecystitis which results in arrest of inspiration when palpating the right upper quadrant

What are the clinical features of cholecystitis?

Right upper quadrant pain, fever, and leukocytosis

What is peritonitis?

Inflammation of the serosal lining of the abdominal cavity that results from infection, injury, or associated with other diseases (eg, spontaneous bacterial peritonitis associated with nephrotic syndrome)

What is the difference between primary and secondary peritonitis?

Primary peritonitis is caused by the hematogenous spread of infection to the peritoneum. Secondary peritonitis is caused by the entry of bacteria or enzymes into the peritoneum from the GI or biliary tract.

What condition is associated with primary peritonitis?

Chronic liver disease

What are the risk factors for secondary peritonitis?

Appendicitis; peptic ulcer disease; cholecystitis; damage to the pancreas; inflammatory bowel disease; intestinal obstruction; peritoneal dialysis; iatrogenic damage to the GI tract

Neoplasm

What is the most common primary liver cancer?

Hepatocellular carcinoma (HCC)

What conditions are associated with HCC?

Hepatitis B and C; chronic alcoholism; Wilson disease, hemochromatosis, and α_1-antitrypsin deficiency; carcinogen exposure (aflatoxin B1)

What is the key laboratory finding in HCC?

Elevation of serum α-fetoprotein (>400-500 ng/mL)

How does HCC spread to other sites of the body?

Hematogenous route

The majority of hepatic malignancies are what type of cancers?

Metastatic cancers usually from the colon

What is the most common liver tumor in childhood?

Hepatoblastoma

What two genetic conditions are associated with hepatoblastoma?

1. Beckwith-Wiedemann syndrome
2. Familial adenomatous polyposis

What is angiosarcoma?

A rare, malignant endothelial tumor of the liver

What are the risk factors for the development of angiosarcoma?

Exposure to vinyl chloride, thorotrast, or arsenic

What are the most common benign neoplasms of the liver?

Cavernous hemangiomas and liver cell (hepatic) adenomas

What are hepatic adenomas?

Benign tumors of hepatocytes that occur mainly in young, female patients. They are often asymptomatic and are often found by chance when imaging a patient for an unrelated problem.

What exposure are hepatic adenomas typically associated with?	Oral contraceptive use
What occasionally complicates hepatic adenomas?	Rupture—spontaneously or following minor trauma, especially during pregnancy
If a patient has a hepatic adenoma, what is his or her risk of developing HCC later in life?	Negligible
What is cholangiocarcinoma?	An adenocarcinoma of the biliary duct system
What is cholangiocarcinoma associated with?	It is associated with liver fluke (*Opisthorchis sinensis*) infestation, primary sclerosing cholangitis, and thorotrast administration.
What is primary sclerosing cholangitis?	A chronic liver disease associated with inflammation and fibrosis of the bile ducts leading to obstruction of bile flow. Alternating stricture and dilation of the bile ducts has appearance of "beading" on ERCP.

PANCREAS

Inflammatory/Autoimmune

What are the most common causes of pancreatitis?	Excessive alcohol intake (most common) and gallstones
What are other causes of pancreatitis?	• Trauma • Hypertriglyceridemia • Endoscopic retrograde cholangiopancreatography (ERCP) • Medications—azathioprine, furosemide, glucocorticoids, and cimetidine • Infections—*Ascaris lumbricoides*, *Opisthorchis sinensis*, and viruses (coxsackie and mumps) • Hypercalcemia • Scorpion stings (ie, *Tityus trinitatis*—rare!)

What are the signs and symptoms of acute pancreatitis?	Epigastric abdominal pain radiating to the back, nausea, vomiting, and anorexia
What are two common complications of acute pancreatitis?	1. Pseudocyst formation 4 to 6 weeks after acute attack 2. Chronic pancreatitis
What is a pancreatic pseudocyst?	A nonepithelialized, encapsulated pancreatic fluid collection that appears several weeks after a bout of acute pancreatitis
What are the key lab findings in patients with acute pancreatitis?	Elevated amylase and lipase (higher specificity) with hypocalcemia
How do you treat acute pancreatitis?	Acute pancreatitis usually resolves on its own. However, patients should refrain from eating and should be supported with pain medications and intravenous fluids. Severe acute pancreatitis can be life-threatening.

Neoplastic

What are the malignancies that affect the pancreas?	Adenocarcinomas, endocrine tumors, carcinoid tumors, lymphomas, and squamous cell carcinomas
What are the key features of pancreatic adenocarcinomas?	Often arises in the head of the pancreas; often silent before widespread dissemination; results in death within 1 year
What are the risk factors that predispose to pancreatic cancer?	Cigarette smoking, chronic pancreatitis, high intake of animal fat, prolonged exposure to petroleum products, and increased body mass index
What are the clinical manifestations of pancreatic cancer?	Weight loss, nausea, vomiting, epigastric pain, obstructive jaundice, generalized malaise, depression, and diabetes or impaired glucose tolerance. Other signs include migratory thrombophlebitis and a palpable gallbladder.
What is the name of the sign associated with painless, palpable enlarged gallbladder?	Courvoisier sign

What is the name of the sign associated with migratory thrombophlebitis that often accompanies pancreatic or other adenocarcinoma?	Trousseau sign
What is a commonly used marker for pancreatic disease?	CA-19-9

INTESTINE

Congenital

What is a Meckel diverticulum?	A congenital "true" diverticulum of the ileum resulting from the incomplete closure of the vitelline duct (the yolk stalk) *Rule of 2s—located 2 ft from the end of the small intestine, is 2 in long, occurs in 2% of the population, is twice as common in males as females, and can contain two types of ectopic tissue—stomach or pancreas
What is cystic dilation of the vitelline duct referred to as?	Omphalomesenteric cyst
In contrast to a Meckel diverticulum, what is a Zenker diverticulum?	A false diverticulum (only contains mucosa) occurring at the junction of the pharynx and esophagus and presents with halitosis and dysphagia
What is an omphalocele?	An abdominal wall defect in which abdominal organs (intestine, liver) are contained in a sac of peritoneum which protrudes through the umbilicus
What is gastroschisis?	An abdominal wall defect in which abdominal organs are present outside of the fetal body but are not contained within a sac of peritoneum
How are omphalocele and gastroschisis treated?	With serial reductions of the organs back into abdomen—sometimes the infant's abdomen is too small to accommodate all the organs because it failed to expand adequately during in utero development

Table 8.4 Omphalocele versus Gastroschisis

Condition	Defect	Location	Surrounding Membrane	Genetic Association
Omphalocele	Herniation of abdominal contents	Umbilical root	Peritoneum	Yes
Gastroschisis	Herniation of abdominal contents	Paramedian abdominal wall	None	No

What is congenital megacolon or Hirschsprung disease?	A disease caused by the absence of parasympathetic ganglion cells in the myenteric plexus and submucosal plexus of the distal colon due to failure of neural crest cell migration
What is a common outcome of Hirschsprung disease?	Large bowel obstruction with significant dilation proximal to the aganglionic segment and abdominal distention
What are some clinical features of Hirschsprung disease?	Failure to pass meconium within the first 48 hours of life, frequent vomiting, and chronic constipation
What other conditions are associated with Hirschsprung disease?	Down syndrome, congenital malrotation, and intestinal atresia

Anatomic

What are the major causes of intestinal obstruction?	Hernias, adhesions, intussusception, paralytic ileus, volvulus, tumors, obstructive gallstones, bowel infarction, foreign bodies, congenital bands, meconium, imperforate anus, myopathies, and neuropathies
What is intussusception?	The telescoping of a proximal segment of the bowel into the immediate distal segment
What are classical symptoms of intussusception?	Bilious vomiting, intermittent colicky abdominal pain, and currant jelly stools

| What is volvulus? | Twisting of a loop of bowel or other structure about its base of attachment |

Vascular

| What is ischemic bowel disease? | A disorder which results from the inadequate flow of oxygenated blood to the intestines |

| What conditions predispose to ischemic bowel disease? | Atherosclerosis and diabetes |

| What are the clinical features of ischemic bowel injury? | Abdominal pain out of proportion to the physical signs and bloody diarrhea |

| What is angiodysplasia of the colon? | Tortuous dilations of submucosal and mucosal blood vessels in the cecum or proximal ascending colon |

| What is a common symptom of angiodysplasia of the colon? | Painless bleeding |

Table 8.5 Hemorrhoids

Classification	Veins	Epithelium	Location	Drainage
Internal	Superior rectal vein	Simple columnar	Above the dentate line	Portal circulation
External	Inferior rectal vein	Stratified squamous	Below the dentate line	Central circulation

| What are hemorrhoids? | Variceal dilations of the anal and perianal submucosal venous plexuses |

| How do you treat both internal and external hemorrhoids? | Treatment varies from noninvasive to surgical and includes stool softeners, diet modification, sitz baths, sclerotherapy, and excision. |

| What are the risk factors for developing hemorrhoids? | Obesity, pregnancy, constipation, portal hypertension, sedentary lifestyle, and heavy lifting |

Infectious

Which infectious organisms of the intestine work through the cAMP pathway?

Vibrio cholerae, Escherichia coli, Bacillus anthracis, and *Bordetella pertussis*

Which infectious organisms of the intestine can be associated with bloody diarrhea?

Campylobacter jejuni, Salmonella, Shigella, Yersinia enterocolitica, Entamoeba histolytica, Clostridium difficile, enterohemorrhagic *E. coli,* enteroinvasive *E. coli*

Which infectious organisms of the intestine are predominately associated with watery diarrhea?

Vibrio cholerae, Clostridium perfringens, enterotoxigenic *E. coli,* protozoal infections, viral infections

Which bacterial infection of the intestine can clinically mimic acute appendicitis?

Yersinia enterocolitica

Which bacterial infection of the intestine is associated with eating improperly canned food?

Clostridium botulinum

Which bacterial infection of the intestine is associated with eating reheated rice?

Bacillus cereus

Which bacterial infection of the intestine is associated with eating contaminated seafood?

Vibrio parahaemolyticus and *Vibrio vulnificus*

How does *Vibrio cholerae* cause diarrhea?

It elaborates an exotoxin that causes the bowel cells to actively secrete electrolytes.

What is the difference in transmission between *Salmonella* and *Shigella*?

Salmonella is usually transmitted via its animal reservoir whereas *Shigella* is said to be transmitted via "food, fingers, feces, and flies."

Name two bacteria which can infect the intestine that are nonlactose fermenters:

1. *Salmonella*
2. *Shigella*

Table 8.6 Causes of Bacterial Enterocolitis

Bacteria	Disease	Classification	Route	Reservoir
Enterotoxigenic *Escherichia coli*	Traveler's diarrhea	Gram-negative rod, lactose-fermenting	Fecal-oral	Small intestine
Enterohemorrhagic *E. coli*	Bloody diarrhea, HUS	Gram-negative rod, lactose-fermenting	Uncooked beef	Large intestine
Enteropathogenic *E. coli*	Childhood diarrhea	Gram-negative rod, lactose-fermenting	Fecal-oral	Small intestine
Shigella	Bloody diarrhea, HUS	Gram-negative rod, nonmotile, nonlactose fermenting	Fecal-oral	Large intestine
Salmonella	Bloody diarrhea, septicemia	Gram-negative rod, motile, nonlactose fermenting	Eggs, chicken	Small intestine
Campylobacter	Bloody diarrhea	Gram-negative rod, motile	Fecal-oral, ingestion of animal products	GI tract of animals and birds
Clostridium difficile	Pseudomembranous enterocolitis	Gram-positive bacilli, motile, anaerobic	Ingestion of spores	Colon
Clostridium perfringens	Diarrhea, food poisoning, gas gangrene	Gram-positive bacilli, anaerobic	Ingestion of spores	GI tract, soil
Vibrio cholerae	Secretory diarrhea	Gram-negative, curved rod, highly motile	Fecal-oral, contaminated water	Small intestine

Abbreviations: GI, gastrointestinal; HUS, hemolytic uremic syndrome

What are three common causes of viral gastroenteritis?

1. Rotavirus
2. Norovirus
3. Adenovirus

What viral infection of the intestine are immunocompromised patients susceptible to acquiring?

Cytomegalovirus infection

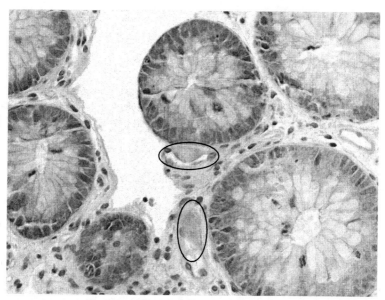

Figure 8.2   Cellular changes due to cytomegalovirus (CMV) infection are identifiable in two endothelial cells in the lamina propria of the colon. Infected cells are enlarged with peripheralized chromatin and glassy cytoplasm. (Reproduced, with permission, from OHSU.)

What organism causes Whipple disease?

Tropheryma whippelii

What is Whipple disease and what are the associated signs and symptoms?

A systemic infection—often associated with malabsorption, abdominal pain, arthralgias, intestinal lipodystrophy, and diarrhea

What are the classic histologic features associated with Whipple disease?

Foamy macrophages with PAS-positive inclusions infiltrating the lamina propria of the colon

Inflammatory/Autoimmune

What is a diverticulum?

An outpouching from a fluid-filled or hollow organ (eg, the bladder, esophagus)

What is the condition called when a patient has diverticula in their colon?

Diverticulosis

Are the "diverticula" in diverticulosis "true" diverticula?

NO! They are protrusions of the inner lining of the intestine through the outer muscular layer. They do not involve all layers of the intestinal wall and are therefore considered "false" diverticula. Bladder diverticula or Meckel diverticula are examples of true diverticula.

Where are the majority of diverticula commonly located?

In the left colon (sigmoid)

What are the risk factors for diverticulosis?

Age >60 years; consumption of low-fiber, high red-meat diet; colonic motility disorders

What are the typical signs and symptoms of diverticulosis?

Most presentations are asymptomatic, but patients can have intermittent left lower quadrant (LLQ) pain, a sensation of incomplete emptying of the rectum, or lower GI bleeding.

What is diverticulitis?

Inflammation of one or more diverticulum

What is the classical clinical presentation?

LLQ tenderness and fever

What are the complications of diverticulitis?

Perforation, fistula formation, pericolic abscess, and peritonitis

Table 8.7 Malabsorption Syndromes

Malabsorption Syndromes	Morphology	Symptoms	Diagnosis	Additional Information	Treatment
Celiac sprue	Flattened intestinal villi, hyperplastic crypts, increased lymphocytes, and plasma cells in lamina propria	Diarrhea, growth retardation, epilepsy, and classic rash (dermatitis herpetiformis)	Biopsy	Gluten sensitivity	Gluten-free diet
Tropical sprue	Villus atrophy	Diarrhea, weight loss, glossitis, stomatitis, and steatorrhea	Clinical	Associated with overgrowth of coliform bacteria	Tetracycline, B₁₂ and folate supplements
Whipple disease	PAS positive macrophages in lamina propria, villus blunting	Diarrhea, anemia, arthralgia, and cardiac/CNS symptoms	Biopsy	Any organ can be affected	Prolonged course of broad-spectrum antibiotics
Lactase deficiency	No characteristic change	Abdominal pain, diarrhea, and bloating after ingestion of diary products	Clinical	Most adults are lactase deficient	Lactose-free diet or use lactase
Intestinal lymphangiectasia	Dilation of lymphatics in small intestine	Diarrhea, hypoproteinemia, and generalized edema	Jejunal biopsy	Congenital or acquired	Supportive

Abbreviations: CNS, central nervous system; PAS, periodic acid-Schiff.

What are the clinical features of acute appendicitis?

Periumbilical discomfort progressing to right lower quadrant (RLQ), tenderness, anorexia, and vomiting

What is the risk of colorectal cancer in inflammatory bowel disease (IBD)?

The risk is slightly increased in Crohn disease, but markedly increased in ulcerative colitis.

What are systemic symptoms of Crohn disease?

Aphthous ulcers; erythema nodosum; uveitis

What findings would be expected on endoscopy gross examination of a partial colectomy specimen from a patient with Crohn disease?

Sharp demarcation of diseased bowel (*skip* lesions); linear ulcers; *cobblestone* mucosa; sinus *tract/* fistula formation; creeping fat around the bowel surface

*The old Crohn *skips* down the *cobblestone tract*

What findings would be expected histologically?

Transmural inflammation of bowel wall; noncaseating granulomas; mucosal damage; ulceration

What gross and histologic features are characteristic of UC?

Continuous involvement beginning at rectum; microabscesses; pseudopolyps; superficial ulceration

What are the complications of ulcerative colitis (UC)?

Colonic adenocarcinoma; toxic megacolon

Table 8.8 Inflammatory Bowel Disease

IBD	Crohn Disease	Ulcerative Colitis
Pathological features	Transmural involvement, skip lesions/irregular pattern, noncaseating granulomas, cobblestoning	Inflammation limited to submucosa, continuous involvement starting at the rectum and limited to the colon, crypt abscesses and pseudopolyps
Symptoms	Diarrhea, crampy abdominal pain	Bloody diarrhea, rectal pain
Complications	Fistulas, abscess, obstruction	Toxic megacolon, perforation, hemorrhage, carcinoma
Radiological findings	Barium x-ray shows wall thickening and narrowed lumen (string sign)	Lead-pipe colon on barium x-ray

Table 8.8 Inflammatory Bowel Disease (Continued)

IBD	Crohn Disease	Ulcerative Colitis
Extraintestinal manifestations	Polyarthritis, uveitis/episcleritis, fatty liver, cholelithiasis, nephrolithiasis, sacroiliitis, erythema nodosum, and pyoderma gangrenosum	Polyarthritis, uveitis/episcleritis, *primary sclerosing cholangitis*, sacroiliitis, erythema nodosum, and pyoderma gangrenosum
Surgical treatment	Only for complications	Complete colectomy—curative

Neoplasm

What is the most common neoplasm of the appendix?	Carcinoid tumors
What are the most common benign tumors of the small intestine?	Polyps, gastrointestinal stromal tumors (GIST), adenomas, and lipomas
What are the most common malignant tumors of the small intestine?	Adenocarcinomas and carcinoid tumors
Where are the most common sites of carcinoid tumors?	The appendix and small intestine (mainly the ileum)
What are the clinical signs and symptoms of carcinoid syndrome?	Cutaneous flushing, diarrhea, asthmatic wheezing, diaphoresis, itching, salivation, color changes (pallor or cyanosis), retroperitoneal fibrosis, and symptoms of valvular heart disease (often right heart)
What are some of the chemical substances produced by carcinoid tumors?	Depending on location, carcinoid tumors can produce: 5-HIAA, 5-hydroxytryptamine (5-HT), histamine, gastrin, and kinins
What are adenomatous polyps (adenomas)?	Benign overgrowths of the intestinal lining of the rectum and rectosigmoid colon that have an increased risk of malignant transformation

How common are adenomatous polyps?

They are found in more than half of patients over age 60 years.

What determines the malignancy risk of an adenomatous polyp?

Polyp size, architecture, and severity of epithelial dysplasia

What are juvenile polyps?

The most common pediatric GI polyps typically characterized as either hamartomatous overgrowths or reactive inflammatory proliferations

Are juvenile polyps usually benign or malignant?

Benign

What is familial adenomatous polyposis (FAP)?

An autosomal dominant colon cancer syndrome where patients develop 500 to 2000 polyps over the entire mucosal surface of the colon

What genetic abnormality causes FAP?

Mutations in the adenomatous polyposis coli (APC) gene which affect the ability of a cell to maintain normal growth and function

Table 8.9 Adenomatous Polyps

Adenomas	Percentage	Morphology	Risk of Malignancy
Tubular	Majority	Small and pedunculated	Rare, especially if <1 cm
Villous	Minority (1%)	Large and sessile	High, especially if >4 cm
Tubulovillous	Intermediate (5%-10%)	Mixed	Intermediate

What is hereditary nonpolyposis colon cancer (HNPCC or Lynch syndrome)?

An autosomal dominant condition that leads to a syndrome which predisposes patients to the malignant transformation of colonic polyps

Why is it called *nonpolyposis* if there are polyps involved in cancerous transformation?

This is to distinguish HNPCC, which causes a small number of polyps to develop, from other colon cancer syndromes where thousands of polyps are involved.

What genetic abnormality results in HNPCC?

Mutations in DNA mismatch repair genes (MSH2, MSH6, MLH1, PMS1, and PMS2) that cause microsatellite instability

What other types of cancers are patients with HNPCC prone to?

Cancers of the stomach, small intestine, liver, gallbladder, upper urinary tract, brain, skin, and prostate

What is Gardner syndrome?

An autosomal dominant syndrome that results from an APC mutation and is associated with osteomas, soft tissue tumors, supernumerary teeth, fibrous dysplasia of the skull, desmoid tumors, and an increased risk of colon cancer

What is Turcot syndrome?

An autosomal dominant condition that is characterized by the association of colonic polyps and CNS system tumors

What are the predominant brain tumors associated with Turcot syndrome?

Medulloblastomas and gliomas

What is Peutz-Jeghers polyposis syndrome?

A rare, dominantly inherited condition characterized by nonneoplastic hamartomas along the intestinal wall and melanotic pigmentation of the mucosal and cutaneous areas of the lips and gums

The majority of cancers in the large intestine are what kind of cancers?

Adenocarcinomas

What are the risk factors for colorectal cancer?

Age >60 years; ulcerative colitis; familial adenomatous polyposis (FAP); HNPCC; high-meat, high-fat, low-fiber diet; diet low in vitamins A, C, and E; first-degree relative with colon cancer

What are the common sites of colorectal cancer metastasis?

Regional lymph nodes, liver, lung, bones

What is the classical presentation of colorectal cancers?

- Proximal colon cancers—iron deficiency anemia, palpitations, fatigue, weakness, and weight loss
- Distal colon cancers—changes in bowel habits, changes in stool caliber, abdominal cramping, obstruction, occult bleeding, and barium x-ray findings of an "apple-core" lesion

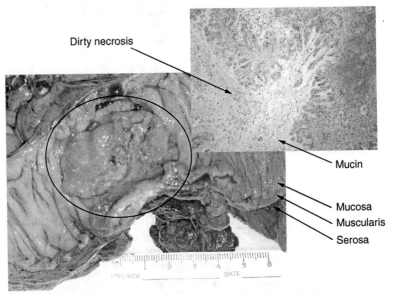

Dirty necrosis

Mucin

Mucosa

Muscularis

Serosa

Figure 8.3   On the left is a polypoid mass in the colon. Microscopic examination reveals colon adenocarcinoma with mucin production and dirty necrosis (neutrophils in the presence of individual tumor cell necrosis). (Reproduced, with permission, from OHSU.)

CLINICAL VIGNETTES

A 22-year-old college student presents with small vesicular lesions on the right corner of the vermillion border of her lip. She reports that these lesions are recurrent and occur mainly when she is under stress. What is the most likely diagnosis?

Herpetic stomatitis, also known as *cold sores* or *fever blisters*

A 35-year-old HIV-positive patient presents with whitish, curd-like plaques on his oral cavity that can be scraped off. What is the most likely diagnosis?

Pseudomembranous candidiasis or oral thrush

A 67-year-old man presents with a flat, velvety, granular, demarcated red patch on the floor of his mouth. He has been smoking cigarettes and chewing tobacco for 37 years. Biopsy of the lesion is obtained which shows significant epithelial dysplasia. What is the likely diagnosis?

Erythroplasia

A 40-year-old woman with history of arthritis complains of dry mouth, dry eyes, difficulty swallowing, and recurrent dental infections. Laboratory results are significant for presence of antibodies to Ro and La. What is the diagnosis?

Sjögren syndrome

A 15-year-old boy presents to the ED with a fluid-filled, fluctuant swelling on his lower lip. He tells you that the swelling followed a mouth injury that resulted when he fell during football practice. What is the likely diagnosis?

Mucocele

A 40-year-old woman complains of fatigue, sore tongue, and difficulty swallowing. Laboratory findings are significant for microcytic, hypochromic anemia. What is the likely diagnosis?

Plummer-Vinson syndrome

A 30-year-old pregnant woman complains of chest pain (worse when she is lying supine and after meals), a sour taste in her mouth, and hypersalivation. What is the most likely diagnosis?

GERD

Everybody on a cruise in the Gulf of Mexico gets diarrhea after eating poorly cooked shrimp and crabmeat. What is the diagnosis?

Vibrio parahaemolyticus infection (halophilic)

A 60-year-old alcoholic fisherman who has cirrhosis of the liver dips his foot in the seawater where he's fishing. Two weeks later he is dead. What happened?

It is likely that this man had chronic liver disease. If also he had an open wound on his foot which became infected with *Vibrio vulnificus*, he would have been especially susceptible to developing fatal septicemia.

*Associate this vibrio with liver cirrhosis

A 34-year-old man presents with a 1-year history of cough, recurrent pneumonia, weight loss, and difficulty swallowing. Barium esophagogram reveals a dilated esophagus with a distal "bird beak" appearance. What is the most likely diagnosis?

Achalasia

A 45-year-old alcoholic man presents with chest pain, upper abdominal pain, and hematemesis. He reportedly had a bout of forceful vomiting prior to the onset of pain. What is the most likely diagnosis?

Mallory-Weiss tear

A 1-month-old infant is brought to the clinic because of forceful vomiting after feeding. The parents say he seems hungry all the time, but cannot keep the food down. Physical examination is significant for signs of dehydration and an olive-shaped mass in midepigastric area. What is the most likely diagnosis?

Pyloric stenosis

A 50-year-old woman suffers from epigastric pain for months and complains of having "too much gas" and feeling bloated. The pain gets better when she uses an antacid. Laboratory studies are positive for *H. pylori* antibodies. What is the most likely diagnosis?

Peptic ulcer disease (PUD)

A 67-year-old man presents with a 10-lb unintentional weight loss over the last 3 weeks. He complains of abdominal pain and nausea. Physical examination is significant for an enlarged, fixed supraclavicular lymph node. The patient has a history of chronic gastritis. What is the most likely diagnosis?

Gastric carcinoma

A 9-year-old boy with recent travel to Mexico presents with an abrupt onset of fever, nausea, vomiting, and abdominal pain. Physical examination is significant for icteric sclera and a yellowish hue to his skin. His brother also suffers from similar signs/symptoms. What is the most likely diagnosis?

Hepatitis A infection

A young boy is brought to the hospital because of jaundice, tremor, and behavioral changes. Physical examination is significant for a ring of greenish-brown pigment at the limbus of cornea, hepatomegaly, and rigidity. What is the likely diagnosis?

Wilson disease

A 45-year-old man with a history of hepatitis C and cirrhosis presents with abdominal pain, worsening edema, and significant weight loss. Physical examination is positive for a palpable abdominal mass, icteric sclera, and ascites. Laboratory data show an increased α-fetoprotein (AFP) level (600 ng/mL), and an ultrasound of the right upper quadrant (RUQ) reveals a hypoechoic lesion. What is the most likely diagnosis?

Hepatocellular carcinoma (HCC)

A 25-year-old woman patient with recent complaints of RUQ fullness and pain is brought to the ER with severe abdominal pain, hypotension, and hypovolemic shock. There is no report of any antecedent trauma. Radiological studies indicate the presence of a hemoperitoneum around the liver. The patient has been on oral contraceptive pills for many years. What is the likely diagnosis?

A ruptured hepatic adenoma

A 55-year-old woman is brought to the hospital because of fever and severe RUQ pain. The patient is tachycardic; has a positive Murphy sign, guarding, and rebound tenderness of the RUQ. Blood tests reveal a leukocytosis. Ultrasound studies show a thickened gallbladder wall, the presence of gallstones, and pericholecystic fluid. What is the most likely diagnosis?

Cholecystitis

A 48-year-old patient with cirrhosis and ascites has abrupt deterioration of hepatic and renal function, fever, and abdominal pain. Paracentesis is performed which reveals 350 polymorphonuclear neutrophil (PMN) cell/mm^3. What is the likely diagnosis?

Spontaneous bacterial peritonitis (SBP)

A 20-year-old man presents with weight loss, diarrhea, steatorrhea, rash, and seizures. Labs are significant for anemia and a decrease in total Ca^{2+}, folic acid, vitamin B_{12}, Fe, Mg^{2+}, and fat-soluble vitamins. Antigliadin and antiendomysial antibodies are positive. What is the most likely diagnosis?

Celiac sprue

A 65-year-old man with history of diverticulosis complains of constant LLQ pain of moderate severity. He is febrile to 101.0°F. The patient has been constipated, but does not report nausea or vomiting. What is the likely diagnosis?

Diverticulitis

A patient with established UC presents to the ER with high fever and symptoms of shock and abdominal distention. What should you suspect?

Toxic megacolon

A 15-month-old boy is brought to the ED with bilious vomiting, lethargy, mucosy stools, and intermittent abdominal pain. Ultrasound of the abdomen shows a *donut sign*. What is likely diagnosis?

Intussusception

For the past several weeks, a 41-year-old man has had frequent facial flushing, palpitations, diaphoresis, colicky diarrhea, and wheezing. His laboratory values show increased level of urinary 5-hydroxyindoleacetic acid (5-HIAA). What is the most likely diagnosis?

Carcinoid tumor

A 53-year-old man complains of hard, itchy lumps around his anus that are painful and often bleed after wiping. On physical examination, swollen lesions are noted on the lateral sides of the anus. What is the likely diagnosis?

External hemorrhoids

A 62-year-old man complains of crampy, lower abdominal pain, constipation, and narrowing of stools. Fecal occult blood test (FOBT) is performed and is positive. Barium x-ray shows an "apple-core" filling defect in the descending colon. What is the most likely diagnosis?

Colorectal cancer

A 45-year-old white man presents with new-onset diabetes and abdominal pain. On physical examination, his skin is tan, and he has hepatosplenomegaly. He also complains of impotence and setting off metal detectors. What is the most likely diagnosis?

Hemochromatosis (bronze diabetes)

A 69-year-old patient presents with new-onset diabetes, weight loss, stomach and back aches, anorexia, and fatigue. His skin appears slightly yellow on examination and he has a painlessly enlarged gallbladder. What is the most likely diagnosis?

Pancreatic carcinoma

CHAPTER 9

Renal Pathology

EMBRYOLOGY

What embryologic structure gives rise to the urinary system?	The nephrogenic cord
What structure gives rise to the nephrogenic cord?	The urogenital ridge
What three sets of nephric structures does the nephrogenic cord develop into?	1. Pronephros 2. Mesonephros 3. Metanephros
Which of the above structures is nonfunctional and regresses completely by week 5 of gestation?	The pronephros
The mesonephros differentiates within the nephrogenic cord to form what two structures?	1. Mesonephric tubules 2. Mesonephric duct (Wolffian duct)
What nephric structure develops into the definitive adult kidney?	The metanephros
When does the metanephros become functional?	At week 10 of development
What undergoes repeated divisions to form the ureters, renal pelvis, major and minor calyces, and collecting ducts?	The ureteric bud
Where is the fetal metanephros located?	In the sacral region

The kidneys ascend from the sacral region in fetal life to vertebral levels T12-L3 in the adult. This upward migration is accompanied by what other event?

The medial rotation of the kidneys by 90°

What is unique about the blood supply to the kidneys?

It varies as the kidneys ascend to their adult position. At approximately the L2 vertebral level, the definitive renal arteries will develop.

What are the arteries formed during ascent called?

Supernumerary arteries

The urinary bladder develops from what structure?

The upper end of the urogenital sinus which is continuous with the allantois

What does the allantois become in the adult human?

The median umbilical ligament (urachus)

What nephric structure becomes incorporated into the posterior wall of the bladder at the trigone?

The mesonephric ducts

An urachal cyst is a remnant of what structure?

The allantois (which later become the urachus)

What forms the female urethra?

The lower end of the urogenital sinus

The transitional epithelium and stratified squamous epithelium lining the female urethra are derived from what embryonic layer?

The endoderm

What are the three parts of the male urethra that are derived from endoderm?

1. The prostatic urethra
2. The membranous urethra
3. The proximal part of the penile urethra

Endodermal outgrowths from what part of the male urethra develop into the prostate gland?

Prostatic urethra

Endodermal outgrowths from what part of the male urethra develop into the bulbourethral glands (Cowper glands)?

Membranous urethra

Endodermal outgrowths from what part of the male urethra develop into Littre glands?

Proximal part of the penile urethra

The distal part of the penile urethra is derived from what ectodermal structure?	The glandular plate
The glandular plate joins the penile urethra and becomes canalized to form what structure?	The navicular fossa
Ectodermal septa lateral to the navicular fossa become canalized themselves to form what structure?	The foreskin

HISTOLOGY

The metanephric vesicles differentiate into various structures that together form a nephron. What are the structures?	1. Glomerulus 2. Bowman capsule 3. Proximal convoluted tubule 4. Loop of Henle 5. Distal convoluted tubule 6. Connecting duct
What are the four histologic "compartments" of the kidney?	1. Glomeruli 2. Tubules 3. Interstitium 4. Vessels
What type of tissue lines the ureter, pelvis, major calyx, and minor calyx?	Transitional epithelium
What type of tissue lines the collecting ducts?	Simple cuboidal epithelium
What type of tissue lines the urinary bladder?	Transitional epithelium

RENAL PATHOPHYSIOLOGY

General Principles

What is renal failure (end-stage nephropathy)?	The inability of the kidneys to excrete wastes and maintain electrolyte balance. It can be broadly divided into acute and chronic renal failure. See Table 9.1 for manifestations of electrolyte abnormalities.

Table 9.1 Serum Electrolyte Abnormalities

	Concentration in Serum	
Electrolyte	**Low**	**High**
Na^+	Disorientation, stupor, coma	Irritability, delirium, coma
Cl^-	Secondary to metabolic alkalosis	Secondary to nonanion gap acidosis
K^+	U waves, flattened T waves, arrhythmias on ECG	Peaked T waves and arrhythmias
Ca^{2+}	Tetany, neuromuscular irritability	Delirium, renal stones, abdominal pain
Mg^{2+}	Neuromuscular irritability and arrhythmias	Delirium, decreased DTRs, cardiac arrest
PO_4^{2-}	Bone loss	Metastatic calcification and renal stones

Abbreviations: DTRs, deep tendon reflexes; ECG, electrocardiogram.

What are the common causes of renal failure?	1. Acute tubular necrosis (ATN) 2. Severe glomerular disease like rapidly progressive glomerular nephritis (RPGN) 3. Diffuse renal vessel disease like polyarteritis nodosa and malignant hypertension 4. Acute papillary necrosis associated with acute pyelonephritis 5. Acute drug-induced interstitial nephritis 6. Diffuse cortical necrosis
What happens in advanced cases of renal failure?	Patients develop uremia which is a clinical syndrome characterized by the buildup of waste products in the blood due to the inability of the kidneys to excrete them.
What are the indications for dialysis in acute renal failure?	1. Hyperkalemia 2. Central fluid overload 3. Metabolic acidosis 4. Severe hyperphosphatemia 5. Severe uremia

What is the definitive treatment of hyperkalemia?

Treatment includes administration of a loop diuretic, administration of Kayexalate (cationic-exchange resin), or emergency dialysis. Glucose, insulin, and bicarbonate can be used as temporizing measures moving potassium into cells (cellular shifts) but do NOT actually decrease total body potassium.

What are the major clinical characteristics of uremia?

Azotemia is caused by abnormally high concentrations of urea and other nitrogenous substances in the blood and can lead to:

- Acidosis from the accumulation of sulfates, phosphates, and organic acids
- Hyperkalemia
- Abnormal control of fluid volume
- Hypocalcemia leading to renal osteodystrophy
- Anemia caused by decreased erythropoietin
- Hypertension due to increased rennin

What are other common clinical manifestations of uremia?

Anorexia, nausea, and vomiting; neurologic manifestations ranging from diminished mental function to convulsions and coma; bleeding from disordered platelet function; accumulation of urochrome and other urinary pigments in the skin; fibrinous pericarditis

What are the nonrenal causes of acute renal failure?

- *Prerenal* azotemia which can result from decreased renal blood flow caused by blood loss, decreased cardiac output, systemic hypovolemia, or septic shock
- *Postrenal* azotemia which can result from bilateral obstruction of urinary flow

What is the step-wise approach to diagnosing acid-base disorders?

1. Is the patient acidemic or alkalemic?
2. Is the primary disturbance respiratory or metabolic?
3. For a respiratory disturbance, is it acute or chronic?
4. For metabolic acidosis, is an anion gap present?
5. If an anion gap is present, are there still other coexistent metabolic disturbances?
6. What is the degree of compensation by the respiratory system for a metabolic disturbance?

How do you determine whether an acute primary disturbance is respiratory or metabolic?

A respiratory disturbance will alter the arterial P_aCO_2 level (normal 40), while a metabolic disturbance will alter the serum HCO_3^- level (normal 24).

What causes anion gap acidosis?

Methanol; Uremia; Diabetic ketoacidosis; Paraldehyde or phenformin; Iron tablets or isoniazid (INH); Lactic acidosis; Ethylene glycol; Salicylates

MUD PILES

What causes nonanion gap acidosis?

Hyperalimentation; adrenal insufficiency; uteroenteric fistula; pancreaticoduodenal fistula; diarrhea; glue sniffing; renal tubular acidosis; hyperchloremia

What causes metabolic alkalosis?

This can result from volume contraction, hypokalemia, alkali ingestion, excess glucocorticoids/mineralocorticoids, or Bartter syndrome. All of these conditions elevate serum bicarbonate levels.

What causes respiratory acidosis (accumulation of CO_2)?

Central nervous system (CNS) depression; pleural disease; lung disease—chronic obstructive pulmonary disease (COPD), pneumonia; musculoskeletal disease—kyphoscoliosis, Guillain-Barre, polio

What causes respiratory alkalosis (excess elimination of CO$_2$)?

CNS hemorrhage; drugs; pregnancy; decreased lung compliance—interstitial lung disease; liver cirrhosis; anxiety

Table 9.2 Acid-Base Physiology

	pH	P$_a$CO$_2$	[HCO$_3^-$]	Potential Cause	Response
Metabolic acidosis	↓	↓	↓*	Diarrhea	Hyperventilation
Respiratory acidosis	↓	↑*	↑	COPD	Renal HCO$_3^-$ reabsorption
Respiratory alkalosis	↑	↓*	↓	High altitude	Renal HCO$_3^-$ secretion
Metabolic alkalosis	↑	↑	↑*	Vomiting	Hypoventilation

Abbreviation: COPD, chronic obstructive pulmonary disease.
*Primary disturbance

What is renal tubular acidosis (RTA)?

A disease that occurs when the kidneys fail to excrete acids into the urine

What is the mechanism of disease in RTA?

Impaired tubular bicarbonate absorption or hydrogen secretion that results in hypochloremic acidosis

What are the major types of RTA?

Type I (classic distal), type II (proximal), and type IV (distal)

What is type III RTA?

It is considered a variant of type I RTA with transient wasting of bicarbonate.

Table 9.3 Features of RTA

	Distinguishing Features of RTA		
	Type I (Classic distal)	Type II (Proximal)	Type IV (Distal)
Defect	H^+ secretion (intercalated cells)	HCO_3^- reabsorption	Aldosterone deficiency/ resistance (principal cells)
Plasma K^+	Variable	Low	High
Urine pH	High (>5.5)	Low (<5.5)	Low (<5.5)
Treatment	Citrate	Citrate	Furosemide, kayexalate
Complications	Nephrolithiasis	Rickets, osteomalacia	Hyperkalemia, arrhythmias

What are the most common etiologies of type I RTA?

Idiopathic, hereditary, collagen vascular disease (ie, Sjögren syndrome and SLE), cirrhosis, and nephrocalcinosis

What are the most common etiologies of type II RTA?

Hereditary, Fanconi syndrome, and carbonic anhydrase inhibitors

What are the most common etiologies of type IV RTA?

Conditions and drugs that impair the action of aldosterone—endocrine abnormalities, hypertension, DM, trimethoprim/pentamidine, nonsteroidal anti-inflammatory drugs (NSAIDs), angiotensin receptor blockers (ARB), angiotensin-converting enzyme (ACE) inhibitors, heparin, and immunosuppressive agents

Congenital

What is renal agenesis?

The failure of development of one (unilateral) or both (bilateral) kidneys

Is renal agenesis compatible with life?

Unilateral renal agenesis is compatible with life because the single kidney hypertrophies to maintain adequate function. However, bilateral renal agenesis is 100% fatal in singleton pregnancies.

What effects does bilateral renal agenesis (BRA) have on the developing fetus?

Fetal kidneys are necessary for amniotic fluid production. As such, there will be less than the normal amount of amniotic fluid present (oligohydramnios) which will subsequently impair pulmonary development.

What is the most common cause of fetal death in BRA?

Pulmonary hypoplasia—fetal urine is essential for development of lung, aiding in alveolar expansion through hydrostatic pressure and providing proline, an essential amino acid to the developing lung.

What is a Potter sequence?

A term used to describe the sequence of events that results in the typical physical appearance of a fetus that develops under conditions of oligohydramnios. Oligohydramnios may be due to several etiologies including bilateral renal agenesis.

What are some clinical features of Potter sequence?

Deformed limbs (*Sirenomelia, "mermaid syndrome,"* clubbed feet and/or bowed legs), redundant/wrinkly skin, abnormal facies, hypoplastic lungs

What is a *pelvic kidney*?

A kidney which fails to ascend to its normal position and remains in the pelvic cavity

What is a *pancake kidney*?

The fusion of two kidneys that are in close proximity in the pelvis due to a limited amount of space within the pelvic cavity

What is a *horseshoe kidney*?

A congenital anomaly that results in the fusion of the inferior poles of the kidneys forming a horseshoe shape

The normal ascent of a horseshoe kidney is arrested by what structure?

The inferior mesenteric artery

What is a common complaint in patients with ectopic ureteric orifices?

Incontinence

In males, where will an ectopic ureter drain?

The neck of the bladder or the prostatic urethra

In females, where will an ectopic ureter drain?

The neck of the bladder or the vestibule of the vagina

What is polycystic kidney disease (PKD)?

A disorder characterized by the growth of numerous fluid-filled cysts in the kidneys. These cysts slowly replace much of the renal parenchyma and result in diminished function with eventual renal failure. The disorder may be inherited in AD or AR pattern or may be the result of an acquired sporadic mutation.

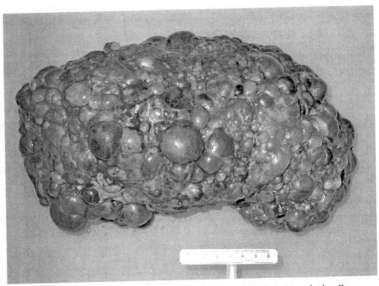

Figure 9.1 Polycystic kidney disease. Numerous fluid-filled cysts replacing the majority of the renal parenchyma. Normally a kidney measures ~12 cm in superior to inferior dimension. This kidney measures greater than 18 cm in superior to inferior dimension. (Reproduced, with permission, Wettach T, et al: *Road Map Pathology*, New York: McGraw-Hill, 2009; fig 10-1b.)

PKD is associated with the formation of cysts in what other organs?

Liver, pancreas, and lungs

Describe the types of PKD:

- Autosomal dominant PKD—a common form of the disease that usually presents in midlife
- Autosomal recessive PKD—a rare form of the disease that usually presents in infancy or early childhood
- Acquired cystic kidney disease (ACKD)—an acquired form of the disease that develops in association with long-term kidney problems, dialysis, and old age

What are the common signs of PKD?

Palpable renal masses; hypertension; headaches; urinary tract infections; hematuria; cysts in the kidneys and other organs

What is the treatment of PKD?

Treatment includes dialysis and kidney transplantation.

What vascular problem is associated with the autosomal dominant form of PKD?

Berry aneurysms (often in the Circle of Willis)

What is a simple renal cyst?

An innocuous serous fluid filled cyst that is a common incidental finding with no clinical significance

What are the radiographic characteristics of a simple cyst?

Renal cysts have smooth contours, are usually avascular, and give fluid signals on ultrasonography.

A patient with end-stage renal disease who has undergone prolonged dialysis is at risk for what condition?

Dialysis-associated acquired cysts

What is nephronophthisis (uremic medullary cystic disease)?

A childhood kidney disease marked by progressive symmetrical destruction of the kidneys with cystic lesions in the medulla, involving both the tubules and glomeruli

What are the clinical signs and symptoms that characterize nephronophthisis?

Anemia, polyuria, polydipsia, isosthenuria (decreased ability to concentrate the urine), progressive renal failure, and death in early childhood

| How does this differ from medullary sponge kidney? | Medullary sponge kidney is characterized by multiple small cysts in the medulla; however, renal failure is uncommon, and it is also associated with renal stones. |

Inflammatory/Autoimmune

Glomerular disease

| What is nephrotic syndrome? | A clinical complex characterized by significant (>3.0 g/day) proteinuria as a result of increased basement membrane permeability due to injury to the capillary walls of the glomeruli |

| What are the clinical manifestations of nephrotic syndrome? | 1. Massive proteinuria with daily loss of more than 3.0 g of low-molecular weight proteins such as albumin 2. Generalized edema from decreased plasma colloid oncotic pressure 3. Hypoalbuminemia as a result of urinary protein losses 4. Hyperlipidemia and hypercholesterolemia secondary to increased hepatic lipoprotein synthesis |

| What are the systemic diseases that cause nephrotic syndrome? | Diabetes mellitus (diabetic nephropathy); systemic lupus erythematosus (lupus nephropathy); renal amyloidosis; preeclampsia |

| What are the primary glomerular diseases that can cause nephrotic syndrome? | Minimal change disease (lipoid nephrosis); focal segmental glomerulosclerosis; membranous glomerulonephritis |

| What are the key characteristics of minimal change disease? | Occurs primarily in children; no visible basement membrane changes on light microscopy (LM); diffuse loss/effacement of podocytes on electron microscopy (EM); lipid accumulation in renal tubular cells; responds well to steroids |

What are the key characteristics of focal segmental glomerulosclerosis (FSGS)?

Sclerosis affects some glomeruli (focal vs diffuse) and involves only segments of each glomerulus (segmental vs global); deposition of hyaline masses (hyalinosis) and lipid droplets on LM; loss of foot processes and epithelial cell detachment on EM; immunofluorescence (IF) reveals deposition of immunoglobin M (IgM) and complement in the mesangium

What are some of the causes of FSGS?

1. Human immunodeficiency virus (HIV) infection
2. Toxins (eg, heroin)
3. Immunoglobin A (IgA) nephropathy
4. Familial forms

What are the key characteristics of membranous glomerulonephritis?

Slowly progressive disease common in adulthood; thickened basement membrane due to subepithelial immune complex deposits (typically IgG or C3); "spike and dome" appearance on EM; IF shows granular appearance; does not respond to steroids

What are the known disorders or agents that are associated with membranous glomerulonephritis?

1. Infections—hepatitis B, syphilis, and malaria
2. Cancers—carcinoma of the lung or colon and melanoma
3. Systemic lupus erythematosus (SLE)
4. Exposure to inorganic salts—gold, mercury
5. Drugs—penicillamine, captopril
6. Metabolic disorders—diabetes mellitus, thyroiditis

What is renal amyloidosis?

A disease characterized by subendothelial and mesangial amyloid deposits

What types of stains can be used to visualize amyloid deposits?

Congo red

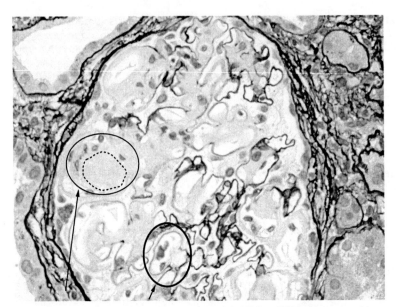

Figure 9.2   Glomerular capillary loops are expanded (thin solid black) compared to normal glomerular capillary loops (thick solid black) by nodular deposits (dashed outline) of amorphous appearing material. With special stains, this material is determined to be amyloid. (Reproduced, with permission, from OHSU.)

What conditions are associated with renal amyloidosis?

Chronic inflammatory diseases like rheumatoid arthritis (RA) and plasma cell disorders like multiple myeloma

What is lupus nephropathy?

The renal component of SLE

What determines the overall prognosis of SLE?

The severity of the renal lesion

How does the World Health Organization (WHO) classify the pattern of renal involvement in SLE?

- Type I—no renal involvement
- Type II—mesangial form characterized by focal and segmental glomerular involvement with an increase in both the number of mesangial cells and mesangial matrix
- Type III—focal proliferative form
- Type IV—diffuse proliferative form with glomerular changes that result in scarring and renal failure. **This is the most common and most severe subtype.
- Type V—membranous form that is indistinguishable from primary membranous glomerulonephritis

What is the most severe form of lupus nephropathy?

Type IV lupus nephropathy because it involves nearly all the glomeruli

What are the key characteristics of diabetic nephropathy?

Increase in glomerular basement membrane thickness with "wire loop appearance"; increase in mesangial matrix resulting in two morphologic patterns—diffuse glomerulosclerosis and nodular glomerulosclerosis

What are the nodular accumulations of mesangial matrix material in diabetic nephropathy called?

Kimmelstiel-Wilson nodules

What is nephritic syndrome?

A clinical complex, usually of acute onset, characterized by inflammatory rupture of the glomerular capillaries with resultant hematuria and minimal to mild proteinuria

What are the key clinical findings?

Oliguria, azotemia, hypertension, and hematuria with red cell casts in urine; proteinuria and edema occur but are usually mild

What are the primary glomerular diseases and systemic diseases that cause nephritic syndrome?

Immunoglobin A (IgA) nephropathy or Berger disease; acute poststreptococcal glomerulonephritis; rapidly progressive (crescentic) glomerulonephritis; membranoproliferative glomerulonephritis; Goodpasture disease; Wegener granulomatosis; Alport syndrome; microscopic polyangiitis

What is acute poststreptococcal glomerulonephritis?

An immune complex disease characterized by an intense inflammatory reaction that often follows or accompanies infection with nephrogenic strains of group A beta-hemolytic streptococci

What are the key morphological characteristics of poststreptococcal glomerulonephritis?

Kidneys have bilateral petechial hemorrhages; glomeruli are enlarged, hypercellular, swollen, and containing neutrophils; basement membrane has normal thickness despite inflammatory reaction; electron-dense "humps" on the epithelial side of the basement membrane (subepithelial localization); "lumpy-bumpy" immunofluorescence (granular deposits of immunoglobin G [IgG] and C3)

What are the key laboratory findings in poststreptococcal glomerulonephritis?

Low serum complement levels (C3); high levels of antistreptolysin O (ASO), anti-DNAase B, and anticationic proteinase titers

What is the prognosis for patients with poststreptococcal glomerulonephritis?

The majority of patients have a complete recovery; however, a small percentage of patients can develop rapidly progressive glomerulonephritis associated with severe oliguria and renal failure.

What is rapidly progressive (crescentic) glomerulonephritis (RPGN)?

It is a clinical syndrome, not related to one specific etiology, characterized by rapid and progressive loss of renal function leading to renal failure within weeks or months.

What histologic feature defines RPGN?

Parietal cell hyperplasia creates "crescents" in Bowman's capsule in the majority of glomeruli. In addition to parietal cell hyperplasia, there is infiltration of the "crescents" by monocytes and macrophages.

Describe the different types of RPGN:

- Type I—anti-GBM (anti-glomerular basement membrane) disease characterized by linear deposits of immunoglobin G (IgG) and C3 (Goodpasture disease)
- Type II—immune-complex mediated disease with "lumpy-bumpy" pattern of staining on IF (SLE, Henoch-Schönlein Purpura [HSP], and postinfectious, eg, poststreptococcal)
- Type III—aka pauci-immune type; is defined by lack of anti-GBM antibodies or immune complexes and are antineutrophil cytoplasmic antibody (ANCA) positive (polyarteritis nodosa [PAN], Wegener granulomatosis)

What is the treatment of RPGN?

Dialysis and transplantation. For patients with RPGN type I, plasmapheresis can remove pathogenic antibodies from circulation leading to some improvement.

What are the two common etiologies of pulmonary-renal syndrome (hemorrhagic pneumonitis and glomerulonephritis)?

1. Goodpasture syndrome
2. Wegener granulomatosis

What are the key characteristics of Goodpasture disease?

1. Antiglomerular basement membrane antibodies directed against antigens in the glomerular and pulmonary alveolar basement membranes (linear immunofluorescence for IgG antibody)
2. Will present with pulmonary hemorrhage and nephritic syndrome
3. Can progress to RPGN
4. Peak incidence in men in the mid-twenties age group

What are the characteristics of Wegener granulomatosis?

1. Small-medium vessel vasculitis of the respiratory tract, kidneys, and sometimes other organs with granuloma formation
2. Can present with pulmonary-renal syndrome
3. Most common in middle age Caucasians, with equal male to female ratio
4. Serology—c-ANCA positive

What is Alport syndrome?

A hereditary nephritis associated with nerve deafness and various eye disorders, including lens dislocation, posterior cataracts, and corneal dystrophy. Patient's often reach end-stage renal disease (ESRD) by 3 years of age.

What mutation is responsible for Alport syndrome?

A mutation in the gene for the α-5 chain of type IV collagen

How is Alport syndrome inherited?

Can be either X-linked or autosomal dominant

What is seen under electron microscopy in Alport syndrome?

Irregular glomerular basement membrane thickening with foci of splitting of the lamina densa

What are the key characteristics of membranoproliferative glomerulonephritis (MPGN)?

Characterized histologically by both basement membrane thickening and cellular proliferation; thickened basement membrane with glomerular capillary walls showing a double contour due to extension of mesangial cells; "tram-track" appearance on silver stains; two forms—types I and II

Describe the two types of MPGN:

1. Type I—immune complex nephritis associated with an unknown antigen
2. Type II—characterized by electron-dense material deposited within the glomerular basement membrane; C3 found adjacent to dense deposits; possibly caused by IgG autoantibody against C3 convertase of the alternate complement pathway

What is IgA nephropathy (Berger disease)?

A condition that affects children and young adults and is characterized by benign recurrent hematuria usually within one week of an upper respiratory infection

What is the pathogenic hallmark of IgA nephropathy?

Deposition of IgA in the mesangium

IgA nephropathy can be a component of which systemic disease?

Henoch-Schönlein purpura

What is Henoch-Schönlein purpura (HSP)?

It is a systemic small-vessel vasculitis most common in the pediatric population, involving the skin (purpuric rash), gastrointestinal tract (abdominal pain), joints (arthritis), and kidneys (hematuria).

What is the prognosis for HSP?

For the majority of patients, HSP is a benign, self-limited disease. However, ~5% will have chronic symptoms and ~1% will progress to ESRD.

Tubulo-interstitial disease

What is tubulointerstitial nephritis (TIN)?

A group of inflammatory diseases of the kidneys that primarily involve the interstitium and tubules. Glomeruli are spared altogether or are affected only late in the course of the disease.

What is TIN caused by a bacterial infection known as?

Pyelonephritis

What is TIN caused by a noninfectious origin called?

Interstitial nephritis

What are some of the noninfectious causes of TIN?

Tubular injury resulting from drugs; metabolic disorders like hypokalemia; physical injury from irradiation; immune reactions

What is acute tubular necrosis (ATN)?

A clinical syndrome that is characterized by the destruction of tubular epithelial cells; it is the most common cause of acute renal injury, which is a reversible injury.

What is the focus of ATN treatment?

Preventing the excess accumulation of fluid and wastes/electrolytes while kidney function is impaired (diuretics, K^+ restriction, dialysis)

Why is proper medical management essential to the prognosis of ATN?

This is because the condition is reversible when patients are treated and maintained on dialysis. Necrotic renal tubular cells will be replaced by new cells in 2 to 3 weeks with complete return of renal function.

When is a patient with ATN most likely to succumb to the syndrome?

Death is most likely to occur during the initial oliguric phase.

What is ATN often associated with?

Renal ischemia (shock); crush injury (myoglobinuria); toxins (ethylene glycol)

What is diffuse cortical necrosis?

An acute generalized ischemic infarction of the cortices of both kidneys that results from the combination of end-organ vasospasm and disseminated intravascular coagulation (DIC)

What is diffuse cortical necrosis often associated with?

Obstetrical catastrophes like abruptio placentae and septic shock

What is Fanconi syndrome?

Generalized dysfunction of the proximal renal tubules characterized by impaired resorption of glucose, amino acids, phosphate, and bicarbonate

What are the clinical manifestations of Fanconi syndrome?

Glycosuria; hyperphosphaturia; hypophosphatemia; aminoaciduria; systemic acidosis

What disease is the result of impaired renal tubular resorption of tryptophan?

Hartnup disease

What symptoms are common to Hartnup disease?

Pellagra-like symptoms including diarrhea, dermatitis, and dementia

What is cystinuria?

An autosomal recessive disorder that causes impaired renal tubular reabsorption of cystine, ornithine, lysine, and arginine

What is nephrocalcinosis?

Diffuse deposition of calcium in the kidney parenchyma that can lead to renal failure. It is often caused by hypercalcemia and hyperphosphatemia.

Collecting system

What is renal papillary necrosis (necrotizing papillitis)?

The ischemic necrosis of the tips of the renal papillae

Renal papillary necrosis is strongly associated with which medical illness?

Diabetes mellitus (DM); it can also occur following severe acute pyelonephritis

Drugs

What is drug-induced interstitial nephritis?	Acute interstitial inflammation that results from a type IV hypersensitivity reaction to certain drugs
What are the drugs most frequently associated with acute tubulointerstitial nephritis?	• Synthetic penicillins—methicillin, ampicillin • Other synthetic antibiotics—rifampin • Diuretics—thiazides • Nonsteroidal inflammatory agents—phenylbutazone • Miscellaneous drugs—phenindione, cimetidine
How is drug-induced interstitial nephritis treated?	It usually resolves on cessation of exposure to the inciting drug.
What is analgesic nephropathy?	Chronic interstitial nephritis that results from the consumption of large amounts of analgesics (Aspirin, NSAIDs)
What condition can result from analgesic nephropathy?	Renal papillary necrosis
What are the common clinical features of analgesic nephropathy?	Chronic renal failure, hypertension, and anemia
Patients who survive the renal failure associated with analgesic nephropathy are at an increased risk of which neoplasm?	Transitional cell carcinoma

Anatomic

What is obstructive uropathy?	Obstruction occurring anywhere along the urinary tract from the kidneys to the urethral meatus
What conditions are associated with obstructive uropathy?	Stones, benign prostatic hyperplasia, tumors, or anatomical abnormalities
What are the clinical sequelae of obstructive uropathy?	Interruption of urinary flow can result in pain, infection, sepsis, and loss of renal function.
What is urolithiasis?	A condition in which crystals combine to form stones in the urinary tract

What are the typical complications of urolithiasis?

Hydronephrosis and pyelonephritis

What is hydronephrosis?

Dilation of the renal pelvis, calices, and sometimes, the collecting ducts secondary to obstruction of urine flow by calculi, tumors, neurologic disorders, or congenital anomalies

If a patient has bilateral hydronephrosis where is the obstructing lesion?

Bilateral hydronephrosis occurs only when the obstruction is below the level of the ureters. If blockage is at the ureters or above, unilateral hydronephrosis would result.

What are the four major types of stones?

1. Calcium
2. Magnesium ammonium phosphate
3. Uric acid
4. Cystine

What are the key characteristics of calcium stones?

Most common type of kidney stone (80%-85%); consist of calcium oxalate, calcium phosphate, or both; are radiolucent; tend to recur

What disorders or conditions cause hypercalcemia and result in hypercalciuria with renal stone formation?

Cancers, increased parathyroid hormone (PTH), increased vitamin D, milk-alkali syndrome, and sarcoidosis—all lead to hypercalcemia and subsequent stone formation

What are the key characteristics of magnesium ammonium phosphate (struvite) stones?

Second most common type of kidney stones; develop in alkaline urine when ammonia is present in the urine; seen with infections caused by urease-positive bacteria (*Proteus, Staphylococcus aureus, Klebsiella pneumoniae*, and *Pseudomonas*); are radiopaque

What are staghorn calculi?

Struvite stones that form casts of the renal pelvis and calyces

What are the key characteristics of uric acid stones?

Strong association with hyperuricemia, often, secondary to gout or diseases marked by increased cell turnover (leukemia and myeloproliferative disorders); are radiolucent

How does the solubility of uric acid affect treatment of uric acid stones?

The solubility of uric acid depends on the acidity or alkalinity of the urine. In acid urine, uric acid crystals precipitate leading to stone formation. In alkaline urine, uric acid remains soluble. Treatment, therefore, involves alkalinization of urine.

What are the key characteristics of cystine stones?

Almost always associated with cystinuria or genetically determined aminoaciduria; are radiolucent

Table 9.4 Distinguishing Features of Urolithiasis

Features	Types			
	Calcium	Struvite	Uric Acid	Cystine
Frequency	80%-85%	5%-10%	5%-10%	1%
Components	Ca^{2+} oxalate	Ammonium	Uric acid	Cystine
	Ca^{2+} phosphate	Phosphate, magnesium phosphate		
Radiology	Radiopaque	Radiolucent	Radiolucent	Radiolucent
Causal conditions	Hypercalciuria	Infection	Hyperuricemia	Cystinuria

Infectious

What are the clinical features of a urinary tract infection (UTI)?

Dysuria, increased urinary frequency, urgency, and suprapubic pain

Why are most infections of the urinary tract and kidney seen in females?

Due to the shorter length of the female urethra

What are the common predisposing factors that increase the risk of urinary tract infection?

Obstruction of urinary flow; surgery on the kidney or urinary tract; catheters inserted through the urethra into the bladder; gynecologic abnormalities; diabetes; pregnancy

What are the common UTI pathogens?

Serratia marcescens
Staphylococcus saprophyticus
Escherichia coli ***most common
Enterobacter cloacae
Klebsiella pneumoniae
Proteus mirabilis
Pseudomonas aeruginosa

*SSEEK PP

What is cystitis?

Inflammation of the bladder, typically due to a bacterial infection, that is characterized by pyuria and hematuria

What is acute pyelonephritis?

Suppurative inflammation/infection of the renal parenchyma, typically the result of an ascending lower UTI

What are the major clinical and laboratory findings associated with acute pyelonephritis?

1. Increased urinary frequency
2. Dysuria (painful urination)
3. Pyuria (WBCs in urine)
4. Hematuria (RBCs in urine)
5. Bacteruria ($>10^5$ organisms/mL)

What are the additional clinical and laboratory findings associated with acute pyelonephritis?

Fever, leukocytosis, flank tenderness, urinary white cells, and white cell casts in the urine

What is chronic pyelonephritis?

Recurrent bouts of renal inflammation and scarring that occur from recurrent infections superimposed on diffuse or localized obstructive lesions

What findings are essential to the diagnosis of chronic pyelonephritis?

Coarse, asymmetric corticomedullary scarring with deformity of the renal pelvis and calyces

What are the stages of interstitial damage in chronic pyelonephritis?

Interstitial inflammatory infiltrate (early); interstitial fibrosis (late); tubular atrophy (late)

What are the sequelae of chronic pyelonephritis?

Renal hypertension and end-stage renal disease

Vascular

What is benign nephrosclerosis?

A term used to describe changes in the kidney that occur as a result of having "benign" hypertension; it involves the hyaline thickening of the walls of small arteries and arterioles which results in the luminal narrowing of the vessels and ischemic atrophy of the kidneys.

Can you have a sclerotic lesion superimposed on a primary kidney disease?

Yes, primary kidney disease can often cause secondary hypertension which can then cause benign nephrosclerosis.

What are the two microangiopathic hemolytic anemic syndromes?

1. Hemolytic uremic syndrome (HUS)
2. Thrombotic thrombocytopenic purpura (TTP)

What is hemolytic uremic syndrome (HUS)?

A childhood condition that consists of hemolytic anemia, thrombocytopenia, and acute renal failure

What condition is HUS highly associated with?

It is highly associated with diarrheal illness caused by *E. coli* 0157:H7.

What is thrombotic thrombocytopenic purpura (TTP)?

A syndrome characterized by microangiopathic hemolytic anemia, thrombocytopenia, neurologic abnormalities, fever, and renal dysfunction

What factors predispose to TTP?

Pregnancy, estrogens, and hormone replacement therapy; bone marrow transplantation and stem cell transplantation; diseases such as HIV, cancer, bacterial infection, and vasculitis; drugs such as ticlopidine, clopidogrel, and cyclosporine A

What causes HUS/TTP?

The exact etiology is unknown. However, a deficiency in the von Willebrand factor cleaving protease (ADAMTS13) is at least a contributing factor. The loss of this enzyme results in large complexes of von Willebrand factor circulating in the blood, which in turn causes platelet clumping and red blood cell destruction. A deficiency of the protease can occur sporadically, as a result of drugs, or secondary to Shiga-like toxins such as that seen in *E. coli* species.

Neoplastic

What is a renal adenoma?	A benign tumor that originates in the renal tubules of the cortex
What is a renal angiomyolipoma?	A benign neoplasm consisting of fat, smooth muscle, and blood vessels
What condition is renal angiomyolipomas associated with?	Tuberous sclerosis
What is a renal cell carcinoma?	The most common renal malignancy arising from the renal tubules
What patient population typically develops renal cell carcinoma?	Males between the ages of 50 and 70 years. There is also an increased incidence in cigarette smokers.
What is the histological appearance of renal cell carcinoma?	Nests and sheets of polygonal tumor cells with abundant clear cytoplasm
What chromosomal abnormalities are frequently associated with renal cell carcinoma?	Gene deletions in chromosome 3 (both in spontaneous cases and those associated with von Hippel-Lindau disease)
How does renal cell carcinoma present clinically?	Flank pain; palpable mass; hematuria It may also present with secondary polycythemia, fever, and ectopic production of hormones/hormone-like substances.
What are the paraneoplastic syndromes induced by renal cell carcinoma?	These include the ectopic production of erythropoietin, adrenocorticotropic hormone (ACTH), parathyroid-like hormone, prolactin, gonadotropins, and renin.
How does renal cell carcinoma typically metastasize?	It often undergoes early hematogenous dissemination through direct invasion of the renal vein and subsequently the inferior vena cava.
How do you treat renal cell carcinoma?	Initial therapy is with surgery—nephrectomy. It is notoriously resistant to radiation therapy and chemotherapy, although some cases do respond to immunotherapy.

What is a Wilms tumor (WT or nephroblastoma)?

The most common malignancy of early childhood (ages 2-4), originating from primitive metanephric tissue

What is the typical clinical presentation of a WT?

Children will present with a large palpable abdominal mass; other signs/symptoms include hypertension, fever from tumor necrosis, hematuria, and anemia.

What are the histologic features of a WT?

It is characterized by triphasic pattern consisting of immature stroma, primitive tubules/glomeruli, and mesenchymal elements such as fibrous connective tissue, cartilage, bone, and striated muscle.

What is the genetic abnormality associated with WT?

Deletion of tumor suppression genes *WT1 (most commonly)* or less commonly *WT2* on the short arm of chromosome 11

What are the genetic syndromes that include WT?

- WAGR syndrome (WT, aniridia, genitourinary malformations, and mental retardation)—WT1 mutation
- Denys-Drash syndrome (WT, pseudohermaphroditism, and glomerulopathy)—WT1 mutation
- Beckwith-Wiedemann syndrome (macroglossia, gigantism, and umbilical hernia)—WT2 mutation

How do you treat a WT?

The tumor is first surgically staged and resected via a radical nephrectomy. Addition of adjunctive chemotherapy and/or radiotherapy depends on initial surgical staging.

What is transitional cell carcinoma?

The most common tumor of the urinary collecting system, including the renal calyces, pelvis, ureter, and bladder.

What is the most common clinical presentation of this type of cancer?

Painless hematuria

What are the risk factors for transitional cell carcinoma?

These include toxic exposures to benzidine or β-naphthylamine (aniline dyes), cigarette smoking, and cyclophosphamide. In the renal pelvis, cancer risk has been associated with phenacetin abuse.

*Problems in your PeeSAC—phenacetin, smoking, aniline dyes, and cyclophosphamide

How does transitional cell carcinoma spread?

Through local extension to the surrounding tissues

Why is follow-up of patients with transitional cell carcinoma important after surgical resection?

There is a high likelihood of recurrence after removal.

Squamous cell carcinoma in the urinary tract is an uncommon malignancy that can result from chronic inflammatory changes. What organism is associated with such an inflammatory process leading to squamous cell carcinoma?

Schistosoma haematobium

CLINICAL VIGNETTES

A 10-year-old boy who is complaining of swollen arms, legs, face, and abdomen is seen by his pediatrician. His urine analysis is positive for protein. What is the clinical syndrome and most likely etiology?

The patient has nephrotic syndrome, most likely secondary to minimal change disease.

A 45-year-old insulin-dependent diabetic man presents to the ED with confusion. Arterial blood gas reveals: pH 7.18, HCO_3 19, and pCO2 18. When his family arrives, they report that he has refused to take insulin for the last 2 weeks and that his morning blood sugar was 438. What other secondary etiology must be considered?

This patient has diabetic ketoacidosis (DKA), likely due to missed insulin doses. However, 40% of DKA presentations may be associated with underlying infection and this secondary etiology should be considered. Treatment for this patient is insulin, IV fluids, and potassium replacement.

A patient has CT of the abdominal/pelvis which shows a heterogenous mass arising from the left kidney including areas of fat and water density. What is the most likely diagnosis? What condition is this diagnosis associated with?

Angiomyolipoma, tuberous sclerosis

A patient arrives to the ED complaining of excruciating colicky pain along his right flank. He also states that he's felt feverish all day and has had trouble urinating. What is the likely diagnosis?

Obstructive uropathy secondary to renal stones

A 30-year-old pregnant woman presents to her family physician for pain with urination. She also complains of having to urinate more frequently. She is afebrile and does not have flank tenderness. A urine analysis is positive for WBCs and bacteria. What are her diagnosis and the most likely causative organism?

Urinary tract infection (UTI), most commonly caused by *E. coli* or other enteric bacteria

A 20-year-old woman with a history of multiple urinary tract infections presents to her doctor. She has had right flank pain, high fevers, nausea and vomiting, and decreased appetite for 2 days. What might you expect to see on her urinalysis? What is a potential diagnosis?

WBC casts, pyelonephritis

An 11-year-old girl falls during a soccer game. Afterward, she complains of abdominal pain. When she is seen by her pediatrician, a large, palpable mass is appreciated in her right abdomen. Biopsy reveals a tumor with triphasic histology. What is the most likely diagnosis?

Wilms tumor

A 12-year-old girl presents to her pediatrician with "dark urine" and mild orbital edema. She reports having a sore throat 1 to 2 weeks ago. A urine analysis confirms hematuria and mild proteinuria. Titers of antistreptolysin O (ASO) and anti-DNAase B are high. What is the diagnosis and what is found on electron microscopy?

Poststreptococcal glomerulonephritis; electron microscopy shows subepithelial "humps" which correspond to IgG and C3 deposits on immunofluorescence.

A 65-year-old man presents to his primary care physician with painless hematuria and recent 10-lb weight loss. He is normotensive and does NOT have an abdominal mass on exam. He has a 50-pack/year smoking history. What is the most likely diagnosis?

Most likely transitional cell carcinoma of the bladder, however, renal cell carcinoma must also be excluded.

CHAPTER 10

Reproductive Pathology

EMBRYOLOGY

When is the genotype of an embryo established?

At fertilization

Define the undifferentiated stage of embryologic development:

A period when the genetically female and male embryos are phenotypically indistinguishable

When does phenotypic sexual differentiation occur?

It begins during week 7 of development and is completed by week 12 when characteristics of the external genitalia can be recognized.

What are the possible phenotypes of sexual differentiation?

Female phenotype, intersex phenotype, or male phenotype

In what sequence do the genital organs develop in utero?

Development begins with the gonads, then the genital ducts, and finally the primordia of the external genitalia.

The gonads of an embryo in the undifferentiated stage develop into what structures?

Either ovaries or testes

Development of ovaries or testes is dependent on the presence of what two hormones?

1. Estrogen
2. Testosterone

What gene on the short arm of the Y chromosome codes for male sex differentiation?

SRY gene

What are the two types of genital ducts found in the undifferentiated embryo?

1. Paramesonephric or mullerian ducts—play a major role in female development
2. Mesonephric or wolffian ducts and tubules—play a major role in male development

The urogenital systems of both males and females develop from what embryologic structure?

Urogenital ridge

What is the name of the thickening along the urogenital ridge from which the gonads develop?

Gonadal ridge

What are primordial germ cells?

Undifferentiated cells that migrate to the gonadal ridge to become either sperm or egg cells

What develops from the gonadal ridge and contains the primordial germ cells?

Primary sex cords

Development of the primary sex cords in females results in the differentiation of an outer cortex and an inner medulla. What part develops into the ovary?

Outer cortex

Primary sex cords also undergo differentiation in males. What part develops into the testes?

Inner medulla

Following primary sex cord development, secondary sex cords arise from the surface epithelium. Primordial germ cells then migrate and incorporate into these structures. In the female, secondary sex cords subsequently break up into smaller cell clusters. What are these clusters called?

Primordial follicles

What do primordial follicles contain?	Primary oocytes surrounded by a layer of simple squamous cells and connective tissue stroma
The gonads initially develop in the abdomen and then descend into the pelvis in females or into the scrotum in males. Which embryologic structure is involved in this descent?	Gubernaculum
The gubernaculum becomes what adult structures in the female?	Ovarian and round ligaments
What function do remnants of the gubernaculum serve in the adult male?	They serve to anchor the testes within the scrotum.
The paramesonephric (müllerian) ducts develop into what structures in the female?	Fallopian tube, uterus, and the upper one-third of the vagina
From which embryologic structure is the lower two-thirds of the vagina derived?	Vaginal plate
What substance suppresses development of the paramesonephric ducts in males?	Müllerian-inhibiting factor
In the female, the mesonephric ducts and tubules become part of the urinary system and eventually regress after the formation of what structure?	Metanephric kidneys
In males, the mesonephric (wolffian) duct and tubules develop into what structures?	Seminal vesicles, epididymis, ejaculatory duct, and ductus deferens *Mesonephric ducts and tubules *SEED*
Some mesonephric tubules in the testes develop into what structures?	The efferent ductules of the testes

Table 10.1 Development of the Male and Female Reproductive Systems

Embryonic Structure	Adult Female (+ Estrogen)	Adult Male (+ DHT)
Gonads	Ovary, primordial follicles, rete ovarii	Tests, seminiferous tubules, tubuli recti, rete testes, Leydig cells
Paramesonephric ducts	Uterine tubes, uterus, cervix, superior one-third of vagina, *hydatid of Morgagni**	*Appendix testes**
Mesonephric ducts	*Appendix vesiculosa, Gartner's duct**	Epididymis, ductus deferens, seminal vesicles, ejaculatory duct
Mesonephric tubules	*Epoophoron, paroophoron**	Efferent ductules, *paradidymis**
Phallus	Clitoris	Glans and body of the penis
Urogenital folds	Labia minora	Penile raphe
Genital swelling	Labia majora, mons pubis	Scrotum and scrotal raphe
Gubernaculum	Ovarian and round ligaments	Gubernaculum testes
Processus vaginalis	—	Tunica vaginalis

Abbreviation: DHT, dihydrotestosterone.
*Vestigial structures

At what stage of embryologic development does separation occur to result in dichorionic-diamniotic twins?	After day 1 to 3—each twin has its own placenta and own amniotic sac
At what stage of embryologic development does separation occur to result in monochorionic-monoamniotic twins?	After day 8 to 13—the twins have a shared placenta and a shared amniotic sac
If separation occurs between days 4 to 7, what sort of shared environment will the twins have?	These twins are likely to be monochorionic-diamniotic and will have a shared placenta but two amniotic sacs.

ANATOMY

Describe the venous drainage of the gonads:	The left ovarian or testicular vein drain to the left gonadal vein which drains to the left renal vein which drains to the inferior vena cava, whereas the right ovarian or testicular vein drains into the right gonadal vein which drains directly into the inferior vena cava.
What vessels are contained in the suspensory ligament (ie, infundibulopelvic or IP ligament) of the ovary?	Ovarian vessels
What vessels are contained in the transverse cervical (cardinal) ligament?	Uterine vessels
Where does spermatogenesis occur?	Spermatogenesis begins in the seminiferous tubules and is completed in the epididymis.
Which part of the autonomic nervous system regulates male erection?	Parasympathetic nervous system
Which part of the autonomic nervous system regulates ejaculation?	Sympathetic nervous system *Point and Shoot
Describe the anatomic pathway followed by sperm in the process of spermatogenesis and ejaculation:	Seminiferous tubules, epididymis, vas deferens, ejaculatory ducts, urethra

HISTOLOGY

What are the histologic components of the ovary?	Germinal epithelium, cortical stroma containing theca and granulosa cells, and follicles containing germ cells
What are the two histologic compartments of the testis?	1. Seminiferous tubules containing germ cells and Sertoli cells 2. Interstitium containing Leydig cells
What are germ cells?	Cells in the ovary or testis which will develop into ova or sperm, respectively
What are Sertoli cells?	Sustentacular cells that nurture the developing germ cells through the various stages of spermatogenesis

What are Leydig cells?

Cells that are found in the interstitium adjacent to the seminiferous tubules and produce testosterone

Leydig cells produce testosterone when stimulated by what hormone?

Luteinizing hormone (LH)

What cells secrete müllerian-inhibiting factor?

Sertoli cells

In males, when do germinal cells differentiate into primary spermatocytes?

Puberty

Describe spermatogenesis:

Germ cells become primary spermatocytes under the hormonal influence of testosterone. Each primary spermatocyte undergoes a meiotic division which results in two haploid secondary spermatocytes. The secondary spermatocytes then divide again forming four spermatids. These spermatids mature into four sperm.

From which cellular structure is the acrosome of sperm derived?

Golgi apparatus

What two events must take place after ejaculation before a sperm can be fully functional and capable of fertilization?

1. Capacitation
2. Acrosome reaction

What is capacitation?

A series of enzymatic and biochemical events which occur while sperm are in the female genital tract prior to fertilization. The result of capacitation is that sperm are hypermotile and have destabilized plasma membranes facilitating initiation of the acrosome reaction.

What is the acrosome reaction?

A reaction that occurs when a sperm contacts the zona pellucida of an ova. During the reaction, enzymes are released from the acrosome of the sperm facilitating penetration of the outer layer of the ova and subsequent fertilization.

Formed ova within primordial follicles arrest at what stage of meiotic division?

First prophase of meiotic division

The first meiotic division is completed before ovulation takes place. The cell then continues onto a second division that is also arrested. At what stage of meiosis does this second arrest occur?

Metaphase

When is the second meiotic division of an oocyte completed?	At fertilization
During meiosis, a primary oocyte will divide into four daughter cells. Of the four daughter cells, only one will become an ovum and the rest will degenerate. What are the cells that degenerate called?	Polar bodies
During the ovulatory cycle, which hormone stimulates endometrial proliferation?	Estrogen
During the ovulatory cycle, which hormone serves to maintain the endometrium to support an implanted embryo?	Progesterone
Loss of stimulation, by which hormone leads to menstruation?	Progesterone

Table 10.2 The Ovulatory Cycle

Follicular (Proliferative) Phase	Luteal (Secretory) Phase
Begins on the first day of menses	Begins with LH surge and ovulation, ends with menses
Characterized by the development of an ovarian follicle	After ovulation follicle known as corpus luteum
FSH secretion from the pituitary increases and stimulates follicle growth	Corpus luteum continues to secrete estradiol and begins to secrete progesterone
Growing ovarian follicle secretes estradiol	Negative feedback loop established where elevated estradiol and progesterone levels suppress FSH and LH secretion
Estradiol without progesterone drives the proliferation of the endometrium	LH and FSH secretion increases as progesterone levels fall at the end of this phase (if no fertilization)
LH secretion increases after a few days	Also causes development of secretory ducts in endometrium
Positive feedback loop established where estradiol increases LH and FSH levels	If no egg is fertilized, deceased LH levels allows the corpus luteum to regress leading to a decline in estradiol and progesterone
Leads to LH and FSH surge	Decline also allows FSH to increase driving follicular growth in the next cycle

Abbreviations: FSH, follicle stimulating hormone; LH, luteinizing hormone.

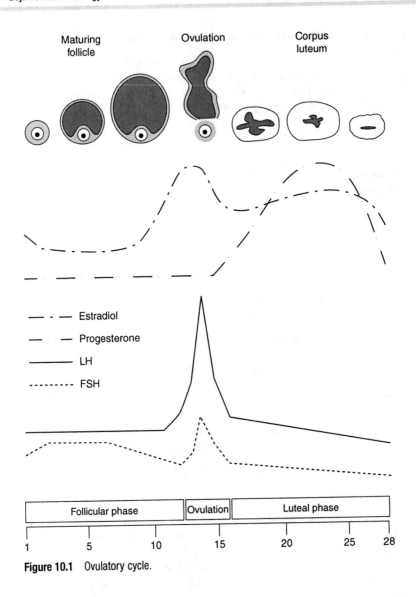

Figure 10.1 Ovulatory cycle.

What hormonal changes result in menopause?	Due to age-related decline in the number of ovarian follicles, estrogen production decreases and is eventually inadequate to stimulate ovulation and endometrial proliferation.
What are the histologic components found in breast tissue?	Glandular epithelium of the terminal duct-lobular unit, fibro-fatty stroma, and adipose tissue

PATHOLOGY

Congenital

What is a double uterus with a double vagina?	A congenital anomaly that results from the complete lack of fusion of the paramesonephric ducts and the sinovaginal bulbs
What is the defect that results in a bicornuate uterus?	The partial fusion of the paramesonephric ducts
What is a bicornuate uterus with a rudimentary horn?	A condition that develops due to the retarded growth of one of the paramesonephric ducts and results in a uterus with one normal and one abnormal horn
What defect results in the absence of the uterus or vagina?	The failure of the paramesonephric ducts and the sinovaginal bulbs to develop
What is atresia of the vagina?	A condition where the vaginal lumen is blocked due to failure of the vaginal plate to canalize and form a lumen
What is an imperforate hymen?	A condition resulting when the vaginal plate fails to canalize resulting in vaginal outflow obstruction
What is gonadal dysgenesis?	A condition that occurs when the primordial germ cells migrate into the gonad but later degenerate resulting in hypoplastic and dysfunctional gonads
What causes gonadal dysgenesis?	Primarily chromosomal abnormalities (eg, Turner syndrome, XX gonadal dysgenesis) which result in absence of both Müllerian-inhibiting factor and testosterone
What is a hypospadia?	A congenital abnormality in males that results in the displacement of the urethral meatus
Where does a hypospadiac urethra usually open?	A hypospadiac urethra opens anywhere along the urethral groove running from the tip along the ventral aspect of the shaft to the junction of the penis and scrotum or perineum.

What is epispadias?	A congenital abnormality more commonly seen in males in which the urethra is on the dorsal surface of the penis (or results in a bifid clitoris in females). Of note, epispadias is *not* a type of hypospadias.
Epispadias is commonly associated with what condition?	Exstrophy of the bladder
What is phimosis and paraphimosis?	• Phimosis—constriction of the opening of the foreskin which prevents it from being pulled back over the head of the penis • Paraphimosis—occurs when the foreskin is retracted behind the corona of the penis and cannot be returned to the unretracted position
What causes phimosis?	Congenital abnormality, inflammation, or trauma
What is a chordee?	A congenital malformation of unknown etiology that results in the downward displacement of the penis
What other congenital abnormality is associated with chordee?	Hypospadias
What is polythelia?	Also known as supernumerary nipple, polythelia is development of a nipple along the "milk line" which extends from bilateral axilla to the groin.
What is polymastia?	Also known as supernumerary breast, polymastia is development of glandular breast tissue with or without an associated nipple and also usually along the "milk line."

Inflammation

What is a Bartholin cyst?	A fluid-filled cyst resulting from an inflammatory obstruction of the Bartholin duct
What is lichen sclerosus?	A benign, chronic inflammatory dermatosis of the vulva that results in a white, patch or plaque with epidermal atrophy

What are the clinical characteristics of lichen sclerosus?

Pruritus and leukoplakia

What are cervical polyps?

Inflammatory proliferations of the cervical mucosa not associated with malignancy

What is balanitis?

A nonspecific inflammation of the glans penis and prepuce that is caused by physical trauma, irritation, or infection

What is chemical epididymitis?

An inflammatory process resulting from the reflux of sterile urine that causes epididymal irritation

Neoplastic

What is the most common gynecologic malignancy in the United States?

Endometrial carcinoma

What is the most common malignant tumor of the vulva?

Squamous cell carcinoma

What skin malignancy may occur on the vulva?

Malignant melanoma

Though primary carcinoma of the vagina is rare, what is the most common type of neoplasm affecting the vagina?

Squamous cell carcinoma

What is vaginal adenosis?

A benign condition characterized by the overgrowth of glandular-type cells in areas normally lined by stratified squamous epithelium

Vaginal adenosis can be a precursor to what condition?

Clear cell adenocarcinoma

If a female patient tells you that she was exposed to diethylstilbestrol (DES) while in utero, what condition is she at risk of developing?

Clear cell adenocarcinoma of the vagina

What is sarcoma botryoides of the genital tract?

A rare variant of rhabdomyosarcoma that arises in the wall of the vagina, usually occurring in females under the age of 8

How does sarcoma botryoides typically present?

It presents as a polypoid mass resembling a "bunch of grapes" that projects into the vagina and may protrude from the vulva.

What is cervical dysplasia?

Disordered squamous epithelial growth marked by the loss of polarity and nuclear hyperchromasia. It is categorized as cervical intraepithelial neoplasia (CIN) 1, 2, and 3.

What is carcinoma in situ?

It is synonymous with CIN 3 and involves dysplastic changes extending through the entire thickness of the epithelium but not invading the basement membrane.

Can cervical dysplasia lead to squamous cell carcinoma of the cervix?

Yes, lower grades of dysplasia can progress to carcinoma in situ (CIS/CIN3) and all have the potential to progress to invasive cancer.

What are the most common types of cervical cancer?

Squamous cell cancer (arising from the ectocervix) and adenocarcinoma (arising from the endocervix)

What are the epidemiologic risk factors for cervical cancer?

Early sexual activity; multiple sexual partners; lower socioeconomic status; cigarette smoking

Which human papillomavirus (HPV) subtypes are most frequently associated with squamous cell carcinoma of the cervix?

HPV types 16, 18, 31, and 33

HPV DNA sequences are often integrated into the genome of dysplastic or malignant cervical epithelial cells. What is the molecular mechanism associated with this process?

HPV viral proteins E6 and E7 bind and inactivate the gene products of *p53* and *Rb*, both tumor suppressor genes, thus allowing the cells to accumulate DNA damage.

What causes endometrial hyperplasia?

Excess estrogen stimulation caused by anovulatory cycles, polycystic ovarian syndrome (PCOS), estrogen-secreting ovarian tumors, and estrogen replacement therapy

Why is endometrial hyperplasia concerning?

Although not considered premalignant, hyperplasia is believed to put a woman at higher risk of developing endometrial carcinoma.

What are the conditions that predispose a woman to endometrial carcinoma?

Nulliparity; older age; prolonged estrogen stimulation; systemic conditions such as obesity, diabetes, and hypertension

Why is obesity associated with endometrial cancer?

Estrogens can be synthesized in peripheral adipose tissue creating an environment of prolonged estrogen stimulation.

What is the most common of all tumor types in females?

Uterine leiomyoma

What is a leiomyoma?

A benign smooth muscle tumor commonly arising in the uterine wall

Leiomyomas are usually estrogen-sensitive. Would you expect tumor size to vary throughout a women's lifetime?

Yes, tumor size would be expected to increase during pregnancy and decrease during menopause.

What is the most common complaint of women with leiomyomas?

Menorrhagia

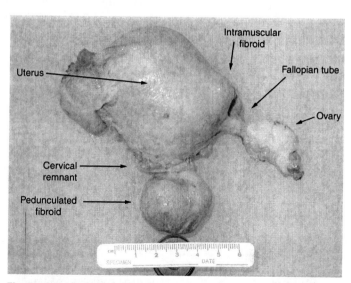

Figure 10.2 Supracervical hysterectomy specimen containing multiple fibroids. Two fibroids are visible—the first near the fallopian tube. The second is a pedunculated fibroid which is attached via a stalk to the left cornu of the uterus but passed through the cervical os and was located in the superior portion of the vagina at the time of resection. (Reproduced, with permission, from OHSU.)

Do leiomyomas commonly transform into malignant neoplasms (leiomyosarcomas)?	No, leiomyosarcomas typically arise de novo and are thought to only very rarely result from malignant transformation.
Describe the gross morphologic characteristics of a leiomyosarcoma:	A bulky mass arising in the uterine wall possibly associated with visible areas of necrosis and hemorrhage
What are two most common tumors that arise in the fallopian tubes?	1. Adenomatoid tumor (benign) 2. Adenocarcinoma
Ovarian tumors are classified into various categories based on what feature determined by the World Health Organization (WHO)?	Cell of tumor origin—epithelial, sex cord-stromal, germ cell
Tumors of surface epithelial origin of the ovary include what types of tumors?	Serous tumors; mucinous tumors; endometrioid tumors; clear cell tumors; Brenner tumors
What is a serous cystadenoma?	A benign cystic tumor lined with fallopian tube-like epithelium (single layer of tall, columnar, ciliated cells) that are frequently bilateral
What is a serous cystadenocarcinoma?	An aggressive, epithelium-lined cystic neoplasm filled with serous fluid that accounts for approximately 50% of all ovarian carcinomas (frequently bilateral)
What is a mucinous cystadenoma?	A benign tumor characterized by multilocular cysts lined by mucus-secreting epithelium
What is a mucinous cystadenocarcinoma?	Malignant tumors that can cause intraperitoneal accumulation of mucinous material (pseudomyxoma peritonei)
What is a Brenner tumor?	A tumor of urothelial-like ovarian surface epithelium
Tumors of germ cell origin typically occur in what age group?	Women younger than 20 years of age
What is a dysgerminoma?	The most common malignant germ cell ovarian neoplasm

A dysgerminoma is homologous to what testicular germ cell tumor?

Testicular seminoma

Yolk sac (endodermal sinus) tumors of the ovaries are homologous to yolk sac tumors of the testes. What tumor marker is typically found in serum?

Alpha-fetoprotein (AFP)

Ovarian choriocarcinoma is a highly malignant tumor that is associated with what tumor marker?

Human chorionic gonadotropin (hCG)—primary ovarian choriocarcinoma is extremely rare, while metastatic choriocarcinoma to the ovary from a uterine primary is more common

What is a teratoma?

A tumor that exhibits evidence of simultaneous differentiation from all three germ layers—endodermal, mesodermal, and ectodermal lines. These elements may be mature or immature.

What tissue types are commonly encountered in teratomas?

Hair, teeth, bone, cartilage, skin, brain, gut, and thyroid

What is the difference in histologic appearance and clinical behavior between immature and mature teratomas?

- Immature teratomas are usually composed of primitive small round blue cells and neural tube-like structures, while mature teratomas generally resemble the normal derivates that they are emulating (skin, hair, thyroid, etc).
- Immature teratomas are typically malignant, while mature teratomas (dermoid cysts) are benign.

What is a struma ovarii tumor?

A teratoma containing thyroid tissue as the predominant tissue type

Tumors of ovarian sex cord-stromal origin include what tumors?

Thecoma-fibroma group tumors, granulosa cell tumors, and Sertoli-Leydig cell tumors

What is a fibroma?

A solid tumor consisting of bundles of spindle-shaped fibroblasts

What is Meigs syndrome?

A syndrome characterized by the triad of ovarian fibroma, ascites, and pleural effusion

What are thecomas?

Solid tumors of spindle-shaped fibroblasts with round, lipid-containing cells

What are granulosa cell tumors?	Estrogen-secreting tumors that often cause precocious puberty in children and are associated with endometrial hyperplasia/carcinoma in adults
What is pathognomonic of granulosa cell tumors?	Call-Exner bodies
What are Call-Exner bodies?	Small spaces filled with eosinophilic fluid and basement membrane material between granulosa cells in both maturing ovarian follicles and ovarian tumors of granulosa cell origin
What are Sertoli-Leydig cell tumors?	Androgen-secreting tumors associated with masculinization
Where are the primary tumors that metastasize to the ovaries usually located?	Gastrointestinal tract, breast, and endometrium
What are Krukenberg tumors?	Ovarian masses caused by metastatic mucin-secreting adenocarcinoma (usually from gastric, pancreatobiliary, or colonic primaries)
What is fibrocystic change (aka fibrocystic disease) of the breast?	The most common disorder of the breast characterized by multifocal fibrosis and cyst formation. It is a painful condition common to patients between the ages of 25 and 50 years.
What are the two histologic types of fibrocystic disease and what are the associated features?	1. Proliferative—associated with adenosis (increased size of breast lobules) and hyperplasia 2. Nonproliferative—associated with fluid-filled cysts, with or without fibrosis
Is fibrocystic disease a premalignant condition?	No—generally, it is considered non-malignant and believed to not indicate increased risk of breast carcinoma.
What is a fibroadenoma?	A benign breast tumor of the intralobular stroma that presents as a firm, rubbery, painless, well-circumscribed mass
What is a phyllodes tumor?	A large, bulky tumor with usually benign behavior, although it can have malignant potential, that arises from intralobular connective tissue of the breast

What is the typical presentation of a papilloma of the breast?

It presents with serous or bloody discharge and a palpable mass.

What is an intraductal papilloma?

A benign proliferation of epithelial and myoepithelial cells on fibrovascular stalks arising in large or small lactiferous ducts

Where do most breast masses occur?

Upper outer quadrant of the breast

Who typically gets breast cancer?

Mostly postmenopausal women and women predisposed by age, positive family history, personal history of breast cancer, early menarche or late menopause, obesity, nulliparity, first pregnancy after age 30, and high animal fat diet

Briefly describe the various histologic types of breast cancer:

1. Invasive ductal carcinoma—firm, fibrous, infiltrating mass, likely preceded by ductal carcinoma in-situ
2. Invasive lobular—multiple foci and may be bilateral, likely preceded by lobular carcinoma in-situ
3. Medullary—fleshy, cellular with lymphocytic infiltrate (good prognosis)
4. Mucinous (Colloid) – gelatinous, pools of mucin surrounding tumor cells (good prognosis)
5. Inflammatory—lymphatic involvement of carcinoma (poor prognosis)
6. Paget disease of the breast— eczematous patches on nipples or areola; represents spread of underlying ductal carcinoma through the breast ducts to the skin of the nipple

Where can breast cancer metastasize to?

Anywhere in the body, but especially the axillary lymph nodes, lung, liver, brain, and bone

What oncogene abnormality is found in some patients with breast cancer?

Amplification of *c-erbV2 (HER-2/neu)*

What are the general treatments available to women with breast cancer?

Surgery (breast-conserving vs mastectomy), radiotherapy, chemotherapy, hormone therapy, and pain management

Hormone therapy is a form of systemic treatment that can be combined with surgery or radiotherapy to destroy undetected cancer cells and cells outside the breast. What are examples of this therapy?

Antiestrogens (tamoxifen), ovarian treatments (ovarian ablation), and aromatase inhibitors

What is extramammary Paget disease?

It is a neoplastic condition clinically similar to Paget disease of the breast characterized by inflammatory, *eczema-like* changes affecting the epidermis of the genital or perianal skin and other nonbreast cutaneous sites.

What is the origin of the neoplastic cells in extramammary Paget disease?

While this is still debated and somewhat controversial, most cases likely arise de novo from the epidermis or within an adnexal structure, either from apocrine gland ducts or keratinocyte stem cells. This is in comparison to mammary Paget disease, where the large majority of cases clearly arise from underlying breast carcinoma.

What is Bowen disease?

A preinvasive form of squamous cell carcinoma that presents as a single erythematous plaque on the shaft of the penis or scrotum

What patient population is frequently affected by Bowen disease?

Uncircumcised men older than 50 years

What are some postulated causes of Bowen disease?

Arsenic ingestion and HPV infection

What is the most frequent cancer affecting the glans penis?

Squamous cell carcinoma

Squamous cell carcinoma is characterized by slow growth and local metastasis. What are the regional lymph nodes typically affected?

Inguinal and iliac lymph nodes

As in cervical carcinoma, squamous cell carcinoma of the penis is associated with what HPV serotypes?

HPV types 16, 18, 31, and 33

What are the two major groups of testicular tumors?

1. Germ cell tumors
2. Nongerm cell tumors

What are the important risk factors associated with testicular tumors?

1. Cryptorchidism
2. Genetic factors
3. Testicular dysgenesis

What is a seminoma?

The most frequently occurring germ cell tumor that presents as painless enlargement of the testis

Testicular seminoma has a peak incidence in males of what age group?

30 to 40 years

What tumor marker can be found in the serum of patients with testicular seminoma?

hCG

A patient newly diagnosed with seminoma asks you about treatment and prognosis. What do you tell him?

Though malignant, seminomas are very radiosensitive and can often be cured.

What is an embryonal carcinoma?

An aggressive germ cell tumor that is characterized by rapid and bulky growth, and often presents with pain and metastasis

Embryonal carcinoma has a peak incidence in males of what age group?

20 to 30 years

What tumor markers can be found in the serum of patients with embryonal carcinoma?

hCG and AFP (only if concomitant yolk sac differentiation occurs)

What is a yolk sac (endodermal sinus) tumor?

A malignant germ cell tumor that accounts for over 80% of the testicular germ cell tumors in children. It is composed of primitive germ cells that form glomeruloid or embryonal-like structures.

What tumor marker can be found in the serum of patients with yolk sac tumors?

AFP

What is a testicular choriocarcinoma?

A highly malignant neoplasm composed of both cytotrophoblastic and syncytiotrophoblastic elements that is often encountered as a component of mixed germ cell tumors

Choriocarcinoma has a peak incidence in males of what age group?	20 to 30 years
What tumor marker can be found in the serum of patients with choriocarcinoma?	hCG
Unlike other germ cell tumors, how do choriocarcinomas metastasize?	Hematogenously
How does the treatment and prognosis of testicular choriocarcinoma differ from other types of germ cell tumors?	Tumors respond poorly to radiation and chemotherapy. Surgery is usually limited to radical orchiectomy for tissue diagnosis; mortality is very high.
What are mixed germ cell tumors?	Tumors that consist of varying combinations of germ cell tumor types. Testicular germ cell tumors are usually mixed and composed of various tumor types, including seminoma, yolk sac, embryonal, choriocarcinoma, and teratoma.
Mixed germ cell tumors have variable prognosis. What feature usually dictates prognosis?	The least mature element making up the mixed germ cell tumor
What are the available treatments for most germ cell tumors?	Treatment usually includes radiation and chemotherapy, depending on the histologic type of the neoplasm. In particular, chemotherapy has dramatically improved the prognosis of nonseminomatous germ cell tumors.
What are the two types of nongerm cell testicular tumors?	1. Leydig cell tumors 2. Sertoli cell tumors
What is a Leydig cell tumor?	A nongerm cell tumor derived from testicular stroma (interstitium) which may elaborate androgens and other steroids
How do patients with Leydig cell tumors typically present?	They usually present with a testicular mass and changes secondary to hormonal abnormalities.
What conditions are Leydig tumors typically associated with?	Precocious puberty in children and gynecomastia in adults

What is a key histologic feature of Leydig cell tumors?

Intracytoplasmic Reinke crystals

What is a Sertoli cell tumor?

A nongerm cell tumor composed of Sertoli cells or a mixture of Sertoli and granulosa cells

Do Sertoli cell tumors secrete any hormones?

They secrete both androgens and estrogens, but rarely in sufficient quantities to produce feminization or precocious puberty.

What is the difference in clinical behavior between mature teratomas in males compared to females?

Mature teratomas in females are benign, but in males they are most often associated with mixed immature elements such as yolk sac and embryonal carcinoma, therefore conferring a worse prognosis.

What is testicular lymphoma?

The most common testicular neoplasm in patients over age 60. Most are diffuse, large cell, non-Hodgkin lymphomas, and disseminate widely with poor outcomes.

What is the most common form of cancer in men?

Carcinoma of the prostate

What tumor marker is associated with prostate cancer?

Serum prostate-specific antigen (PSA)

What zone of the prostate is most frequently involved in prostate cancer?

Peripheral zone

Where does prostate cancer metastasize?

It frequently metastasizes to bone causing osteoblastic lesions.

What laboratory test would be an indicator of osteoblastic lesions?

Elevations in serum alkaline phosphatase

How is prostate cancer treated?

Localized disease may be treated with surgery and/or radiotherapy. Hormonal treatment with orchiectomy or administration of estrogens is generally reserved for patients with advanced disease.

Infectious

What is condyloma acuminatum?	A wart-like, verrucous lesion that can occur on the vulva, perineum, vagina, cervix, penis, or scrotum
What causes condyloma acuminatum?	Human papilloma virus (HPV) infection, frequently types 6 and 11
What is the key histological feature of condyloma acuminatum?	Koilocytosis (expanded epithelial cells with perinuclear clearing)
What flagellated protozoan parasite can cause cervicitis or urethritis?	*Trichomonas vaginalis*
Describe the cervix infected with trichomonas:	*Strawberry cervix*, red mucosa with creamy exudate
How can one diagnose trichomonas?	Do a wet preparation to visualize the trophozoite.
Describe trichomonas urethritis:	Mucosal itching, burning, redness, frothy exudates, or may be asymptomatic
What is candidiasis?	The most common form of vaginitis, caused by *Candida albicans*
What conditions are frequently associated with candidiasis?	Diabetes mellitus, pregnancy, broad-spectrum antibiotic therapy, oral contraceptive use, and immunosuppression
How does candidiasis typically present?	With a thick, white discharge and vulvovaginal pruritus
What is trichomoniasis?	A sexually transmitted type of vaginitis caused by *Trichomonas vaginalis*
What vaginal infection is known for its fishy odor and can be treated with metronidazole?	Bacterial vaginosis (*Gardnerella vaginalis*)
What is characteristically found on a smear preparation in bacterial vaginosis?	Clue cells

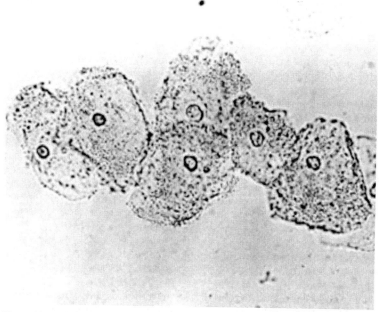

Figure 10.3   Clue cells of bacterial vaginosis. (Reproduced, with permission, from DeCherney AH, Nathan L: *Current Diagnosis and Treatment Obstetrics and Gynecology,* 10th ed, New York: McGraw Hill: 2006; fig 37-4.)

What is toxic shock syndrome (TSS)?	A syndrome that occurs secondary to exotoxin release by *Staphylococcus aureus,* usually associated with prolonged use of tampons
What is the clinical presentation of TSS?	Fever, diarrhea, nausea, diffuse erythema, and shock
What is the common presentation for a gonococcal sexually transmitted infection (STI)?	• Females—often asymptomatic, but can present with vaginal itching, discharge, itching, burning with urination, or vaginal bleeding • Males—burning with urination and purulent penile discharge (urethritis)
Patients with gonorrhea are usually coinfected with what other organism?	*Chlamydia trachomatis*
What is the best way to manage a patient with gonorrhea?	Treat the gonorrheal infection with ceftriaxone, and add doxycycline to cover a possible concurrent chlamydial infection. Ensure that all sexual partners are tested and treated (infections are often asymptomatic).

How does gonorrhea spread?

N. gonorrhea has pili that facilitate adherence to epithelial cells of the cervix.

Describe the clinical features of disseminated gonorrhea:

Septic arthritis, fever, and hemorrhagic rash of pustules and papules

What is the name for the conjunctivitis associated with gonorrhea observed in newborns?

Ophthalmia neonatorum, acquired from the mother during birth

How do you treat ophthalmia neonatorum?

Treat with silver nitrate or antibiotics in the newborn's eyes.

What are the extragenital infections associated with gonorrhea?

Pharyngitis, proctitis, purulent arthritis, and in the newborn, ophthalmia neonatorum

What is the most common sexually transmitted disease?

Chlamydia trachomatis

What is a serious sequela of untreated chlamydial infection?

Pelvic inflammatory disease with the potential for infertility

Which bacteria is the leading cause of blindness worldwide?

Chlamydia trachomatis

What is special about *Chlamydia* compared to other bacteria?

It is an obligate intracellular parasite, therefore, it may not be detected even in purulent urethral or cervical discharge.

What is Reiter syndrome?

A reactive arthritis triad including uveitis/conjunctivitis, urethritis, and large joint inflammatory arthritis*, associated with HLA-B27 and most commonly triggered by *Chlamydia trachomatis* infections (urethritis)

*"Can't see, can't pee, can't climb a tree"

What is lymphogranuloma venereum?

A chronic, ulcerative form of infection by the L-serotypes of *Chlamydia trachomatis* (L1, L2, or L3) that causes a genital papule followed by tender, fluctuant lymph nodes (2-6 weeks later)

Which of the herpes simplex viruses is associated with genital herpes and spreads via sexual contact?

Herpes simplex virus (HSV) type 2

What is the key cytologic feature of HSV infections?

Multinucleated giant cells with viral inclusions

How can one diagnose herpes?

Tzanck smear, monoclonal antibodies, and rapid antigen detection

*Tzanck goodness I don't have Herpes!"

What are the key features of the three stages of syphilis?

- Primary syphilis—chancre formation
- Secondary syphilis—rash (75%-100%), lymphadenopathy (50%-85%), condyloma lata (10%-20%)
- Tertiary syphilis—gumma formation in any tissue and neurosyphilis

What is a syphilic chancre?

An elevated, painless, superficially ulcerated papule

What is the preferred treatment for primary syphilis?

Penicillin G

What is chancroid?

A sexually transmitted disease caused by *Haemophilus ducreyi* that is characterized by painful, ulcerated lesions

What does a chancroid-scraping look like microscopically?

"School of fish" or "railroad tracks"

What is granuloma inguinale?

A sexually transmitted infection caused by *Donovania granulomatosis*, a gram-negative rod

What is the key histopathologic feature of granuloma inguinale?

The presence of Donovan bodies, or large histiocytes containing multiple organisms

Define cervicitis:

An inflammation of the cervix caused by a number of different organisms including staphylococci, enterococci, *Gardnerella vaginalis, Candida albicans, Trichomonas vaginalis, Chlamydia trachomatis,* and *Neisseria gonorrhoeae*

What are the symptoms of cervicitis?

Vaginal discharge, bleeding, itching/irritation of the external genitalia, pain during intercourse, and lower back pain

How is cervicitis diagnosed?

A Pap smear and culture for causative organisms is performed.

What is the treatment for cervicitis?

It depends on the causative organism, but initially involves broad-spectrum antibiotics.

What is endometritis?

Inflammation of the endometrium secondary to intrauterine trauma from instrumentation, intrauterine devices (IUDs), or complications of pregnancy

What bacteria are most often associated with endometritis?

Staphylococcus, streptococcus, clostridium species, and *actinomyces*

What is salpingitis?

Inflammation of the fallopian tubes secondary to infection, trauma, or surgical manipulation

Salpingitis can result from infections caused by what organisms?

Neisseria gonorrhea, C. trachomatis, various anaerobic bacteria, and other pyogenic organisms (*Staphylococcus* and *Streptococcus*)

What are the common complications of salpingitis?

Pyosalpinx (tube filled with pus), hydrosalpinx (tube filled with watery fluid), and tubo-ovarian abscess

What bacteria should all pregnant women be tested for at approximately 36 weeks gestation? Why?

Streptococcus agalactiae (group B streptococci). This is because transfer during delivery can result in neonatal sepsis and meningitis.

What is acute mastitis?

A breast abscess that develops due to infection frequently with *Staphylococcus aureus,* acquired through cracks in the nipple that develop during breast feeding

What is orchitis?

Swelling/inflammation of the testes secondary to viral or bacterial infection. When viral, it is most often due to mumps; when bacterial, it is often associated with epididymitis.

Is sterility a common sequela of orchitis?

Not when orchitis presents with unilateral testicular involvement. If orchitis is bilateral, however, sterility may result due to atrophy of the seminiferous tubules in both testes.

What is epididymitis?

An inflammation or infection of the epididymis due to the retrograde extension of organisms from the vas deferens

Organisms that cause epididymitis will vary with the age of the patient. List the organisms and the typical age groups they affect.	• *Escherichia coli* and other coliforms—prepubertal males and older males • *Mycobacterium tuberculosis*—prepubertal males and older males • *Neisseria gonorrhoeae*—sexually active males under 35 • *Chlamydia trachomatis*—sexually active males under 35
What is acute bacterial prostatitis?	Inflammation of the prostate gland of sudden onset due to a bacterial infection
What causes acute bacterial prostatitis?	Organisms associated with urinary tract infections which reach the prostate via direct extension from the urethra or urinary bladder
What is the typical presentation of acute bacterial prostatitis?	Fever, chills, body aches, dysuria, and a boggy, tender prostate
How is a clinical diagnosis made?	Diagnosis is made based on clinical features and urine culture.
What is chronic bacterial prostatitis?	A slow, indolent infection that persists beyond 3 months and presents with symptomatic bacteriuria despite adequate antibiotic treatment
What is chronic abacterial prostatitis?	A condition that affects sexually active males and presents with symptoms of prostatitis without positive urine cultures
What causes chronic abacterial prostatitis?	The etiology is uncertain, although potential pathogens include *Ureaplasma urealyticum* and *C. trachomatis*.

Anatomic

What is endometriosis?	A nonneoplastic condition caused by the ectopic dissemination of endometrial tissue to the ovaries or other structures outside the uterus
What are the ectopic endometrial foci sensitive to?	Hormonal variations in the menstrual cycle
What are chocolate cysts?	Blood-filled cysts in the ovaries that occur because of menstrual-type bleeding from ectopic endometrium

What is often associated with endometriosis?

Infertility and painful menstrual periods

What is adenomyosis?

A condition characterized by the extension or presence of ectopic endometrial tissue in the myometrium

A woman in her late forties comes to the clinic complaining of prolonged uterine bleeding. What is a reasonable diagnosis to consider in this patient?

Endometrial polyps

What are endometrial polyps?

Small, sessile projections of the endometrium that are composed of edematous stroma and cystically dilated glands

What causes follicular cysts?

Distention of an unruptured graafian follicle

What are follicular cysts associated with?

Hyperestrinism and endometrial hyperplasia

What causes corpus luteum cysts?

Hemorrhage into a persistent mature corpus luteum

A patient with a corpus luteum cyst would likely present with what sign or symptom?

Menstrual irregularity

What causes a theca-lutein cyst?

Gonadotropin stimulation

What are the clinical characteristics of polycystic ovarian syndrome (PCOS)?

Amenorrhea, infertility, obesity, and hirsutism

What causes PCOS?

The etiology is not completely understood, but poor regulation of a variety of enzymes involved in androgen biosynthesis, insulin resistance, excess luteinizing hormone, and hyperandrogenism are believed to play a role.

Women who present with PCOS are at an increased risk of developing what disease?

Type II diabetes mellitus due to increased insulin resistance

How is PCOS described morphologically?

Enlarged ovary with thickened varian capsule; multiple small follicular cysts; cortical stromal fibrosis

What is priapism?

A persistent, abnormal, and painful erection of the penis that develops when blood becomes trapped and is unable to drain

What condition is frequently associated with priapism, especially in the pediatric population?

Sickle cell disease

What are some of the available treatments for priapism?

External perineal compression; alpha agonists; oral terbutaline; aspiration of blood from the corpora; injection of phenylephrine into the corpora; surgical treatment

What are the long-term sequelae of untreated priapism?

Scarring and permanent erectile dysfunction

What is Peyronie disease?

A condition that occurs secondary to subcutaneous fibrosis in the erectile tissue of the penis, causing painful and curved erections

What is cryptorchidism?

Failure of one or both of the testicles to descend into the scrotum

What are the main adverse outcomes of cryptorchidism?

Sterility and cancer

What is cryptorchidism usually associated with?

Congenital inguinal hernias

What is a congenital inguinal hernia?

A condition that results from a large patency in the processus vaginalis

What is a hydrocele?

A painless swelling of the scrotum caused by a collection of fluid around the testicle which results from a small patency in the processus vaginalis

What is a chylocele?

An accumulation of lymphatic fluid within the tunica vaginalis secondary to lymphatic obstruction

What is a hematocele?

The abnormal accumulation of blood distending the tunica vaginalis of the testis, often secondary to trauma or tumor

What is a varicocele?

A dilatation of the veins associated with the spermatic cord in the testes

What is a spermatocele?

A cyst of the epididymis containing sperm

What is testicular atrophy?

A condition in which the male testes are decreased in size and function

List some conditions associated with testicular atrophy:

Mumps orchitis; trauma; hormonal excess or deficiency secondary to pituitary disorders, hormonal therapy, or liver cirrhosis; cryptorchidism; Klinefelter syndrome; chronic disease; old age

What is testicular torsion?

A twisting of the spermatic cord with resultant venous obstruction that typically occurs in males younger than 30 years, often secondary to trauma or activity

Why is it important to differentiate between testicular torsion and other conditions that may result in unilateral testicular pain/swelling?

Testicular torsion is a urologic emergency that must be treated with surgery in order to salvage the testicle.

What is the typical clinical presentation of testicular torsion?

The involved testicle is painful to palpation, frequently elevated in position when compared to the other side, and may have a horizontal lie.

What are other signs and symptoms in testicular torsion?

Scrotal erythema with edema, ipsilateral loss of the cremasteric reflex, and no relief of pain upon elevation of the scrotum (negative Prehn sign)

What is a Prehn sign?

A technique used to discriminate between bacterial epididymitis and testicular torsion. Scrotal elevation relieves pain in epididymitis but not in torsion.

What is benign prostatic hyperplasia (BPH)?	A common disorder of men over age 50 that is characterized by hyperplasia of both glandular and fibromuscular prostatic elements
What causes BPH?	An age-related increase in estrogens which promotes expression of receptors for residual dihydrotestosterone (DHT) and encourages prostatic growth, even in the face of decreased testosterone
What are the symptoms of BPH?	Common symptoms include nocturia, hematuria, dribbling, frequency, urgency, interrupted urine stream, and incontinence
What causes the symptoms of urinary obstruction in BPH?	An enlarged prostate compressing the urethra
What lobes are typically involved in BPH?	The anterior and middle lobes, formerly called the periurethral and transitional zones of the prostate
What are the common complications of BPH?	Urinary tract infections due to incomplete bladder emptying, bladder distention, and muscular hypertrophy of the bladder behind the obstruction caused by the enlarged prostate. Hydroureter and hydronephrosis are also common.

Obstetrical

What is a placental abruption (abruptio placentae)?	The premature detachment of the placenta from the wall of the uterus causing severe antepartum bleeding and potentially fetal death
What are common risk factors for placental abruption?	Trauma, preeclampsia, and drug use (eg, cocaine use)
What condition is associated with placental abruption?	Disseminated intravascular coagulation (DIC)
What is a placenta accreta?	The abnormal attachment of the placenta directly into the myometrium due to a defective decidual layer
What conditions typically predispose to a placenta accreta?	Prior cesarean section and endometrial inflammation

What will you see after delivery of a baby in a patient with placenta accreta?	Massive hemorrhage
What is a placenta previa?	The abnormal attachment of the placenta to the lower part of the uterus, partially or completely covering the cervical os
How does placenta previa usually present?	Painless bleeding in any trimester
How can you verify that an ectopic pregnancy is present?	Ultrasound, serial hCG
What are the complications of an ectopic pregnancy?	Hemosalpinx and tubal rupture

Table 10.3 Obstetric Complications

Classification of Spontaneous Abortions			
Type of Abortion	History	Viability of Pregnancy	Treatment
Threatened	Bleeding	Uncertain	Ultrasound/follow hCG levels
Inevitable	Cramping, bleeding	Abortion inevitable	D&C
Incomplete	Cramping, bleeding with some passage of tissue	Nonviable	D&C
Complete	Cramping, history of bleeding, and passage of all tissue	Nonviable	Follow hCG levels to negative
Missed	No symptoms	Nonviable	D&C

Abbreviations: D&C, dilation and curettage; hCG, human chorionic gonadotropin.

What is preeclampsia?	A condition that is clinically characterized by the triad of hypertension, proteinuria, and edema developing after the twentieth week of gestation. The etiology of this condition is not completely known.
What is the definitive treatment of severe preeclampsia?	Delivery of the fetus as soon as viable

What is HELLP syndrome?	A condition that is often associated with preeclampsia and includes *H*emolysis, *E*levated LFTs, and *L*ow *P*latelets **HELLP*
What are other clinical features associated with preeclampsia?	Headache, blurred vision, abdominal pain, edema of the face and extremities, altered mental status, and hyperreflexia
What are the common lab findings in preeclampsia?	Thrombocytopenia and hyperuricemia
What is eclampsia?	A severe form of preeclampsia associated with seizures
How do you treat eclampsia?	It is a medical emergency that requires intravenous (IV) magnesium sulfate and diazepam for seizures.
What is a hydatidiform mole?	A pathologic fertilization of either two male sperm and no maternal DNA or two sperm and one haploid copy of maternal DNA, leading to edematous and hyperplastic chorionic villi that present grossly as cystic grape-like clusters
What are the genotypes of complete hydatidiform moles and partial hydatidiform moles?	The genotype of a *complete mole* is 46,XX, and is *completely paternal tissue* (no associated fetus). The genotype of a *partial mole* is triploid (two copies of paternal DNA and one copy of maternal) and therefore a fetus may sometimes be identified.
What tumor marker do hydatidiform moles secrete?	hCG
Hydatidiform moles are precursors of what cancer?	Choriocarcinoma
What is choriocarcinoma?	A highly malignant neoplasm that arises from the cells in the chorion layer of the placenta. It is typically composed of both cytotrophoblastic and syncytiotrophoblastic elements.
What is preterm labor (PTL)?	Labor before 37 weeks gestation

What is the most common identifiable etiology of PTL?

Infection—often ascending infection from the lower vaginal tract after prolonged rupture of membranes, associated with 20% to 60% of cases

What is the predominant inflammatory cell type observed in the placenta in cases of chorioamnionitis?

Neutrophils

What fetal conditions are associated with polyhydramnios?

Conditions which impair fetal ability to swallow amniotic fluid—esophageal atresia, duodenal atresia, anencephaly, or result in excess urine production

What fetal conditions are associated with oligohydramnios?

Conditions which impair fetal ability to excrete urine—renal agenesis, posterior urethral valves in males

Intersex Conditions

What is intersexuality (hermaphroditism)?

A condition that results when a fetus fails to progress toward either of the two usual phenotypes and remains in an intermediate stage

How is intersexuality classified?

It is classified according to the histologic appearance of the gonad and phenotypic appearance of external genitalia.

What is true intersexuality (true hermaphroditism)?

A condition that occurs when an individual has both ovarian and testicular tissue with ambiguous genitalia

What is the genotype of individuals with true intersexuality?

It is usually 46,XY genotype.

What is female pseudointersexuality (female pseudohermaphroditism)?

A condition that occurs when an individual has only ovarian tissue (XX genotype) but with masculinization of the external genitalia

What is the most common cause of female pseudointersexuality?

Congenital adrenal hyperplasia, a condition in which a fetus produces excess androgens leading to virilization of the external genitalia

What is male pseudointersexuality (male pseudohermaphroditism)?

A condition that occurs when an individual has only testicular tissue (XY genotype) and stunted development of the external genitalia

What is the most common cause of male pseudointersexuality?

Inadequate production of testosterone and mullerian inhibiting factor (MIF) by the fetal testes

What is complete androgen insensitivity (testicular feminization)?

A condition that occurs when a fetus with a 46,XY genotype develops testes and female external genitalia with a rudimentary vagina

What is the most common cause of this condition?

Lack of androgen receptors in the urethral folds and genital swellings

What must be done with testes that are found in the labia majora of a patient with complete androgen insensitivity?

They must be removed to circumvent malignant tumor formation.

CLINICAL VIGNETTES

A 32-year-old woman presents for evaluation of infertility. Imaging studies reveal a uterus with 2 horns entering a common vagina. What is this condition called?

Bicornuate uterus, the most common congenital uterine anomaly

A 16-year-old girl presents to your clinic concerned about her lack of menstruation and breast development. Upon examination, you notice that she possesses infantile secondary sexual characteristics and has a webbed neck. What condition is this patient likely to have?

Turner syndrome

A 12-week-G1P0 with a history of pelvic inflammatory disease (PID) presents to the ED with severe lower abdominal pain. Ultrasound fails to reveal an intrauterine pregnancy. There is no history of bleeding. What is the likely diagnosis?

Ectopic pregnancy, most often in the fallopian tubes

A 16-week-G2P1 presents to the ED with high blood pressure, proteinuria, and edema. What is the likely diagnosis?

Hydatidiform mole; preeclamptic symptoms prior to 20 weeks should raise your index of suspicion for molar pregnancy.

A 65-year-old man discretely asks you about his painful and curved erections. He is interested in learning about his condition and any treatment options available. What do you tell him?

Peyronie disease is a condition that occurs in about 1% of men, ages 40 to 65. It has an unknown etiology, but is not known to be malignant. Treatment other than surgery is usually ineffective. Surgical intervention is limited to penile deformities that prevent intercourse.

A woman in her first trimester of pregnancy is exposed to a child who has a "slapped cheek appearance" for a few days. The fetus dies from hydrops fetalis. What virus caused this?

Parvovirus B19 (fifth disease)

A sexually active 17-year-old boy noticed some dysuria but it "went away." Now he has fever, pain, and swelling in his scrotal area. What happened?

Untreated gonorrhea infection likely spread from the patient's urethra to his prostate and epididymis, causing epididymitis

A 32-year-old woman is having trouble conceiving. An exploratory laparotomy shows extensive scarring and damage to her fallopian tubes. What is the diagnosis?

Pelvic inflammatory disease (PID) secondary to chlamydial or gonorrheal infection

A term neonate begins having respiratory distress at about 2 hours of life, requires oxygen, and eventually requires intubation. What is the diagnosis?

Group B streptococci sepsis

A 3-week-old infant, the product of a term vaginal delivery, begins wheezing, having respiratory problems, and decreased oral intake. The mother had no prenatal care. What is the diagnosis?

Chlamydia pneumonia acquired from the birth canal of infected mother

A 22-year-old man had nongonococcal urethritis a few weeks ago for which he was not treated. Now he has arthritis symptoms. What is the diagnosis?

Reiter syndrome with a triad of urethritis, arthritis, and conjunctivitis—often associated with HLA type B27
* "Can't see, can't pee, can't climb a tree!"

A 65-year-old man presents with multiple rough papules on the shaft of his penis. He reports three new sexual partners in the last 6 months and endorses only infrequent condom use. What is the diagnosis?

Condyloma accuminatum (associated with HPV types 6 and 11)

A 6-year-old girl is brought to her pediatrician because her mother noticed a mass protruding from the girl's vagina. On examination, the mass has the appearance of a cluster of grapes. What is the diagnosis?

Sarcoma botryoides

A 53-year-old man presents to his doctor concerned that he has started to urinate much more frequently. He also notes that he has a difficult time initiating urination and often will continue to dribble urine after he has finished urinating. What might this patient be at higher risk of developing than another man without these symptoms?

The patient likely has benign prostatic hyperplasia (BPH). As such, he is at higher risk of developing urinary tract infections due to urinary retention and incomplete bladder emptying. BPH is not considered a premalignant lesion; therefore he is not at higher risk of prostatic carcinoma.

A 34-year-old woman who is breast-feeding presents with low-grade fever and breast tenderness. On examination, her breast is warm to the touch and erythematous. What organism is likely responsible for this infection?

The patient likely has acute mastitis, most often caused by *Staphylococcus aureus*.

A 47-year-old woman undergoes surgery to remove an ovarian mass. During surgery, it is observed that the woman's abdomen is full of mucinous material. What is the most likely diagnosis of the ovarian mass?

The woman has pseudomyxoma peritonei, and the mass is likely a mucinous cystadenocarcinoma.

A male patient complains of pain on urination and copious, purulent discharge from his penis. A Gram stain of this fluid demonstrates gram-negative diplococci. What is the likely diagnosis?

Neisseria gonorrhoeae infection

A child who prior to puberty is described as phenotypically female, experiences amenorrhea, virilization, and develops male secondary sexual characteristics at puberty. What is this patient's likely genotype and diagnosis?

46,XY and 5 alpha-reductase deficiency. This is the enzyme responsible for converting testosterone to dihydrotestosterone (DHT) in peripheral tissues.

CHAPTER 11

Endocrine Pathology

PITUITARY

General Principles

Where is the pituitary gland located?	In the sella turcica near the optic chiasm and cavernous sinus
What are the two distinct parts of the pituitary gland?	1. Anterior lobe (adenohypophysis) 2. Posterior lobe (neurohypophysis)
What is the origin of the anterior lobe?	Rathke pouch—oral cavity
What is the portal vascular system of the anterior pituitary?	A transport system for circulating hormones between the hypothalamus and anterior pituitary
What are the major cell types in the anterior pituitary?	Somatotrophs; lactotrophs; corticotrophs; thyrotrophs; gonadotrophs

Table 11.1 Pituitary Hormones

Cell Type	Hormone	Hypothalamic Regulator
Somatotroph	GH	GHRH+
Lactotroph	Prolactin	Dopamine–, TRH+
Corticotroph	ACTH, MSH	CRH+
Thyrotroph	TSH	TRH+
Gonadotroph	FSH	GnRH+
	LH	GnRH+

Abbreviations: GH, growth hormone; ACTH, adrenocorticotropic hormone; MSH, melanocyte stimulating hormone; TSH, thyroid stimulating hormone; FSH, follicle stimulating hormone; LH, luteinizing hormone; GHRH, growth hormone-releasing hormone; TRH, thyrotropin releasing hormone; CRH, corticotropin releasing hormone; GnRH, gonadotropin releasing hormone.

How is prolactin regulated?	Prolactin release has a negative feedback mechanism—prolactin increases dopamine release from the hypothalamus, dopamine then inhibits prolactin secretion. Therefore, an increase in dopamine results in a decrease in prolactin, and a decrease in dopamine (as seen with many antipsychotics) results in an increase in prolactin.
What is the embryologic origin of the posterior pituitary?	Neuroectoderm—outpouching of the third ventricle with modified glial and axonal components from supraoptic and paraventricular nuclei
What hormones are produced in the hypothalamus and stored in the posterior pituitary?	Oxytocin; vasopressin (antidiuretic hormone [ADH])
What are the effects of oxytocin on the human body?	Contracts the uterus and lactiferous ducts in mammary glands
When is vasopressin secreted from the posterior pituitary?	Decreased blood volume; increased osmolarity
What role does vasopressin play in the kidney?	Saves water by increasing permeability at collecting ducts, ie, *antidiuretic hormone*

Anterior Pituitary Pathology

What is the visual field defect that occurs in patients with pituitary adenomas?	Bitemporal hemianopsia
What is the field defect caused by?	Compression of the optic nerve at the optic chiasm
What do pituitary adenomas look like histologically?	Uniform monoclonal polygonal cells in cords or sheets
What is the most common type of hyperfunctioning pituitary adenoma?	Prolactinoma
What are the symptoms associated with a prolactinoma?	Amenorrhea, galactorrhea, erectile dysfunction (in males), ± visual field deficit

Why do these symptoms occur?	Elevated levels of prolactin suppress secretion of follicle stimulating hormone (FSH) and luteinizing hormone (LH)
What are the histologic findings consistent with prolactinoma?	Lactotroph hyperplasia with secretory granules on immunohistochemical staining
What are other causes of hyperprolactinemia?	Medications; cirrhosis; hypothyroidism; stress
Which drugs can cause galactorrhea?	Neuroleptics/antipsychotics (eg, haloperidol); reserpine (antihypertensive); phenothiazines; metoclopramide
By what mechanism do most drugs cause galactorrhea?	Blocking dopamine receptors thereby releasing inhibition of prolactin
What is the treatment for galactorrhea?	Bromocriptine (dopamine agonist)
What is acromegaly?	The result of continued stimulation by excess growth hormone (GH) after closure of the epiphyseal plates (ie, adults), characterized by frontal bossing (prominent forehead), large head, nose, hands, protruding jaw, thick tongue, and deepening of the voice
What syndrome is caused by growth hormone adenoma of the pituitary in a child who is still growing (epiphyses have not closed)?	Gigantism
What oncogene is associated with growth hormone adenomas?	GSP oncogene
What is the treatment for growth hormone adenomas?	Surgical removal of tumor or radiation
What is Cushing disease?	Elevated serum cortisol secondary to corticotroph cell (ACTH releasing) pituitary adenoma, resulting in weight gain, truncal obesity, abdominal striae, buffalo hump, headaches, hypertension, irregular menses, hyperpigmentation of the skin

What is Cushing syndrome?

Also an increase in serum cortisol with similar symptoms (except for hyperpigmentation), but secondary to an adrenal adenoma or carcinoma releasing cortisol

Is Cushing disease or syndrome more common?

Cushing disease—accounting for ~70% of cases

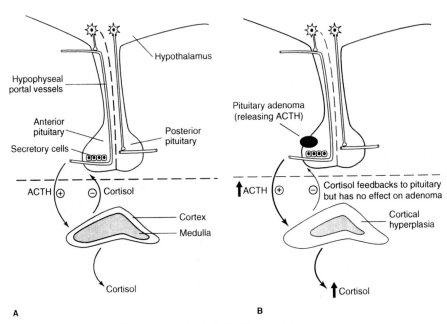

Figure 11.1   A. Normal pituitary-adrenal axis. **B.** Cushing disease.

What is the syndrome that is associated with pituitary microadenoma, bitemporal hemianopsia, hyperpigmentation, and Cushing syndrome?

Nelson syndrome

What is the cause of Nelson syndrome?

The loss of the inhibitory effect of corticosteroids on a corticotroph adenoma of the pituitary. The adenoma increases in size after removal of bilateral adrenal glands for treatment of Cushing syndrome.

What are the symptoms of a gonadotroph adenoma of the pituitary gland?

No recognizable syndrome; decreased libido; amenorrhea

What are the symptoms of a thyrotroph adenoma of the pituitary gland?

Tachycardia, palpitations, weight loss, and diarrhea

What are null-cell adenomas of the pituitary?

Nonfunctional adenomas, a cause of hypopituitarism

What is pituitary apoplexy?

Sudden hemorrhage into a pituitary adenoma which can result in pan-hypopituitarism

What is the treatment for the symptoms of hypopituitarism that occur with pituitary apoplexy?

Glucocorticoids and thyroid hormones

What is Sheehan syndrome?

Postpartum ischemic necrosis of the pituitary, often resulting in pan-hypopituitarism

What is the cause for Sheehan syndrome?

During pregnancy the size of the pituitary gland increases. At delivery, severe hemorrhage or shock causes anoxic injury of the anterior pituitary.

What is the treatment for Sheehan syndrome?

Give glucocorticoids due to decreased ACTH and thyroid hormones due to decreased thyroid-stimulating hormone (TSH).

Posterior Pituitary Pathology

What are the classic features of central diabetes insipidus (DI)?

Increased frequency and volume of urination; increased thirst; polydipsia

What will serum and urine lab tests find in patients with central DI?

- Serum—increased sodium and osmolarity
- Urine—negative glucose and low osmolarity

What is the underlying cause for central DI?

Damage to posterior pituitary

What hormone is lacking in central DI?

ADH

What are the common causes of central DI?

Head trauma (including surgery or radiation); tumor; sarcoidosis

What is the treatment for central DI?	Vasopressin/desmopressin
What is the other mechanism/form of diabetes insipidus?	Nephrogenic DI—renal tubules are unresponsive to ADH
Are ADH levels increased, decreased, or normal in nephrogenic DI?	Normal to increased levels
What drugs can cause nephrogenic DI?	Lithium; demeclocycline; methoxyflurane
What is the treatment for nephrogenic DI?	Thiazides
What is the most common presentation of syndrome of inappropriate secretion of antidiuretic hormone (SIADH)?	Altered mental status
What are the common causes of SIADH?	Neoplasm (paraneoplastic syndrome, especially associated with small cell carcinoma of the lung); infections—(meningitis, encephalitis, pneumonia); pain and nausea (especially in perioperative period); mediations (narcotics, carbamazepine); pituitary injury (release of oxytocin)
What is the urine like in patients with SIADH?	Inappropriately concentrated urine
What are the treatments for SIADH?	Fluid restriction; demeclocycline—inhibits ADH effect on renal tubules
What is the dreaded complication that may occur with rapid correction of sodium levels in a patient with SIADH?	Central pontine myelinolysis—acute, noninflammatory demyelination of neurons occurring predominately within the pons of the brain stem

THYROID

General Principles

What is the embryologic origin of the thyroid?	Pharyngeal epithelium

Table 11.2 Thyroid Hormones

Gland/Cell	Hormone
Hypothalamus	TRH
Anterior pituitary	TSH
Thyroid follicles	T_3 and T_4
Parafollicular cells of thyroid	Calcitonin

Abbreviations: TSH, thyroid-stimulating hormone; TRH, thyrotropin-releasing hormone; T_4, thyroxine; T_3, triiodothyronine.

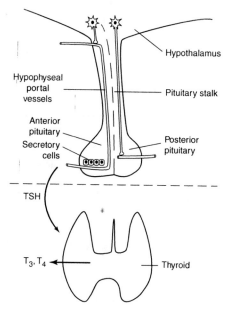

Figure 11.2 Normal thyroid (euthyroid).

What is the role of thyroid hormones in the body?	Increase basal metabolic rate; β-adrenergic effects; bone growth (along with GH); central nervous system (CNS) maturity
What mineral is necessary for thyroid hormone synthesis?	Iodine
What transports thyroid hormone (T_3/T_4) in the blood?	Thyroxine-binding globulin (TBG); only the free, unbound hormone is active

| Which is more potent T_3 or T_4? | T_3 binds to receptors with greater affinity than T_4; however, T_4 is the major product of the thyroid, which is then converted to T_3 peripherally |

Hyperthyroidism

| What are the symptoms of hyperthyroidism? | Palpitations, weakness, nervousness/anxiety, weight loss, diarrhea, intolerance to heat, tremor |

| What are the common causes of hyperthyroidism? | Grave disease; exogenous thyroid hormone; hyperfunctional goiter (multinodular goiter) or thyroid adenoma; thyroiditis |

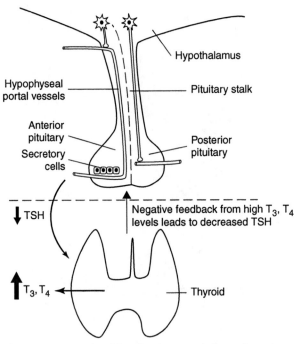

Figure 11.3   Hyperthyroidism (most commonly Grave disease).

| What are the less common causes of hyperthyroidism? | Struma ovarii; TSH-secreting pituitary adenoma; choriocarcinoma/hydatidiform mole |

| What is the most common cause of endogenous hyperthyroidism? | Grave disease |

What is the triad of Grave disease?

*H*yperthyroidism; *O*phthalmic pathology (exophthalmos); *P*retibial myxedema

*Grave disease makes you *HOP*

What is pretibial myxedema?

Skin that overlies shins is thick and indurated, resembling an orange peel. (Rare complication of Grave disease.)

What are other abnormal physical examination findings associated with Grave disease?

Bruit over enlarged thyroid; lid lag; proptosis; weak extraocular muscles

What is the cause of Grave disease?

Development of an autoantibody which stimulates the TSH receptor

What type of immunoglobulin is the autoantibody?

Immunoglobulin G (IgG)

What HLA types are associated with Grave disease?

HLA-DR3 and HLA-B8

What other diseases are commonly found in people with Grave disease?

Systemic lupus erythematosus (SLE); pernicious anemia; diabetes mellitus (DM) type I; Addison disease

What is the morphology of the thyroid gland in Grave disease?

Diffusely enlarged gland, with hypertrophy and hyperplasia

What lab abnormalities are seen in Grave disease?

Increased T_3 and T_4; decreased TSH

What is the treatment for Grave disease?

Propylthiouracil (PTU); ablation by radiation; surgical removal

What cause of hyperthyroidism most commonly occurs in postpartum women and histologic findings on biopsy show a lymphocytic infiltrate?

Subacute lymphocytic thyroiditis

What are the other names for subacute lymphocytic thyroiditis?

Silent or painless thyroiditis

Which HLA types are associated with subacute lymphocytic thyroiditis?

HLA-DR3 and HLA-DR5

What rare cause of thyroiditis is characterized by extensive fibrosis of the thyroid gland?

Riedel thyroiditis

What syndrome consists of hyperthyroidism with goiter but lacks the ophthalmic and dermatologic characteristics of Grave disease?

Plummer syndrome

What causes thyroid goiters to form?

Impaired synthesis of thyroid hormones

Do multinodular goiters cause hyperthyroidism, hypothyroidism, both, or neither?

Most are euthyroid, but a small percentage are hyperfunctioning

Hypothyroidism

What are the signs and symptoms of hypothyroidism?

Weight gain, cold intolerance, fatigue, depression, constipation, brittle hair, cool skin, and decrease deep tendon reflexes (DTRs)

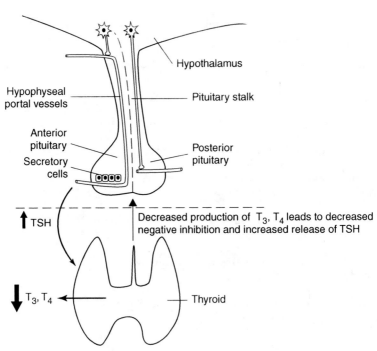

Figure 11.4   Hypothyroidism (most commonly Hashimoto thyroiditis).

What drugs can cause hypothyroidism?	Lithium; amiodarone; propylthiouracil (PTU)
What diseases are associated with hypothyroidism?	Sarcoidosis; amyloidosis; carpal tunnel syndrome
What dietary deficiency can result in thyroid goiters and hypothyroidism?	Iodine deficiency
Iodine deficiency in utero results in what disease?	Congenital hypothyroidism (formerly known as cretinism), typically picked up on newborn screening but can present with mental retardation, short stature, hypotonia, and macroglossia
What is the most common cause of hypothyroidism?	Hashimoto thyroiditis
What physical examination finding of the thyroid is associated with Hashimoto thyroiditis?	Rubbery, nontender diffusely enlarged thyroid
What is the typical presentation of Hashimoto thyroiditis?	Transient hyperthyroidism followed by chronic hypothyroidism
What is the cause of Hashimoto thyroiditis?	Autoimmune destruction of the thyroid gland
What are the histologic features of Hashimoto thyroiditis?	Extensive lymphocytic cell infiltrate, atrophic lymphoid follicles, and Hürthle cell metaplasia
What human leukocyte antigen (HLA) type is associated with Hashimoto thyroiditis?	HLA-DR3 and HLA-DR5
What are some of the autoantibodies (AB) associated with Hashimoto thyroiditis?	Antimicrosomal antibody; anti-TSH receptor antibody
What other autoimmune diseases are seen in patients with Hashimoto thyroiditis?	Systemic lupus erythematosus (SLE); rheumatoid arthritis (RA); Sjögren syndrome; pernicious anemia; autoimmune adrenalitis; type I diabetes
For what type of cancers are people with Hashimoto thyroiditis at higher risk?	B-cell lymphomas of the thyroid gland

What are other names for de Quervain thyroiditis?	Subacute granulomatous thyroiditis
What makes de Quervain thyroiditis unique?	"Painful" thyroid compared to subacute lymphocytic thyroiditis which is classically "painless"; may be preceded by viral upper respiratory infection
What viruses have been associated with de Quervain thyroiditis?	Mumps; coxsackie virus; adenovirus
What HLA type is associated with de Quervain thyroiditis?	HLA-B35
What does de Quervain thyroiditis show microscopically?	Multinucleate giant cells, granulomatous inflammation

Neoplastic

A young adult, female patient has a solitary, painless neck mass. What is the most likely diagnosis?	Thyroid adenoma
True or False? The vast majority (>90%) of discrete solitary masses of the thyroid are benign:	True
What are some features that make a lesion of the thyroid suspicious for cancer?	Solitary lesion; radiation history; cold nodule; female sex
What are some features that are poor prognostic factors?	Age >45 years; male sex; extension of tumor beyond the thyroid; metastasis
When a solitary lesion is detected, what is the next step in diagnosis?	Fine needle aspiration (FNA)
What is the most common type of thyroid cancer?	Papillary carcinoma *Papillary is the most Popular
What microscopic findings distinguish papillary carcinoma from other types?	Psammoma bodies; glandular cells are arranged in a papillary architecture; orphan Annie nuclei; nuclear grooves

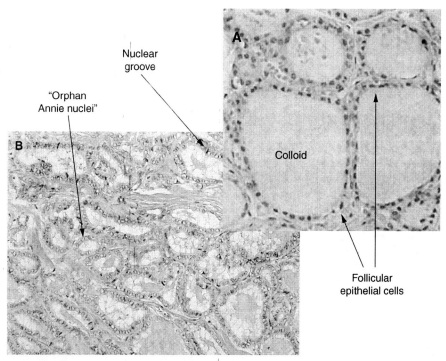

Figure 11.5   A. Benign thyroid tissue composed of colloid-producing follicles. Parafollicular C cells are located in the interstitium. **B.** Papillary thyroid carcinoma with nuclear grooves, intranuclear inclusions (not really visible at this magnification), empty appearing nuclei ("orphan Annie nuclei"), and back-to-back follicles with little intervening interstitium. (Reproduced, with permission, from Wettach T, et al: *Road Map Pathology*, New York: McGraw-Hill, 2009; fig 11-2.)

What familial syndromes have an increased risk of developing papillary carcinomas?	Gardner syndrome; familial adenomatous polyposis (FAP); Cowden syndrome (familial goiter/skin hamartomas)
What is the second most common type of thyroid carcinoma (10%-20%)?	Follicular carcinoma
What is seen microscopically in follicular carcinoma?	Microfollicular hyperplasia with invasion into surrounding thyroid tissue (as opposed to adenoma, which has microfollicular hyperplasia but is encapsulated and does not invade)
What is the third most common type of thyroid carcinoma (5%)?	Medullary carcinoma
What cell type is associated with medullary carcinoma?	Parafollicular C cells

What is seen microscopically in medullary carcinoma?	Neuroendocrine cells arranged in nests or neuroendocrine spindle cells invading into surrounding normal thyroid tissue. Tumor cells immunostain for TTF-1 and calcitonin. Amyloid deposits are often present.
What substance do the parafollicular C cells normally secrete?	Calcitonin
What other substances do medullary carcinomas of the thyroid secrete besides large amounts of calcitonin?	Serotonin; vasoactive intestinal peptide (VIP); somatostatin
What familial syndrome is associated with an increased risk of medullary thyroid carcinoma?	Multiple endocrine neoplasia (MEN) 2A and 2B
What are the three most important things to remember about medullary carcinoma?	1. *MEN* syndromes 2A and 2B 2. *Amyloid* 3. *C*-cells/Calcitonin *MED* student named *MAC*
What is the least common type of thyroid carcinoma?	Anaplastic carcinoma
What is unique about anaplastic thyroid carcinoma?	Very aggressive; poorly differentiated microscopically; metastasizes to lungs

PARATHYROID

General Principles

From what embryologic structure are the parathyroid glands derived?	The superior parathyroids are derived from the fourth pharyngeal pouch, while the inferior parathyroids are derived from the third pharyngeal pouch.
Where are the parathyroid glands?	In the anterior neck around or within the thyroid tissue
What do the parathyroid glands produce?	Parathyroid hormone (PTH)
What does PTH regulate?	Serum calcium
What does increased PTH do to calcium?	Increases serum calcium

How does PTH regulate calcium in the bone?	Mobilizes calcium by activating osteoclasts
How does PTH regulate calcium in the kidney?	Increases calcium reabsorption; increases conversion of active vitamin D; increases excretion of phosphorus
How does PTH regulate calcium in the gastrointestinal (GI) tract?	Increases calcium absorption

Hyperparathyroidism

What are the clinical symptoms of primary hyperparathyroidism?	Fatigue; hypercalcemia symptoms—"stones, bones, groans, and psychiatric overtones"
What are the causes of primary hyperparathyroidism?	Parathyroid adenoma; parathyroid hyperplasia; parathyroid carcinoma (very rare)
What is the most common cause of primary hyperparathyroidism?	Parathyroid adenoma
What are the laboratory findings of primary hyperparathyroidism?	Increased PTH and alkaline phosphatase; hypercalcemia; decreased serum phosphorus
What is the cause of secondary hyperparathyroidism?	Hypocalcemia/hyperphosphatemia, most commonly due to chronic renal disease
What are the lab findings in secondary hyperparathyroidism?	Hypocalcemia; increased PTH and serum phosphorus
What is renal osteodystrophy?	Bone changes due to secondary hyperparathyroidism occurring as a result of renal disease
What disease is characterized by decreased absorbed calcium due to impaired hydroxylation of a precursor of vitamin D and increased PTH secretion?	Vitamin D-dependent rickets
What are the symptoms of hypercalcemia?	• Kidney—stones, polyuria, renal insufficiency • Cardiac—valve calcifications • Bone—osteoporosis/osteitis fibrosa cystica • GI—constipation, ulcers, gallstones • CNS—fatigue *Stones, bones, GI groans with psychological overtones

What electrocardiogram (ECG) change is associated with increased calcium levels?	Short QT interval
What tumors secrete PTH-related peptide resulting in symptoms of hyperparathyroidism?	Bronchogenic squamous cell carcinoma; renal cell carcinoma
What disease that causes hypercalcemia is associated with bilateral hilar lymphadenopathy and noncaseating granulomas, and is more commonly seen in African American populations?	Sarcoidosis
What disease is associated with hypercalcemia, bone pain, renal failure, and clonal proliferation of plasma cells in the bone marrow?	Multiple myeloma

Hypoparathyroidism

What are symptoms of hypoparathyroidism due to?	Hypocalcemia
What are the symptoms of hypocalcemia?	Tetany; CNS (paresthesias); cardiac (prolonged QT)
What is tetany?	Neuromuscular spasm/irritability
What are the two classic clinical signs of hypocalcemia?	1. Chvostek sign—facial nerve spasm 2. Trousseau sign—carpal nerve spasm
What is the most common cause of hypoparathyroidism?	Accidental removal of parathyroid glands by surgical excision during thyroidectomy or lymph node dissection
What is the syndrome associated with congenital thymic hypoplasia or absence, hypoparathyroidism, and cardiac abnormalities?	DiGeorge syndrome
DiGeorge syndrome is caused by the failure of what structures to develop normally?	Third and fourth pharyngeal pouches
What structures fail to form in the fetus due DiGeorge syndrome?	Thymus; parathyroid glands
What immune defect is associated with DiGeorge syndrome?	T-cell deficiency

What is the chromosomal abnormality associated with DiGeorge syndrome?	22q11 deletion
What are the clinical manifestations of pseudohypoparathyroidism?	It typically presents with hypocalcemia in a child of short stature, with rounded facies and shortened metacarpals and metatarsals.
What is the mode of inheritance in pseudohypoparathyroidism?	Autosomal recessive

ADRENAL GLANDS

Embryology

The adrenal cortex is derived from what primitive cell layer?	Mesoderm
At what age does the fetal cortex regress?	Usually by the second postnatal month
When does the definitive adult cortex appear?	It is present at birth, but not fully formed until age 3.
The adrenal medulla is derived from what cell type?	Neural crest cells
Neural crest cells differentiate into what type of cells?	Chromaffin cells which produce catecholamines (epinephrine and norepinephrine)

General Principles

What are the two parts of the adrenal glands?	1. Adrenal cortex 2. Adrenal medulla
What are the three parts of the adrenal cortex?	1. Zona glomerulosa 2. Zona fasciculate 3. Zona reticularis *"G, F, R"
What substances do each portion secrete?	Mineralocorticoids (aldosterone), glucocorticoids (cortisol), androgens (DHEA—dehydroepiandrosterone) *From outer most to inner most layer: "salt, sugar, sex"

Table 11.3 Zones of the Adrenal Gland

Zone of the Adrenal Gland	Hormones Produced
Zona glomerulosa	Mineralocorticoids (aldosterone)
Zona fasciculate	Glucocorticoids (cortisol)
Zona reticularis	Sex steroids (estrogen/androgens)
Adrenal medulla	Catecholamines (epinephrine)

Congenital

What are the classic features of congenital adrenal hyperplasia (CAH)?	Ambiguous genitalia or virilization (in female infants), low blood pressure, hyperkalemia, and hyponatremia
What is the most common form of CAH?	21-hydroxylase deficiency
Which enzymatic step in the cortisol pathway is 21-hydroxylase involved in?	Progesterone conversion to 11-deoxycorticosterone
What is the consequence of this deficiency?	Decrease in cortisol; increased ACTH (to raise cortisol levels); adrenal hyperplasia
What is the treatment for CAH?	Cortisol and mineralocorticoids if needed

Hypercortisolism

What is the hormone abnormality causing Cushing syndrome?	Excess cortisol production
What are the classic clinical findings associated with Cushing syndrome?	Weight gain, hypertension, truncal obesity, moon facies, abdominal striae, and accumulation of fat on the posterior neck
What is the technical term for the accumulation of fat on the posterior neck in Cushing syndrome?	Buffalo hump
What is the most common cause of Cushing syndrome?	Exogenous steroid administration (drugs)

What are the causes of endogenous Cushing syndrome?

Hypothalamic/pituitary origin; adrenal origin; ectopic ACTH from nonendocrine neoplasm

What is Cushing disease?

Cushing symptoms associated with pituitary adenoma

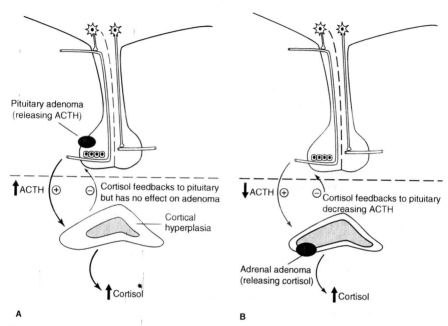

A

B

Figure 11.6 **A.** Cushing disease, by definition from a pituitary adenoma. **B.** Cushing syndrome, resulting from an adrenal adenoma.

What lab values are associated with Cushing disease?

Increased ACTH (hypersecretion); suppression of ACTH with high levels of dexamethasone

What lab values distinguish an adrenal origin of Cushing syndrome from other causes?

Decreased ACTH (feedback); increased cortisol

What are some adrenal causes for Cushing syndrome?

Adrenal adenoma; adrenal hyperplasia; adrenal carcinoma

What lab values suggest that Cushing syndrome is due to ectopic ACTH from a nonendocrine neoplastic origin?

Increased ACTH; no suppression of ACTH with any level of dexamethasone

What neoplasms frequently secrete ACTH-like substances?

Small cell carcinoma of lung; carcinoid tumors; medullary carcinomas of thyroid

Hyperaldosteronism

What are the clinical findings, including lab values, associated with hyperaldosteronism?

Hypertension, water retention (weight gain ± edema), muscle wasting, paresthesias; labs—hypokalemia, hypernatremia, and metabolic alkalosis

What is the most likely cause of primary hyperaldosteronism?

Adrenal adenoma (aldosterone secreting)

What is the syndrome associated with aldosterone-secreting adrenal adenoma?

Conn syndrome

What lab values support a diagnosis of Conn syndrome?

Increased Na^+; decreased K^+ and renin level

What is the medical (nonsurgical) treatment for Conn syndrome?

Spironolactone

By what mechanism does spironolactone work?

Inhibits aldosterone at distal tubule, spares K^+

What are the causes of secondary hyperaldosteronism?

Renal failure; congestive heart failure (CHF); cirrhosis

What is the underlying cause of secondary hyperaldosteronism?

Activation of the renin-angiotensin system

What is the distinguishing lab value that separates secondary hyperaldosteronism from primary hyperaldosteronism?

Renin is increased in secondary aldosteronism

Adrenal Insufficiency

How might a patient with Addison disease present?

With nausea, vomiting, hypotension, increased pigmentation of the skin

What lab values would support the diagnosis of Addison disease?

Decreased serum sodium, chloride, glucose, and bicarbonate; increase serum potassium; decreased serum cortisol and aldosterone; increased ACTH

What are the synonyms for Addison disease?

Primary chronic adrenocortical deficiency or adrenal atrophy

What is the most common cause of Addison disease?	Autoimmune lymphocytic adrenalitis
What HLA types are associated with the autoimmune form of Addison disease?	HLA-B8 and HLA-DR3
What other syndromes are associated with Addison disease?	Hashimoto; DM type I; pernicious anemia
What are other less common causes of Addison disease?	Infectious—tuberculosis, histoplasmosis, coccidioidomycosis; metastatic cancer
Why is the skin pigmentation increased in Addison disease?	Increased ACTH stimulates melanocytes
What is secondary adrenocortical deficiency?	Decreased secretion of stimulatory hormones at the level of hypothalamus or pituitary gland
In secondary adrenocortical deficiency, what are the lab values?	Decreased ACTH; decreased cortisol; decreased androgens; normal aldosterone and melanin
What is the major difference that sets secondary adrenocortical deficiency apart from primary?	ACTH level decreased; no pigmentation
What are the reasons for an acute primary adrenal insufficiency?	Stress; withdrawal of exogenous steroid medicines; adrenal hemorrhage
What is Waterhouse-Friderichsen syndrome?	Hemorrhagic necrosis of the adrenal cortex often due to meningococcemia or other infection

Neoplastic

What is the most common tumor of the adrenal gland?	Adrenal adenoma, as mentioned above, these can be hyperfunctioning secreting either cortisol or aldosterone, producing Cushing or Conn syndrome respectively
What other tumors occur in the adrenal cortex?	Adrenal cortical carcinoma, metastases (particularly from lung primary)
What are the two most common tumors of the adrenal medulla?	Pheochromocytoma and neuroblastoma

What is a pheochromocytoma?	A tumor of chromaffin cells of the adrenal medulla
How would a patient with a pheochromocytoma present?	With severe (sometimes episodic) hypertension, headaches, chest pain, sweating, tremor
What lab tests diagnose pheochromocytoma?	Increased urine epinephrine; increased urine metanephrine; increased urine vanillylmandelic acid (VMA)
What is the 10% rule with pheochromocytomas?	10% of pheochromocytomas are malignant, familial, bilateral, and extraabdominal
What familial syndromes are associated with pheochromocytomas?	MEN2A; MEN2B; neurofibromatosis 1; Von Hippel-Lindau; Sturge-Webber
What is the treatment for pheochromocytoma?	Surgical removal with alpha blockade (lower blood pressure) followed by beta- blocker (to oppose reflex tachycardia)
What is a neuroblastoma?	Malignant neuroendocrine tumor of childhood, arising from neural crest cells, that most commonly originates in adrenal medulla (~50%) but can arise from any neural tissue; most common solid tumor in infancy (most common extracranial solid tumor of childhood)
What oncogene is often amplified in neuroblastoma?	N-myc

PANCREAS

General Principles

What are the two pancreatic parenchymal tissue types and corresponding functions?	1. Islet of Langerhans—endocrine function (hormone production and secretion) 2. Pancreatic acini—exocrine function (digestive enzyme production and secretion)

What are the cellular components of the Islet of Langerhans?	α, β, and δ endocrine cells
What does each cell type produce and secrete?	α = glucagon; β = insulin; δ = somatostatin

Diabetes Mellitus

What are the common presenting symptoms of diabetes mellitus (DM)?	Polydipsia, polyphagia, polyuria, weight loss
What is the defect associated with DM type I?	Failure of insulin synthesis by pancreatic beta cells
What causes the failure of insulin synthesis?	External environmental factors causing insulitis (autoimmune destruction of pancreas), coupled with a genetic predisposition
What microscopic change is seen in patients with insulitis?	Lymphocytic infiltration of pancreatic islets
Which HLA types are associated with type I DM?	HLA-DR3 and HLA-DR4
What is an older term/name for type I DM?	Juvenile diabetes, because the large majority of cases present in childhood/adolescence
What life-threatening condition is associated with DM type I?	Diabetic ketoacidosis (DKA)
What are the symptoms of DKA?	Fruity odor of breath, hyperglycemia, and Kussmaul breathing
What is the biochemical significance of DKA?	Increased catabolism of fats, producing ketone bodies
What are the three ketone bodies produced from DKA?	1. β-Hydroxybutyric acid 2. Acetoacetic acid 3. Acetone
What is the rapid and deep breathing found in DM type I known as?	Kussmaul breathing
What is the first-line treatment in DM type I?	Insulin and hydration

What sinus/respiratory infections are patients with DKA at risk of contracting?	Life-threatening invasive *Mucor* and *Rhizopus* fungal infections
What is the mechanism of DM type II?	Increased insulin resistance
What modifiable risk factor is associated with DM type II?	Obesity
Which type of diabetes is associated more strongly with family history of diabetes?	DM type II
What is the first-line of treatment for a borderline diabetic?	Diet and exercise
What is the treatment of choice if diet and exercise do not lower fasting glucose levels?	Oral hypoglycemic agents
What are the lab values that lead to a diagnosis of DM?	Fasting glucose >126; random glucose >200; HbA1c >7
What organ systems are especially at risk with DM types I and II?	Cardiovascular; kidney; eye (retina); nervous system
What are patients with DM at higher risk for which affects the blood vessels and coronary arteries?	Atherosclerosis
What are the complications from atherosclerosis that increase morbidity and mortality in diabetics?	Myocardial infarction and peripheral vascular disease
What nervous system changes are consequences of long-standing DM?	Peripheral neuropathy
What gastrointestinal consequence of DM results in nausea, vomiting, and early satiety after meals?	Gastroparesis
What is the earliest sign of DM in the kidney?	Increased thickening of the basement membrane (BM)
What histologic finding is a late feature in the course of diabetic nephropathy?	Kimmelstiel-Wilson nodules (glomerulosclerosis)
What are Armanni-Ebstein lesions of the kidney?	Deposition of glycogen from prolonged hyperglycemia

NEOPLASMS

What are the symptoms of carcinoid syndrome?	About 70% of carcinoid syndrome patients experience flushing of the face and neck. Other symptoms may include abdominal pain, cyanosis, diarrhea, erectile dysfunction, fever, heart damage, skin lesions, and wheezing.
What causes carcinoid syndrome?	Neuroendocrine tumor, usually in gastrointestinal tract, releasing excessive amounts of neuroendocrine hormones into the circulation
What is the most common site of carcinoid tumor?	Appendix
What do carcinoid tumors secrete?	Serotonin (5-hydroxytryptamine [HT]), histamine, and prostaglandins
What do lab values show in patients with carcinoid tumors?	Increased 5-hydroxy indole acetic acid (HIAA) (serotonin metabolite)
What is the rule of one-third with carcinoid tumors?	One-third of carcinoids are multiple and one-third metastasize
What is the treatment for carcinoid tumors?	Surgical removal and treatment with octreotide (biological agent)
What are the three categories of multiple endocrine neoplasia syndromes?	1. MEN1 2. MEN2A 3. MEN2B or MEN3
What is the other name for MEN1?	Wermer syndrome
What chromosome is affected with MEN1?	11q13
What organs/glands are affected by MEN1?	Pancreas; parathyroid; pituitary *MEN1 involves the three Ps
What pathology is seen in the parathyroid in those with MEN1?	Hyperparathyroidism (adenoma)
What pathology is seen in the pancreas with MEN1?	Islet cell tumors—VIPoma, glucagonoma, insulinoma, and gastrinoma (Zollinger-Ellison) *One (MEN1) VIP has a gig

What pathology is seen in the pituitary in MEN1?	Prolactinoma
What is the eponym for MEN2A?	*Sipple* syndrome *Take 2 *sipps*
What organs/glands are affected by MEN2A?	• *Medulla* (adrenal)—pheochromocytoma • *Medullary* carcinoma of *thyroid* • *Parathyroid* (hyper) *MEN2A has problems with a pair of medullas and parathyroids!
What glands/organs are affected by MEN3 (MEN2B)?	• Medullary carcinoma of thyroid • Adrenal medulla (pheochromocytoma) • Neuroma *2B a strong *MAN* is equal to 3 *MEN*
What are the unique things about MEN3?	Neuromas
What is MEN3 lacking that the other MEN syndromes have?	Hyperparathyroidism
What is the protooncogene responsible for the MEN3 syndrome?	RET oncogene

Table 11.4 Review of MEN Syndromes

Which MEN syndrome deals with parathyroid, pancreas, and pituitary?	MEN1
Which MEN syndrome has neuromas?	MEN3 (2B)
Which MEN syndrome has pheochromocytoma, medullary carcinoma of the thyroid, and parathyroid hyperplasia?	MEN2A
Which MEN syndrome does not have pheochromocytoma?	MEN1
Which MEN syndrome does not have parathyroid hyperplasia?	MEN3

What disease is characterized by renal cell carcinoma, pheochromocytoma, angiomas, cerebellar hemangioblastomas, and cysts of the pancreas and liver?	Von Hippel-Lindau

What disease is characterized by café au lait spots, schwannomas, meningioma, glioma, and pheochromocytoma?	Von Recklinghausen (Neurofibromatosis 1)
What disease is characterized by cavernous hemangiomas and pheochromocytoma?	Sturge-Weber syndrome
What syndrome is associated with recurrent peptic ulcer, diarrhea, hypercalcemia, and increased gastrin levels?	Zollinger-Ellison (gastrinoma)
What tumor is associated with Whipple triad: (1) episodic hyperinsulinemia and hypoglycemia, (2) CNS abnormality—confusion, convulsion, or coma, (3) all problems reversed with glucose administration?	Insulinoma
In insulinoma, is the C peptide high or low?	High
What syndrome is associated with hypoglycemia in a health-care worker who also has a low C peptide?	Munchausen syndrome (psychiatric disorder)—giving self-insulin injections
What tumor is associated with DM and necrolytic migratory erythema?	Glucagonoma (alpha-cell tumor)
What tumor is associated with watery diarrhea, hypokalemia, and achlorhydria (WDHA) and is associated with increased levels of VIP?	VIPoma
What other names are associated with the symptoms of VIPoma?	WDHA syndrome; Verner-Morrison syndrome; pancreatic cholera

CLINICAL VIGNETTES

A 42-year-old woman presents with increasing nausea, vomiting, and headache for the past month. On physical examination, she has abnormal vision in the temporal fields. What is the most likely diagnosis?

Pituitary adenoma

A 28-year-old woman presents with amenorrhea, galactorrhea, nausea, vomiting, and fatigue. What common laboratory test should be included in the initial diagnostic work-up?

Beta-human chorionic gonadotropin (β-HCG)/urine pregnancy test

A 28-year-old woman presents with amenorrhea, galactorrhea, and fatigue. Physical examination reveals a visual field defect. β-HCG is negative. Magnetic resonance imaging (MRI) shows a small lesion in the pituitary gland. What is the most likely diagnosis?

Prolactinoma

A 28-year-old man in the county psychiatric hospital presents with galactorrhea. What is the most likely cause of the galactorrhea?

Neuroleptic drugs

A 35-year-old woman presents with headaches and generalized aches and pains. She comments that she does not look the same as she did when she was younger, and that her voice has changed and is now deeper. On physical examination, she has a large head with protruding jaw, thick tongue, and overly large hands and feet. What is the most likely diagnosis?

Growth hormone adenoma with acromegaly

A 45-year-old woman presents with weight gain, headaches, hypertension, and menstrual abnormalities. On physical examination, she has a buffalo hump, truncal obesity, and abdominal striae. Lab values show that her adrenocorticotropic hormone (ACTH) and cortisol are markedly elevated. What is the most likely diagnosis?

Cushing disease due to corticotroph cell adenoma of pituitary

A 38-year-old woman with a history of a "benign pituitary adenoma" presents to the ER with a sudden excruciating headache, double vision, and weakness. Her blood pressure is 89/58. What is the most likely diagnosis?

Pituitary apoplexy (sudden hemorrhage)

A 28-year-old G1P1 woman presents to the ER with a headache, dizziness, fatigue, and low blood pressure. She had a difficult delivery 1 week ago that required a transfusion. On physical examination, she appears diaphoretic and pale. What is the most likely diagnosis?

Sheehan syndrome (postpartum necrosis of the anterior pituitary)

A 45-year-old G5P5 woman complains of headaches, fatigue, and high blood pressure. On physical examination, she is obese and has a visual field defect. MRI shows cerebrospinal fluid (CSF) where the pituitary should be. What is the most likely diagnosis?

Empty sella syndrome

A 26-year-old man with a recent history of head trauma presents with increased volume and frequency of urination, thirst, and polydipsia. Urinalysis (UA) is negative for glucose and shows low osmolarity. What is the most likely diagnosis?

Central diabetes insipidus (DI)

A 43-year-old patient with history of bipolar disorder complains of polyuria, polydipsia, and increased thirst. Lab values reveal hypernatremia, serum osmolarity >290, and dilute urine. What is the most likely diagnosis?

Nephrogenic DI likely due to chronic lithium exposure

A 69-year-old smoker is found restless and confused. Labs show hyponatremia, low serum osmolarity, and elevated ADH levels. There is cerebral edema evident on computed tomography (CT). What is the most likely diagnosis?

Syndrome of inappropriate secretion of antidiuretic hormone (SIADH)

What is the mechanism of SIADH in the 69-year-old smoker?

Ectopic ADH secretion from small cell carcinoma of the lung

A 32-year-old woman presents with palpitations, nervousness, weight loss despite increased appetite, diarrhea, heat intolerance, and fine tremor of the hand. What is the most likely diagnosis?

Hyperthyroidism

A 45-year-old woman presents with fatigue, depression, constipation, cold intolerance, and weight gain. On physical examination, she is found to have decreased reflexes, cool skin, and brittle hair. What is the most likely diagnosis?

Hypothyroidism

A 35-year-old postpartum woman presents with palpitations, tachycardia, fatigue, and tremor. Labs show increased T_3 and T_4 with decreased TSH. The thyroid is slightly enlarged and a biopsy shows many small lymphocytes. What is the most likely diagnosis?

Subacute lymphocytic thyroiditis

A 26-year-old woman presents with weight loss, palpitations, anxiety, and thinning of hair. On physical examination, she has tachycardia, exophthalmos, increased reflexes, and moist skin. What is the most likely diagnosis?

Hyperthyroidism—Grave disease

A 20-year-old woman presents with a painless lump in her neck. She denies any symptoms of palpitations, racing heart, or nervousness. On physical examination, the thyroid is diffusely enlarged without nodularity. What is the most likely diagnosis?

Simple diffuse (nontoxic) goiter

A 20-year-old woman presents with a painless lump in her neck. She denies any symptoms of palpitations, racing heart, or nervousness. On physical examination, the thyroid is irregularly and asymmetrically enlarged with palpable nodularity. What is the most likely diagnosis?

Multinodular goiter

A 5-year-old recently adopted child presents to clinic with mental retardation, short stature, and umbilical hernia. On examination, the child has coarse facial features and protruding tongue. What is the most likely diagnosis?

Congenital hypothyroidism

A 45-year-old white woman presents with fatigue, weight gain, and depression. She recalls that a few weeks ago, she felt very nervous, jittery, and had palpitations. Lab values show that her TSH is elevated and T_3 and T_4 are decreased. What is the most likely diagnosis?

Hashimoto thyroiditis—it often is preceded by a transient hyperthyroid flare followed by chronic hypothyroidism

A 35-year-old female presents with fatigue and pain in the neck, jaw, and throat. She has symptoms of hypothyroidism and had symptoms of hyperthyroidism 1 week ago. She reports that she just recovered from an upper respiratory tract infection (URI). What is the most likely diagnosis?

de Quervain thyroiditis

A 68-year-old man presents with hoarse voice, dysphagia, and cough. He mentions that he was exposed to radiation from the Chernobyl plant explosion several decades ago. On physical examination, a small solitary mass is detected in the thyroid. What is the most likely diagnosis?

Thyroid carcinoma

A 2-year-old child with abnormal facies presents with tetany due to hypocalcemia and frequent fungal and viral infections. He has known cardiac abnormalities. What is the most likely diagnosis?

DiGeorge syndrome

A 3-year-old boy presents with hypocalcemia. On physical examination, he exhibits short stature, round facies, and short metacarpals and metatarsals. What is the most likely diagnosis?

Pseudohypoparathyroidism (Albright hereditary osteodystrophy)

A 42-year-old woman presents with hypertension, weight gain, new-onset diabetes, easy bruising, and menstrual abnormalities. On physical examination, she has truncal obesity, moon facies, an accumulation of fat on the posterior neck and abdominal striae. What is the most likely diagnosis?

Cushing syndrome

A 45-year-old man presents with hypertension, water retention, muscle wasting, and paresthesias. Lab values show hypokalemia, hypernatremia, and a metabolic alkalosis. What is the most likely diagnosis?

Hyperaldosteronism

A term female infant is born with ambiguous genitalia and low blood pressure. Labs show increased serum potassium and hyponatremia. What is the most likely diagnosis?

Congenital adrenal hyperplasia (CAH)

A 62-year-old woman presents with hypotension, nausea, vomiting, and increased pigmentation of the skin. Labs show decreased serum sodium, chloride, glucose, and bicarbonate, but increased potassium. What is the most likely diagnosis?

Addison disease

A 17-year-old boy presents with signs of meningitis. His lumbar puncture (LP) shows meningococcemia and he is immediately started on several intravenous (IV) antibiotics. Hours after his admission, his blood pressure drops and adrenal insufficiency is diagnosed. What is the most likely diagnosis?

Waterhouse-Friderichsen syndrome

A 67-year-old man presents with severe hypertension, headaches, chest pain, sweating, and tremor. Work up for myocardial infarction is negative, but lab values show increased urinary excretion of catecholamines and their metabolites. What is the most likely diagnosis?

Pheochromocytoma

A 65-year-old man presents with diarrhea, cutaneous flushing, asthmatic wheezing, and chest pain. ECG shows right-sided valvular disease. What is the most likely diagnosis?

Carcinoid syndrome

A 14-year-old girl presents with weight loss of 10 lb in the last few weeks, fatigue, polydipsia, polyphagia, and polyuria. On physical examination, the patient appears dehydrated and is breathing rapidly and deeply. She has fruity odor on her breath. What is the most likely diagnosis?

DM type I

A 56-year-old woman presents with polyuria. On physical examination, she is moderately obese and has acanthosis nigricans on her posterior neck. Lab values show fasting hyperglycemia and HBA1c of 8.1. What is the most likely diagnosis?

DM type II

A 2-year-old child presents with an abdominal mass and elevated blood pressure. Increased urine catecholamines are detected. What is the most likely diagnosis?

Neuroblastoma

CHAPTER 12

Neuropathology

EMBRYOLOGY

What structures or cells related to the nervous system are derived from neuroectoderm?	The pineal gland, neurons of the central nervous system, oligodendrocytes, and astrocytes
What structures or cells related to the nervous system are derived from neural crest?	Schwann cells, dorsal root ganglia, autonomic ganglia, and pia mater
From which embryologic tissue type is dura mater derived?	Mesoderm
What structure induces ectoderm to form neuroectoderm?	Notochord

ANATOMY

What are the anatomic components of the central nervous system (CNS)?	The brain and the spinal cord
What are the anatomic components of the peripheral nervous system (PNS)?	Peripheral nerves and nerve roots—divided into sensory and motor divisions. The PNS is composed the somatic and autonomic nervous system; the autonomic nervous system is then further divided into the sympathetic, parasympathetic, and enteric nervous systems.
Name the three layers of meninges:	1. Dura mater 2. Arachnoid mater 3. Pia mater Together, the arachnoid and pia mater are referred to as leptomeninges.

Where is the subdural space?	Between the dura mater and arachnoid mater
Where is the subarachnoid space?	Between the arachnoid mater and pia mater
Where is the choroid plexus?	It is located in all parts of the ventricular system excluding the occipital and frontal horns of the lateral ventricles and cerebral aqueduct.
What is the function of the choroid plexus?	To produce cerebrospinal fluid (CSF) which acts as a mechanical buffer and immunologic barrier for the nervous system
Where is cerebrospinal fluid (CSF) located?	CSF fills spaces in the nervous system including the ventricles, sulci, cisterns, and the central canal of the spinal cord. CSF is then reabsorbed through the arachnoid granulations into the venous system.
Describe the arterial blood supply to the brain:	The internal carotid arteries give rise to the anterior and middle cerebral arteries which form an anastomosis (the Circle of Willis) with the posterior cerebral arteries arising from the vertebral arteries.
Describe the venous drainage of the brain:	Cerebral veins (eg, great cerebral vein, superior ophthalmic vein) drain into venous sinuses (eg, superior sagittal sinus, transverse sinus) located between the meningeal and periosteal layers of the dura mater which drain into the internal jugular veins.
Name two locations in the nervous system which lack a blood-brain barrier:	1. Area postrema 2. Posterior pituitary
How many spinal nerves do humans have?	31—8 cervical spinal nerves, 12 thoracic spinal nerves, 5 lumbar spinal nerves, 5 sacral spinal nerves, and 1 coccygeal spinal nerve

Name the three major spinal tracts and describe the type of transmitted information:	1. Lateral corticospinal tract—voluntary movement (motor) of contralateral limb
	2. Dorsal column-medial lemniscal pathway—pressure, vibration, light touch sensation, and proprioception
	3. Spinothalamic tract—pain and temperature sensation
What is the function of the basal ganglia?	Coordination of voluntary movements and posture
Which are the nuclei composing the basal ganglia?	Caudate, putamen, subthalamic, globus pallidus, and substantia nigra
What are the functions of the thalamus?	To relay afferent (ascending) sensory, special sensory, and motor information to the cerebral cortex and to regulate degree of consciousness
What are the functions of the hypothalamus?	Regulation of body temperature, hunger, sexual urges and emotions, circadian rhythms, thirst and water balance, and the autonomic nervous system
Where is the visual cortex?	Occipital lobe
What is the function of the vestibular apparatus?	Spatial orientation
What is the function of the cochlea?	Hearing—the base of the cochlea detects high-frequency sounds while the apex detects low-frequency sounds

HISTOLOGY

What are the major supporting cells of the brain?	Astrocytes
What cells form myelin sheets around axons in the brain?	Oligodendrocytes
What is the predominate cell type found in white matter?	Oligodendrocytes
What cells form myelin sheets around axons in the peripheral nervous system?	Schwann cells

What cells in the brain become phagocytic in response to tissue damage?

Microglia

What are ependymal cells?

Low cuboidal epithelial cells composing the choroid plexus; they may be ciliated which facilitates movement of cerebrospinal fluid.

Which three structures constitute the blood-brain barrier?

1. Capillary endothelial cells and tight junctions between the cells
2. Basement membrane
3. Astrocyte processes

Describe the layers of a peripheral nerve:

The epineurium surrounds an entire nerve. Each fascicle of nerve fibers within a single nerve is surrounded by perineurium. Endoneurium surrounds each single nerve fiber within a fascicle.

What is the function of Meissner corpuscles?

Sensation of light discriminatory touch in skin of palms, soles, and digits

What is the function of Pacinian corpuscles?

Sensation of pressure, coarse touch, vibration, and tension in deep skin, joint capsules, serous membranes, and mesenteries

NEUROPATHOLOGY

General Principles

What is the range of normal values for intracranial pressure (ICP)?

0 to 15 mm Hg

Is the normal range of ICP low or high relative to mean arterial pressure (MAP)?

Low. Increases in ICP (eg, by mass lesions, increased amount of CSF, or bleeding) can quickly cause neurologic compromise.

What are the potential causes of elevated intracranial pressure?

Because the skull is a defined physical space, anything causing increased volume in the confined space will increase pressure, including mass lesions (eg, tumors, blood, abscesses), increased CSF (eg, due to obstructed flow or decreased absorption), or cerebral edema.

What are the main types of cerebral edema?	Vasogenic, cytotoxic, osmotic, and interstitial
Which type of cerebral edema stems from disruption of the blood-brain barrier?	Vasogenic edema—disruption of the blood-brain barrier can result from physical effects of processes such as hypertension or trauma on endothelial cell tight junctions or from release of vasoactive and inflammatory substances by certain tumors.
Where in the brain is vasogenic edema mostly seen?	White matter
What type of edema results from the influx of sodium and water in the neural cells?	Cytotoxic edema—which is due to inadequate function of the sodium-potassium pump in glial cells. The blood-brain barrier remains intact.
Where in the brain is cytotoxic edema most likely to be found?	Gray matter
What is the most common cause of cytotoxic edema?	Hypoxia/ischemia
What is a potential life-threatening complication of increased intracranial pressure?	Increased ICP may result in brain herniation compromising blood flow and/or brain activity, leading to death.
Which cerebral artery can be compressed in a cingulate herniation?	Anterior cerebral artery
What cranial nerve can be compressed in an uncal herniation?	Cranial nerve III

Table 12.1 Types of Herniation

Type	Description
Cingulate or subfalcine	Herniation of the cingulate gyrus beneath the falx cerebri
Transtentorial or uncal	Medial temporal lobe herniation over the free edge of the tentorium cerebelli
Tonsillar	Inferomedial cerebellum caudally displaced into the foramen magnum
Fungus cerebri	Herniation of edematous brain through a skull defect

What is tearing of the penetrating vessels of the midbrain and pons called in a tonsillar herniation?

Duret hemorrhages

What surgical intervention can be used to relieve increased intracranial pressure?

Resection or evacuation of a space-occupying lesion or craniotomy to allow the brain additional room to expand

What is hydrocephalus?

A condition in which there is increased fluid within the skull

Table 12.2 Types of Hydrocephalus

Type of Hydrocephalus	Clinical Feature
Communicating hydrocephalus	Obstruction is distal to the outlet foramina of the fourth ventricle
Normal pressure hydrocephalus	Slowly evolving with clinical triad of dementia, urinary incontinence, and ataxia
Hydrocephalus ex vacuo or compensatory hydrocephalus	Occurs as a result of atrophy and loss of brain tissue
Noncommunicating hydrocephalus	Obstruction is intraventricular or at the foramen of Monro

Congenital

What condition in a newborn is caused by failure of the vertebral arches to close and clinically may present with a tuft of hair at the lower lumber region?

Spina bifida occulta

What is the condition called if in addition to failed closure of the vertebral arches, the meninges are herniated through the defect in the spine?

Meningocele

What is the condition called if in addition to failed closure of the vertebral arches, the spinal cord and meninges are herniated through the defect in the spine?

Meningomyelocele

What clinical findings in a newborn might make a physician suspicious of a congenital viral infection?

Microcephaly, focal cerebral calcification, and an infant whose weight is small for gestational age

What are the common pathogens involved in congenital infections?

Toxoplasma; Other—human immunodeficiency virus (HIV), *Varicella, Listeria*; Rubella; Cytomegalovirus; Herpes; e; Syphilis (*Treponema pallidum*)

TORCHeS

What common manifestations do the TORCHeS infections share?

With any of these infections, patients may present with microcephaly, chorioretinitis, and focal cerebral calcifications.

What is a common household reservoir for toxoplasmosis?

Cat feces

What congenital syndrome is associated with the development of early Alzheimer disease?

Down syndrome

What is microcephaly?

Head circumference smaller than two standard deviations below the mean for age and sex; there are numerous etiologies for microcephaly including infectious and genetic causes and maternal alcohol use.

What is macrocephaly?

Head circumference larger than two standard deviations above the mean for age and sex; there are numerous etiologies for macrocephaly including hydrocephalus and genetic, infectious, and environmental causes.

What is anencephaly?

Absence of a large part of the brain and skull; results when the cephalic end of the neural tube fails to close (around day 23-26 of gestation)

What are the typical clinical findings of Klüver-Bucy syndrome?

Hypersexuality, uninhibited behavior, visual agnosia, and hyperorality

What part of the brain is affected in Klüver-Bucy syndrome?

Bilateral amygdalae

Anatomic

What visual field defect will a patient experience if a lesion involving the right optic nerve is present?	Right anopia (blindness of the right temporal and right nasal visual fields)
What visual field defect will a patient experience if a lesion involving the optic chiasm is present?	Bitemporal hemianopia (blindness of the left temporal and right temporal visual fields)
What visual field defect will a patient experience if a lesion involving the right optic tract is present?	Left homonymous hemianopsia (blindness of the left temporal and right nasal visual fields)
What visual field defect will a patient experience if a lesion involving Meyer loop is present?	Left upper quadrantanopsia
What visual field defect will a patient experience if a lesion involving the dorsal optic radiation is present?	Left lower quadrantanopsia
What are the signs of a complete cranial nerve III lesion?	No pupillary light reflex; dilation of pupil; no accommodation of lens; ptosis of upper eyelid; inability to gaze downward and outward

Table 12.3 Cranial Nerves

Name	Function
Cranial nerve I (olfactory)	Smell
Cranial nerve II (optic)	Sight
Cranial nerve III (oculomotor)	Innervates superior, medial, and inferior recti muscles and the levator palpebrae superioris muscle of the upper eyelid; pupillary constriction
Cranial nerve IV (trochlear)	Innervates the superior oblique muscle
Cranial nerve V (trigeminal)	Corneal reflex; sensory information from head/neck; muscles of mastication
Cranial nerve VI (abducens)	Innervates the lateral rectus muscle
Cranial nerve VII (facial)	Taste sensation to anterior two-thirds of tongue; muscles of facial expression; all glands except parotid gland
Cranial nerve VIII (vestibulocochlear)	Hearing and balance

Table 12.3 Cranial Nerves (Continued)

Name	Function
Cranial nerve IX (glossopharyngeal)	Sensory from carotid sinus and carotid body; taste/sensory to the posterior one-third of the tongue; parotid gland
Cranial nerve X (vagus)	Parasympathetic innervation to thoracic and abdominal viscera; muscles of pharynx and larynx
Cranial nerve XI (accessory)	Movement of sternocleidomastoid and trapezius muscles
Cranial nerve XII (hypoglossal)	Controls muscles of the tongue (except palatoglossal)

What other functions does cranial nerve VII have?	Taste to the anterior two-thirds of tongue; sensory to the external ear and muscles of facial expression; parasympathetic to submandibular, sublingual, and lacrimal glands
What nerve is entrapped in carpal tunnel syndrome?	Median nerve
Tingling along the median nerve distribution reproduced by tapping on the palmaris longus tendon at the wrist is known as what sign?	Tinel sign
Tingling along the median nerve distribution reproduced by opposing the dorsal aspects of the hands is known as what sign?	Phalen sign
What is the treatment of carpal tunnel syndrome?	NSAIDs, wrist splints, ergonomics, and carpal tunnel release surgery
Injury to which upper extremity nerve will result in "wrist drop"?	Radial nerve
What clinical findings are associated with Arnold-Chiari malformation?	Due to downward displacement of the cerebellar vermis and medulla, patients may develop headaches which worsen with Valsalva maneuver, syringomyelia, facial pain, muscle weakness, and hearing problems.

What is the diagnostic test of choice to evaluate for possible Arnold-Chiari malformation?	MRI
What is the treatment?	Surgery for symptomatic patients (usually a suboccipital craniectomy)
What is a seizure?	A transient condition of excessive or synchronous neuronal activity in the brain
What is epilepsy?	A disorder in which a patient experiences recurrent seizures (does not include febrile seizures)
What is the difference between a partial and a generalized seizure?	Partial seizures affect only one, localized part of the brain, therefore the clinical symptoms will be specific to the area of affected brain. Generalized seizures affect the brain diffusely, therefore the clinical symptoms will be generalized and nonlocalizing.
What is the difference between a simple and a complex seizure?	Simple and complex seizures are subtypes of partial seizures. A complex partial seizure is one that starts localized (as a simple partial seizure) but then secondarily generalizes thereby *impairing consciousness*. There is no alteration of consciousness in a simple seizure.
What is status epilepticus?	A condition in which the brain is in a state of persistent seizure
What is the first-line drug therapy for patients in status epilepticus?	Benzodiazepines (diazepam or lorazepam)
Which medication is first-line prophylaxis for status epilepticus?	Phenytoin
For which type of seizure is ethosuximide the recommended first-line drug therapy?	Absence seizures
Which medications may be used as first-line therapy in patients with generalized tonic-clonic seizures?	Phenytoin, carbamazepine, or valproic acid
Which medication may be used in pregnant women and children who have seizures?	Phenobarbital, however, if a pregnant woman has eclampsia, magnesium sulfate is the first-line therapy.

Neoplastic

What are the common presenting features of patients with brain tumors?	Patients may present with a variety of symptoms including nausea, headache, seizures, focal findings (eg, compression of a single cranial nerve), and/or altered mental status/confusion.
What is the most common adult brain tumor?	Metastases (eg, lung, breast, melanoma)
Within the skull, where are adult brain tumors most often located?	Superior to the tentorium—"supratentorial"
Within the skull, where are pediatric brain tumors most often located?	Inferior to the tentorium—"infratentorial"
What is the most common primary brain tumor in adults?	Glioblastoma multiforme (GBM)
What is a "glioma"?	A glioma is a relatively nonspecific term applied to any brain tumor derived from glial cells which include astrocytes, oligodendrocytes, and microglia.
From what cell type does glioblastoma multiforme (GBM) arise?	Astrocytes—GBM is a term applied to a grade IV astrocytoma
How would a GBM appear microscopically?	Tumor cells in GBM are often described as "pseudopalisading" and forming a border around central areas of hemorrhage and necrosis.
What is the classic radiological finding for GBM?	Ring-enhancing lesion with surrounding edema
Why might a GBM be referred to as "butterfly glioma"?	When detected, GBMs may already have crossed the corpus callosum and will be involving both cerebral hemispheres. Radiographically, this may appear as the shape of a butterfly.
What is the treatment of GBM?	Surgical removal, radiation, and chemotherapy, but the prognosis remains very poor
What primary brain neoplasm originates from the dura mater or arachnoid?	Meningioma

How would a meningioma appear microscopically?

The tumor is composed of spindled cells arranged in a whorled pattern and may contain "psammoma bodies" which are laminated calcifications.

From what cell type are acoustic neuromas derived?

Schwann cells, although termed acoustic neuroma because they are often localized to cranial nerve VIII

What neurocutaneous syndrome is associated with bilateral acoustic neuromas?

Neurofibromatosis 2

What is the most common location for a tumor developing from oligodendrocytes to arise?

Oligodendrogliomas most often arise in the frontal lobes

What physical examination finding is associated with pituitary adenoma?

Bitemporal hemianopia due to compression of the optic chiasm

Among pituitary adenoma, what is the most common secreted hormone?

Prolactin

What tumor is common in children, located in the cerebellum or third ventricle, and histologically has brightly eosinophilic Rosenthal fibers?

Pilocytic (low-grade) astrocytoma

What is the most common supratentorial brain tumor in children?

Craniopharyngioma—histologically, composed of nests and trabeculae of squamous epithelium, often with abundant keratin resembling a follicular cyst

What physical examination finding is associated with craniopharyngioma?

Bitemporal hemianopia due to compression of the optic chiasm (may be confused clinically with pituitary adenoma)

The clinical findings of retinal angiomas and polycythemia in a child with a brain tumor might make a physician suspicious of which type of pediatric brain tumor?

Hemangioblastoma

What clinical syndrome might the physician want to consider in a patient with retinal angiomas and hemangioblastoma?

von Hippel-Lindau syndrome

Finding cells arranged in a "rosette" pattern on microscopic evaluation of a pediatric cerebellar tumor would suggest the diagnosis of what?	Medulloblastoma
How might medulloblastomas cause increased ICP?	By mass effect of the tumor or by compression of the fourth ventricle and resulting obstructive hydrocephalus
What neurologic findings are associated with tuberous sclerosis?	Clinically, patients may present with seizures, developmental delay, and behavioral problems. Within the CNS, patients develop cortical/subcortical tubers which are believed to be foci of abnormal neural migration, subependymal nodules, and giant cell astrocytomas.

Vascular

What are the common causes of intracranial hemorrhage?	Berry aneurysm, arteriovenous malformation, and hypertension
What are the possible locations of intracranial hemorrhage?	Hemorrhage can occur into essentially any space in the CNS including: epidural, subdural, subarachnoid, intraventricular, and parenchymal spaces.
How do you initially evaluate a subarachnoid hemorrhage?	Computed tomography (CT) without contrast
How does blood appear on a noncontrast CT?	White
How is a subarachnoid hemorrhage (SAH) treated?	Nimodipine to prevent vasospasm, phenytoin to prevent seizures, lowering ICP by hyperventilation, raising the head greater than 30 degrees, possible clipping or radiological coiling of a ruptured aneurysm
Injury to which artery is usually the cause of an epidural hematoma?	Middle meningeal artery
What is initially used for evaluation of a possible cranial/intracranial bleed?	CT without contrast
In what shape does an epidural hematoma classically appear on a noncontrast CT?	Convex, lens-shaped *Epidural = Elliptical

How is an epidural hematoma treated? Surgical evacuation

By what mechanism do subdural hematomas occur? Tearing of the bridging veins within the subdural space (between the dura mater and arachnoid mater)

In what shape does a subdural hematoma appear on noncontrast CT? Concave, crescent-shaped

How is a subdural hematoma treated? Surgical evacuation if symptomatic or may resolve on its own

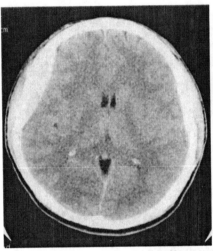 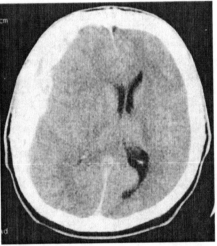

A   B

Figure 12.1 Epidural (A) and subdural (B) hematoma CT images. (Reproduced, with permission, from Ropper AH, Samuels MA: *Adams & Victor's Princples of Neurology*, 9th ed, New York: McGraw Hill; figs. 35-8 and 35-9.)

What feature about a patient is important to determine when attempting to localize the area of brain affected by a stroke? Handedness—95% of right-handed people are left hemisphere dominant, as many as 60% of left-handed people are also left hemisphere dominant

What symptoms are common with middle cerebral artery strokes? Contralateral hemiplegia, eye deviation toward the side of the lesion, contralateral hemianopia, and contralateral hemianesthesia. If involving the dominant hemisphere, will include aphasia, and if involving the nondominant hemisphere will cause anosognosia.

A stroke involving which area of the brain results in expressive aphasia?

Broca area—posterior inferior frontal gyrus of the dominant hemisphere

A stroke involving which area of the brain results in receptive aphasia?

Wernicke area—posterior superior temporal gyrus of the dominant hemisphere

A stroke involving which artery may present with Horner syndrome?

Posterior inferior cerebellar artery

Patients with a stroke involving the vertebrobasilar system will have which clinical features?

Cerebellar signs (eg, dysmetria, ataxia), ipsilateral cranial nerve palsy, contralateral corticospinal tract symptoms, dysarthria or dysphagia, and dissociated sensory loss

Table 12.4 Features of Cerebral Artery Stoke Presentations

Clinical Manifestation	Artery Affected
Paralysis and sensory loss of the contralateral foot/leg	Anterior cerebral
Expressive aphasia	Middle cerebral
Paralysis of the contralateral arm	Middle cerebral
Hemisensory loss	Posterior cerebral

Table 12.5 Presentations of Common Headaches

Clinical Manifestation	Headache Type
Associated with auras, photophobia, and nausea, often unilateral frontal pain	Classic migraine
Band-like pain often in occipital region	Tension headaches
Periorbital pain, ipsilateral tearing, nasal discharge	Cluster headaches

What are the main abortive therapies for migraines?

NSAIDs and triptans

What are the options for prophylactic therapy for migraines?

Beta blockers (propranolol), calcium channel blockers, tricyclic antidepressants (amitriptyline), and antiepileptic medications (topiramate, gabapentin, valproic acid)

Inflammatory/Autoimmune

What is the proposed mechanism of disease in Guillain-Barré syndrome (aka acute idiopathic polyneuritis)?	Immune attack of peripheral myelin resulting in inflammation and demyelination of peripheral nerves and motor fibers
What clinical features are associated with Guillain-Barré syndrome?	Ascending paralysis, muscle weakness, facial diplegia, autonomic dysfunction, and papilledema
What laboratory findings are associated with Guillain-Barré syndrome?	Albuminocytologic dissociation in the CSF—meaning the cell count in the CSF will be normal but CSF protein will be elevated
With which microorganisms is Guillain-Barré syndrome associated?	*Campylobacter jejuni* and herpesvirus; but the link with these pathogens is not considered definitive.
What is potentially life-threatening about Guillain-Barré syndrome?	Respiratory failure—secondary to paralysis of the muscles of respiration
What is considered first-line treatment for Guillain-Barré syndrome?	Intravenous immunoglobulin (IVIG) and plasmapheresis
Describe the classic ophthalmologic examination finding associated with multiple sclerosis (MS):	Internuclear ophthalmoplegia (INO) (also called medial longitudinal fasciculus [MLF] syndrome) occurs when a multiple sclerosis patient has a demyelinating lesion involving the MLF. If the left MLF were affected, then a left medial rectus palsy would result and while in right lateral gaze, the left eye will fail to abduct and nystagmus may be observed in the right eye.
What microscopic findings would be associated with CNS lesions in MS?	Oligodendrocyte loss and reactive gliosis, axons will be preserved.
What CSF finding is present in MS?	Increased IgG
What are the treatments for MS?	Beta interferon, immunoglobulins, methotrexate, and corticosteroids
What demyelinating disease occurs after viral infection and, unlike MS, is self-limited?	Acute disseminated encephalomyelitis

What demyelinating disease is specifically associated with JC virus?	Progressive multifocal leukoencephalopathy (PML)
What demyelinating disease occurs in some AIDS patients?	Progressive multifocal leukoencephalopathy (PML) due to reactivation of JC virus infection
What is myasthenia gravis?	An autoimmune disease resulting from circulating autoantibodies which block the acetylcholine receptors in neuromuscular junctions
What are the presenting signs and symptoms of myasthenia gravis?	Muscle weakness and easy fatigability—key words "fatigable weakness"
What are the available treatments for myasthenia gravis?	Acetylcholinesterase inhibitors, immunosuppressants, occasionally thymectomy

Infectious

What is meningitis?	An inflammatory process of the leptomeninges and cerebrospinal fluid (CSF) located within the subarachnoid space, usually associated with an infectious organism
What are the common causative agents of bacterial meningitis in the neonate?	*Escherichia coli*, group B *streptococcus*, *Listeria monocytogenes*
Against which organism are infants now vaccinated that previously was the cause of many cases of bacterial meningitis?	*Haemophilus influenza* type B
In adolescents and young adults, what is the most common causative organism of bacterial meningitis?	*Neisseria meningitides*
In the elderly, what is the most common causative organism of bacterial meningitis?	*Streptococcus pneumonia, Listeria monocytogenes*, gram-negative bacilli
Describe the CSF composition of bacterial meningitis:	High white blood cells (WBCs)—mostly neutrophils (ie, neutrophilic pleocytosis), low glucose, high protein
What are the clinical signs and symptoms of bacterial meningitis?	Headache, neck stiffness, altered mental status, and fever

What characterizes the CSF in aseptic (viral) meningitis?

Lymphocytic pleocytosis, normal glucose, and only moderate protein elevation

What virus is associated with 70% to 80% of aseptic meningitis?

Enterovirus

Name two ways a patient can acquire a brain abscess:

1. Local extension from nearby infection such as sinusitis or mastoiditis
2. Hematogenous spread (from site in the lungs or heart usually)

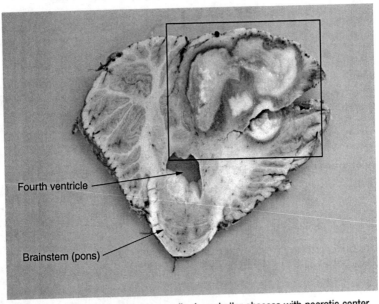

Fourth ventricle

Brainstem (pons)

Figure 12.2 Multifocal, well-circumscribed cerebellar abscess with necrotic center. (Reproduced, with permission, from OHSU.)

What is a local infection of the subdural space that usually spreads from infection of the sinuses or skull bones?

Subdural empyema

What characterizes the CSF of tuberculous meningitis?

Mild-to-moderate pleocytosis; very elevated protein level; moderately reduced or normal glucose; may visualize acid-fast bacilli

Describe the gross and microscopic findings associated with tuberculosis meningitis:

Gelatinous exudates at base of brain, granulomatous inflammation, caseous necrosis, and giant cells

What is the tertiary form of syphilis called?	Neurosyphilis
What percent of untreated patients with primary syphilis will develop tertiary syphilis?	10%
Name the three forms of neurosyphilis:	1. Meningovascular neurosyphilis 2. Paretic neurosyphilis 3. Tabes dorsalis
Which form of neurosyphilis may have obliterative endarteritis and cerebral gummas?	Meningovascular neurosyphilis
Which form of neurosyphilis is characterized by mood changes, severe dementia, gliosis, and iron deposits?	Paretic neurosyphilis
Which form of neurosyphilis involves dorsal root ganglia and posterior spinal columns?	Tabes dorsalis
In tertiary syphilis, a patient may have a pupil defect called Argyll Robertson pupil. What is the defect?	Pupil that reacts to accommodation, but not to light
What microscopic findings are characteristic of herpes encephalitis?	Hemorrhagic necrosis of the temporal lobes and orbital gyri with Cowdry type A inclusion bodies in neurons and glia
What viral encephalitis, affecting fetuses and the immunocompromised, shows prominent intranuclear and intracytoplasmic inclusions, especially in the paraventricular and subependymal regions of the brain?	Cytomegalovirus (CMV)
Which picornavirus attacks the ventral horns, often causing loss of neurons and prominent neuronophagia?	Polio virus
What is postpolio syndrome?	Progressive weakness and pain developing about 30 years after the original diagnosis
What viral infection produces paresthesias, headache, fever, central nervous system (CNS) excitability, foaming at the mouth, and paralysis?	Rabies virus

Name the neuronal eosinophilic cytoplasmic inclusions found in the hippocampus and cerebellum of a rabies victim:

Negri bodies

What characterizes human immunodeficiency virus (HIV) meningoencephalitis?

Microglial nodules, reactive gliosis, and multinucleated giant cells

What is the rare syndrome associated with a previous measles infection?

Subacute sclerosing panencephalitis (SSPE)

What characterizes SSPE?

Mental decline, seizures, spasticity of limbs, gliosis, myelin degeneration, and neurofibrillary tangles

Name two fungal brain infections:

1. *Cryptococcus*
2. *Candida* meningitis; many others are possible

How can one diagnose cryptococcal meningitis?

Lumbar puncture. The CSF will usually show encapsulated yeasts when India ink preparations are used. Cryptococcal antigen testing is also available.

What is the classic computed tomography (CT) or magnetic resonance imaging (MRI) finding associated with cerebral toxoplasmosis?

Multiple ring-enhancing lesions

What forms of *Toxoplasma* are seen on histology?

Free tachyzoites and encysted bradyzoites can be seen around the necrotic foci.

What brain infection is characterized by multiple calcified cysts at the gray-white interface?

Cysticercosis (from uncooked pork)

What is the classic histologic triad seen in spongiform encephalopathies?

Spongiosis—microvacuolation of cortex and gray matter; cortical astrogliosis and neuronal loss; kuru plaques—composed of aggregates of prion protein

What is the infectious agent in Creutzfeldt-Jakob disease?

Prions—a misfolded, infectious protein. Normal prion protein is folded in α-helix conformation, when pathologic the protein is folded in β-pleated sheets.

What are the chances of surviving a prion disease?

It can have a long incubation period, but once dementia begins, most patients die within 7 months.

What are the some common infectious causes of viral encephalitis?	Human immunodeficiency virus, Herpes simplex virus, West Nile virus, Rabies virus, and JC virus

Degenerative

What location of the brain is affected in Huntington disease?	Basal ganglia—specifically the caudate nucleus (GABAergic neurons)
What are the common clinical features observed in Huntington disease?	Chorea and dementia
What is the mode of inheritance of Huntington disease?	Autosomal dominant, may also display anticipation
What is the genetic mutation of this disease?	Expansion of CAG trinucleotide repeats on chromosome 4
What are common clinical features observed in Parkinson disease?	Rest tremor, rigidity, akinesia, and postural instability with shuffling gait
What is the mechanism causing this disease?	Dopamine depletion in the substantia nigra
What gross and histologic findings may be present at autopsy in Parkinson disease?	Depigmentation of the substantia nigra and Lewy bodies
What is the primary component of Lewy bodies?	Alpha-synuclein
What are the treatments for Parkinson disease?	Levodopa/carbidopa; dopamine agonists (bromocriptine); Selegiline; Amantadine; deep brain stimulation of globus pallidus interna and subthalamic nucleus
What are the two most common causes of dementia in elderly patients?	1. Alzheimer disease 2. Multi-infarct (vascular) dementia
What are the classic microscopic findings in Alzheimer disease?	Senile plaques and neurofibrillary tangles; may also be associated with findings of amyloid angiopathy
What is the composition of a neurofibrillary tangle?	Abnormally phosphorylated tau protein
What is the anatomic distribution of Pick disease?	Frontal and temporal lobes of the brain

What is the classic microscopic finding in Pick disease?

Pick body—also composed of abnormally phosphorylated tau protein

Among the degenerative neurological diseases, which disease presents clinically with both upper and lower motor neuron signs and no sensory deficits?

Amyotrophic lateral sclerosis (ALS)

Which infectious disease causes degeneration of the anterior horns but only presents with lower motor neuron signs?

Polio

What do spinocerebellar ataxia, Friedreich ataxia, and Huntington disease have in common?

They are neurodegenerative diseases caused by trinucleotide repeat expansions.

Table 12.6 Upper Motor Neuron and Lower Motor Neuron Symptom Localization

Clinical Manifestation	Location
Wasting of muscles	LMN
Fasciculations	LMN
Hyperactive reflexes	UMN
Clonus (jerking with passive stretching)	UMN
Loss of reflexes	LMN
Caused by nerve damage	LMN
Damage to corticospinal tract	UMN
Extensor plantar response	UMN

Abbreviations: LMN, lower motor neuron; UMN, upper motor neuron.

Traumatic

Traumatic injury of which artery is associated with epidural bleeding?

Middle meningeal artery—because it underlies the pterion, a relatively weak area of the skull, this artery is particularly susceptible to trauma.

Why do epidural bleeds have a "convex" appearance on CT and/ or MRI?

Bleeding into the epidural space is limited by borders established where the dura mater attaches to the skull along the skull sutures.

What are the symptoms of traumatic brain injury (TBI)?

Symptoms of increased intracranial pressure (ICP)—decreased level of consciousness, unilateral paralysis or weakness, blown or sluggish papillary response to light, anisocoria, Cushing triad, or abnormal posturing

What system is responsible for regulation of degree of consciousness after trauma?

Reticular activating system

What is a Cushing triad?

Irregular respirations/respiratory depression, hypertension, and bradycardia—indicating increased ICP

Describe decorticate posturing:

A patient will exhibit muscle rigidity in a specific pattern including elbow flexion, wrist and finger flexion, and leg extension. The arms and hands are held on the chest.

Describe decerebrate posturing:

A patient will exhibit muscle rigidity in a specific pattern including elbow extension, wrist and finger flexion, foot extension, leg extension, and neck and back extension.

What is Brown-Séquard syndrome?

A clinical syndrome that results from a neurologic lesion which causes hemisection of the spinal cord affecting the corticospinal tract, dorsal columns, and spinothalamic tracts.

What are the clinical features of Brown-Séquard syndrome?

Ipsilateral upper motor neuron signs below the level of the lesion; contralateral pain and temperature loss below the lesion; ipsilateral loss of proprioceptive, vibratory, and tactile sensation below the lesion; ipsilateral loss of all sensation at the level of the lesion; lower motor neuron (LMN) signs at the level of the lesion

When will a person with hemisection of the spinal cord present with features of Horner syndrome?

When the hemisection occurs above the level of T1

What are the features of Horner syndrome?

Ptosis, miosis, and anhidrosis

What does the presence of a Babinski sign indicate? | A localizing upper motor neuron (UMN) lesion

When is a Babinski sign a normal finding? | In infants less than 1 year old

If shoulder dystocia occurs during delivery of a newborn infant, what nerve injury is the infant at risk of sustaining? | Stress on the neck and shoulder during delivery may result in tearing of the C5 and C6 roots of the brachial plexus (aka Erb-Duchenne palsy); this can result in upper extremity abductor and lateral rotator paralysis and paralysis of the biceps brachii.

What is shaken baby syndrome? | A collection of clinical symptoms that are believed to be the result of acceleration-deceleration injury that occurs when a baby is shaken. Neurologic symptoms may include retinal hemorrhages, subdural hematomas, subarachnoid hemorrhages, and cerebral edema.

Environmental/Toxins

What syndrome is characterized by confabulation and retrograde amnesia? | Wernicke-Korsakoff syndrome

What vitamin deficiency is usually present? | Thiamine

What part of the brain is most likely affected? | Mammillary bodies

What is the principal neurological lesion of B_{12} deficiency? | Demyelination of the posterior columns of the spinal cord

What is niacin (Vitamin B_3) deficiency called? | Pellagra

What are the clinical manifestations of niacin deficiency? | Diarrhea, dementia, and dermatitis
*Three Ds

Carbon monoxide poisoning affects what part of the brain? | Globus pallidus (medial basal ganglia)

Methanol affects what part of the brain? | Putamen and claustra (lateral basal ganglia)

What clinical signs are seen with methanol poisoning?	Blindness, central nervous system depression, and metabolic acidosis
What are two possible treatments for methanol poisoning?	Ethanol and fomepizole. Presently, ethanol is used as a temporary treatment until the patient can be taken to a hospital that has fomepizole available.
What are the clinical features of opioid intoxication?	Respiratory depression, constipation, miosis, CNS depression
What are some withdrawal symptoms?	Tachycardia, hypertension, piloerection, mydriasis, lacrimation, and body aches
Which opioid antagonist is used to treat opioid overdose?	Naloxone
What is central pontine myelinolysis?	An iatrogenic condition in which damage to myelin sheaths of neurons located in the pons results from rapid correction of hyponatremia

CLINICAL VIGNETTES

A 12-year-old boy was involved in a motor vehicle accident (MVA) and sustained head trauma. Evaluation of his neurological status revealed a mean arterial pressure (MAP) of 70 mm Hg and intracranial pressure (ICP) of 30 mm Hg. What is cerebral perfusion pressure (CPP)?

40 mm Hg (CPP = MAP – ICP)

A 65-year-old man presents with alcohol on his breath, ataxia, nystagmus, ophthalmoplegia, and mental confusion. What is the likely diagnosis?

Wernicke encephalopathy

A 40-year-old alcoholic is found to be hyponatremic (low serum sodium). His sodium level is corrected from 120 to 155 mEq/L in 1 hour, and he develops flaccid quadriplegia with mental status changes. What is the diagnosis?

Central pontine myelinolysis

A 60-year-old woman with a prior gastrectomy complains of symmetric numbness, tingling, and unsteady gait. What vitamin is she likely deficient in?

B_{12} (cobalamin)

A 27-year-old woman gives birth to a full-term (40 weeks) baby boy with a neural tube defect. What is most likely the vitamin deficiency that contributed to this birth defect?

Folic acid

A 20-year-old woman with a history of intravenous (IV) drug abuse and immunosuppression gives birth to a 34-week infant with intrauterine growth retardation (IUGR), microcephaly, and focal cerebral calcifications. What infection does the newborn most likely have?

Cytomegalovirus infection

A 55-year-old man is no longer able to speak, but can comprehend what you are saying. What area of the brain is affected?

Broca area

A 60-year-old woman can speak, but her words make no sense. Where is the brain lesion?

Wernicke area

A newborn baby has a *blueberry muffin* rash, a patent ductus arteriosus, and cataracts. What congenital infection might he have?

Rubella

A 45-year-old woman has had multiple car wrecks because she states she has lost her peripheral vision. Where is the lesion?

Optic chiasm

A 40-year-old woman with a recent head injury has diplopia and difficulty looking down when walking downstairs. Which cranial nerve is affected?

Cranial nerve IV (trochlear)

A 20-year-old man had right-sided facial droop after sustaining a knife wound to the right jaw and cheek. What cranial nerve is affected?

Cranial nerve VII (facial)

A 61-year-old man has sudden, excruciating pain that shoots down the side of his jaw. What condition does he have?

Trigeminal neuralgia

A 60-year-old man with a 6-month history of headaches gets an magnetic resonance imaging (MRI) of the brain which shows an irregular, contrast-enhancing lesion, edema adjacent to the lesion, hemorrhage, and necrosis. What tumor is most likely present?

Glioblastoma multiforme (GBM)

A 50-year-old man develops ipsilateral hearing loss, tinnitus, vertigo, and cerebellar dysfunction. What is the diagnosis?

Acoustic neuroma (schwannoma)

A 1-year-old girl develops seizures, *ash-leaf* pigmented lesions on the trunk, sebaceous adenomas, and a shagreen patch (flesh-colored soft plaque) on her lumbosacral region. What is the diagnosis?

Tuberous sclerosis

A 45-year-old man presents with a sudden onset, intensely painful headache, neck stiffness, nausea, and vomiting. He says, "This is the worse headache of my life." What is the diagnosis?

Subarachnoid hemorrhage (SAH)

A 20-year-old man is hit in the side of the head with a baseball. He has a 30-minute lucid interval followed by headache and decreased level of consciousness. What is his diagnosis?

Epidural hematoma

A 90-year-old man trips and falls. A few days later, he develops mental status changes and contralateral hemiparesis. What is his diagnosis?

Subdural hematoma

A 4-month-old infant is brought to the ER by his stepfather. The infant has multiple contusions on his body, multiple long bone fractures, and is crying uncontrollably. The stepfather states the infant fell off the couch. What is the diagnosis?

Shaken baby syndrome

A 15-year-old girl suddenly loses consciousness and begins extending her back and extremities followed by repetitive movements. What is the likely diagnosis?

Tonic-clonic seizure

A 6-year-old girl has multiple episodes of a motionless stare throughout the day and has been told to stop "daydreaming" in class. What is her diagnosis?

Absence seizure

A 10-year-old boy has sudden spells where he falls to the ground with complete loss of muscle tone. What is the diagnosis?

Atonic seizure

A 30-year-old man has progressive jerking of his arm without loss of consciousness. What is his diagnosis?

Simple partial seizure (jacksonian)

A 41-year-old man shows up to the ER with symptoms of euphoria, decreased appetite, and increased motor activity. On physical examination, you find a perforated nasal septum. What is the diagnosis?

Cocaine abuse

A 25-year-old woman shows up to the ER and says, "spiders are crawling on my legs." She also states she is having flashbacks. What is the diagnosis?

D-Lysergic acid diethylamide (LSD) abuse

A 24-year-old man enters the ER with respiratory depression, altered mental status, pinpoint pupils, and an indifference to pain. What is the diagnosis?

Opioid abuse

A 24-year-old man presents with rapid, ascending paralysis. He said he was sick a couple of weeks ago. What is the diagnosis?

Guillain-Barré syndrome

A 31-year-old woman has intermittent exacerbations and remissions of visual disturbances, upper and lower extremity weakness, paresthesias of the face, and urinary incontinence. What is the diagnosis?

Multiple sclerosis (MS)

A 45-year-old executive assistant complains of tingling in the thumb, index, middle, and half of the ring finger. What is the diagnosis?

Carpal tunnel syndrome

A 45-year-old man complains of progressive weakness in his arms and legs, speech difficulty, and multiple areas of small involuntary muscle contractions. What is the diagnosis?

Amyotrophic lateral sclerosis (Lou Gehrig disease)

A 41-year-old man complains of involuntary writing movements which began about 6 months ago. He has become irritable, depressed, and cannot remember things. What is his diagnosis?

Huntington disease

A 62-year-old man develops a resting tremor, expressionless facies, slowed movements, stooped posture, and rigidity. What is his diagnosis?

Parkinson disease

A 70-year-old woman has progressive impairment of memory. Over the last 5 years, she has forgotten family members' names, and on several occasions, has forgotten where she lives. What is the diagnosis?

Alzheimer disease

A 32-year-old man complains of gait abnormalities which have gotten worse over the last 6 months. On physical examination, you notice impaired proprioception and vibratory sense. What is your diagnosis?

Tabes dorsalis

A 40-year-old woman complains of occipital headaches, weakness/numbness in her hands and feet, and has downbeat nystagmus on physical examination. An MRI shows tonsillar herniation below the foramen magnum. What is the diagnosis?

Arnold-Chiari malformation or Chiari malformation

A 60-year-old man complains of problems walking, decreased vibration and position sense in the right foot, and poor localization of tactile touch on the right from the pectoralis major muscle down. Temperature and pain senses are normal. What somatosensory pathway is affected?

Medial lemniscal pathway

A 70-year-old woman presents with a badly burned leg and says she has decreased pain and temperature feeling on the right side of her body from her breast down. On examination, her proprioception and discriminative touch are normal. What somatosensory pathway is affected?

Spinothalamic pathway

A 31-year-old man has right-sided proprioception and discriminative touch sensory loss, and left-sided pain and temperature sensory loss from hemisection of his sixth thoracic vertebrae. What is the syndrome called?

Brown-Séquard syndrome

A 56-year-old man develops a loss of pain and temperature sense in a belt pattern around his stomach. Sensation above and below is normal. Where is the lesion?

Anterior white commissure

A 45-year-old woman complains of right-sided temperature and pain loss and left-sided facial sensory loss. An angiography shows an infarct involving the left posterior inferior cerebellar artery (PICA). What is the syndrome?

Wallenberg syndrome

A 46-year-old patient has anhydrosis, miosis, and ptosis on one side of the face. What syndrome is present?

Horner syndrome

CHAPTER 13

Dermatopathology

EMBRYOLOGY

From what embryologic tissue type is the epidermis derived?

Surface ectoderm

From what embryologic tissue type is the dermis derived?

Mesoderm—depending on location in the embryo dermis may be derived from dermatome, lateral somatic, or neural crest tissue

What is the embryologic origin of cutaneous melanocytes?

Neural crest mesoderm

ANATOMY/HISTOLOGY

What are the three layers of the skin?

1. Epidermis
2. Dermis
3. Subcutaneous tissue

What types of epithelium is the epidermis?

Keratinized stratified squamous epithelium

What are the five layers of the epidermis?

1. Stratum corneum
2. Stratum lucidum
3. Stratum granulosum
4. Stratum spinosum
5. Stratum basalis

What types of cells compose the stratum basalis?

Squamous cells which have a basophilic, cuboidal to columnar appearance distinct from the eosinophilic, mature-appearing squamous cells of the upper layers in the epidermis

What are the two layers of the dermis?

1. Papillary layer
2. Reticular layer

What are the small, encapsulated sensory receptors found in the dermis of the palms, soles, and digits of the skin (hint: they are also involved in light discriminatory touch of hairless skin)?	Meissner corpuscles
What is the name of tactile disks that mediate light crude touch?	Merkel corpuscles
What are the large encapsulated sensory receptors found in deeper layers of skin that are involved in pressure, coarse touch, vibration, and tension?	Pacinian corpuscles
Where else are Pacinian corpuscles found?	Joint capsules; serous membranes; mesenteries
What structure connects epidermal basal cells to the underlying extracellular matrix of the basement membrane?	Hemidesmosomes
What structures join adjacent squamous cells together and provide anchoring points for intermediate filaments?	Desmosomes (macula adherens)
What is the function of Langerhans cells?	Antigen-presenting cells; main inducers of antibody response
From where does the epidermis regrow after trauma or removal?	From epidermally derived hair follicles and sweat glands in the dermis

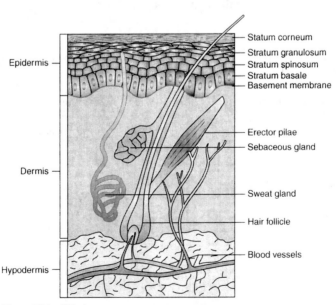

Figure 13.1   Skin layers.

PATHOLOGY

General Principles

What is a macule?	Flat, discolored (hypo- or hyper-pigmented) area of skin <1 cm in diameter
What is a patch?	Flat, discolored area of skin >1 cm in diameter
What is a papule?	Raised area of skin of any color that is <1 cm in diameter
What is a plaque?	Raised area of skin of any color that is >1 cm in diameter
What is a nodule?	A palpable, roughly round lesion arising in the dermis or subcutaneous tissues
What is a vesicle?	A raised, fluid-filled blister measuring <0.5 cm in diameter
What is a bulla?	A raised, fluid-filled blister measuring >0.5 cm in diameter
What is a pustule?	A blister that is filled with pus (generally bacteria and necrotic debris)
What is a wheal?	A "hive," generally a round lesion resulting from edema in the dermis
What is the term for dilated, superficial blood vessels?	Telangiectasia
What are petechiae?	Nonblanchable pin-point foci of hemorrhage in the skin
What is purpura?	A larger area of hemorrhage in the skin, may be palpable
Which test is designed to ascertain whether a skin lesion will blanch as a result of pressure?	Diascopy
What is an erosion?	The skin lesion that results when all or part of the epidermis is removed (ie, abraded), will not leave a scar

What is an ulcer?

Full-thickness loss of epidermis and loss of all or part of the epidermis, will leave a scar

Define hyperkeratosis:

Excessive keratin production leading to thickening of the stratum corneum

Define lichenification:

Visual appearance of thickened skin with prominent skin markings that occurs secondary to chronic scratching of itchy skin, can be associated with atopic dermatitis

Define ichthyosis:

Excessive cornification of the skin, giving it a scaly appearance

Define hypertrichosis:

Excessive hairiness due to increased formation of hair follicles, may be regional or generalized

What is meant when describing a rash as "annular"?

The rash has a ring-like, possibly targetoid appearance. Lesions may be singular or multiple.

What is meant when describing a rash as "herpetiform"?

That the rash is distributed as grouped papules or vesicles, similar to a herpes simplex rash, but does not necessarily indicate a specific etiology

What is meant when describing a rash as "zosteriform"?

That the rash is distributed as clustered papules or vesicles in a dermatomal distribution, similar to a herpes zoster rash, but does not necessarily indicate a specific etiology

What is meant when describing a rash as "morbilliform"?

That the rash appears as erythematous maculopapules, similar to a measles rash, but does not necessarily indicate a specific etiology

What is meant when describing a rash as having "flexor distribution"? Give examples of this type of rash.

Flexor distribution (aka intertriginous) means that the rash is distributed over the body primarily involving skin covering flexor muscle groups (ie, anterior arm including wrist and elbow crease, posterior legs including knee crease, and femoral crease). Examples include: atopic dermatitis and inverse psoriasis.

What is meant when describing a rash as having "extensor distribution"? Give a classic example of this type of rash.

Extensor distribution means that the rash is distributed over the body primarily involving skin covering extensor surface of limbs (ie, elbows, knees). Psoriasis is classically described as involving extensor surfaces.

What is meant when describing a rash as having a "photosensitive" distribution?

That the rash is distributed over the body in a distribution primarily involving sun-exposed skin while sparing areas covered by clothing or shaded by other body parts (ie, nose or chin)

What is meant when describing a rash as having an "acral" distribution?

That the rash is distributed over the body primarily involving distal portions of the limbs (ie, hands, feet) and head (ie, ears, nose)

Congenital/Inherited

What are nevi?

A nevus is any congenital lesion of the skin. Most often applied to melanocytic nevi (moles) which can be either congenital or acquired. Large congenital nevi (>20 cm) are associated with an increased risk of melanoma later in life.

What is a hemangioma?

The most common tumor of infancy, hemangiomas are benign vascular proliferations which can appear in the skin (most often on the face or scalp). Flat, larger lesions may be referred to as port-wine stains.

What are phakomatoses?

Phakomatoses are a family of neurocutaneous syndromes which have disorders of the central nervous system as well as the skin and retina. The five classic phakomatoses include: neurofibromatosis, tuberous sclerosis, ataxia telangiectasia, Sturge-Weber syndrome, and von Hippel-Lindau disease. Depending on the source, this group may also include incontinentia pigmenti and nevoid basal cell carcinoma syndrome.

What is the most common neurocutaneous disorder?

Neurofibromatosis

What are the multiple, light-brown, freckle-like lesions found in neurofibromatosis?	Café au lait spots
Café au lait spots usually grow along what structures?	Peripheral nerves
On what chromosome is the mutation associated with NF type I found?	Chromosome 17
What are other manifestations associated with NF type I?	Optic gliomas; bone abnormalities; freckling of the axillary or genital area
Hypopigmented macules or *ash-leaf spots* on the trunk or lower extremities are associated with what disease?	Tuberous sclerosis
What is the tuberous sclerosis triad?	Mental retardation; epilepsy; multiple angiofibromas
A unilateral port-wine stain of the forehead and upper eyelid is associated with what condition?	Sturge-Weber syndrome (encephalotrigeminal angiomatosis)
Which nerve is associated with Sturge-Weber syndrome?	Ophthalmic branch of the trigeminal nerve
How is alkaptonuria inherited?	Autosomal recessive inheritance
What accounts for the discoloration of the skin and urine in alkaptonuria?	Deposition of homogentisic acid
Hemochromatosis has what manifestation in the skin?	Hyperpigmented bronze skin
Which connective tissue disorder is associated with hyperextensible fragile skin, loose joints, and a tendency toward easy bruising and bleeding?	Ehlers-Danlos syndrome
What are possible life-threatening complications associated with Ehlers-Danlos disease?	Arterial or intestinal rupture
What is the name of the group of autosomal recessive diseases of premature aging?	Progeria
Marfan syndrome is due to a defect in which gene?	Fibrillin-1 (*FBN1*)

On which chromosome is the mutation associated with Marfan syndrome located?	15q21
What is the most common cause of death in a Marfan patient?	Ascending aortic dissection
How is albinism generally inherited?	Autosomal recessive inheritance
What is lacking in the epidermis of albino patients?	Melanin
What condition is associated with multiple neuromas on the eyelid, lips, distal tongue, and/or oral mucosa?	MEN, type 2B
Epidermolysis bullosa acquisita (EBA) is associated with which disease?	Inflammatory bowel disease, especially Crohn disease
What haplotype is frequently found in patients with EBA?	HLA-DR2
Which type of collagen is defective in osteogenesis imperfecta?	Type I collagen

Inflammatory/Autoimmune

Which rash often described as a target lesion that has a red center, pale zone, and a dark outer ring (targetoid)?	Erythema multiforme
What are the common causes of erythema multiforme?	Infections; antibiotics; radiation; chemicals; malignancy
What are the most common causes of nonscarring alopecia?	Telogen effluvium; androgenic alopecia; alopecia areata; tinea capitis; traumatic alopecia
What are the most common causes of scarring alopecia?	Cutaneous lupus; lichen planus; folliculitis planus; linear scleroderma
What is the treatment for rosacea?	Avoid precipitating factors; topical metronidazole; sulfur lotions; oral tetracyclines; isotretinoin
What condition has whitish-red nodules especially on digits and over joints, and is associated with uric acid accumulation?	Gout; the classic gouty tophus of the great toe is called podagra.

What is the most likely cause of xanthomas?	Hyperlipidemia
Sharply demarcated, silvery-white plaques on a patient's elbows and knees (extensor surfaces) are most likely a manifestation of what disorder?	Psoriasis
What conditions can trigger psoriasis?	Trauma; infection; drugs
Which major histocompatibility markers are associated with psoriasis?	HLA-CW6; B13; B17; B27
What disorder has scaly, thickened plaques that develop in response to persistent rubbing of pruritic sites?	Lichen simplex chronicus
Which disease results from the deposition of collagen in skin that causes a "hardened" and "thickened" appearance and is associated with Raynaud phenomenon?	Scleroderma
What is scleroderma?	Also known as systemic sclerosis, scleroderma is a chronic disease characterized by accumulation of fibrous tissue in the skin and other organs. The etiology is unknown.
Which antibodies are associated with scleroderma?	Scl-70 (diffuse); anticentromere antibodies (localized)
What other conditions are associated with scleroderma?	Hypertension; gastrointestinal disease; pulmonary fibrosis; kidney disease
Which disease is associated with a rash on the face, particularly the malar areas?	Systemic lupus erythematosus (SLE)
Atopic dermatitis is associated with what conditions?	Asthma and allergic rhinitis. These three features together complete the "allergic triad."
Which test is often helpful in the evaluation of patients with chronic contact dermatitis?	Patch test—small amounts of potential irritants are topically applied to the skin and evaluated over a period of 4 to 7 days for an inflammatory reaction.
What is the most common presentation of contact dermatitis?	Hand eczema, most likely due to occupational exposure

Contact dermatitis is what type of hypersensitivity reaction?

Type IV (delayed hypersensitivity)

What is Reiter syndrome?

Classified as a seronegative spondyloarthropathy, Reiter syndrome is a form of rheumatoid-factor negative arthritis classically associated with urethritis, conjunctivitis, and anterior uveitis.

Eruptive forms of what condition may be associated with Reiter syndrome?

Psoriasis

Which human leukocyte antigen (HLA) types are increased in frequency in patients with dermatitis herpetiformis?

HLA-B8; HLA-DR3; HLA-DQW2

Which rheumatologic disease is associated with a diffuse red rash of the trunk, periungual telangiectasis, proximal muscle weakness, myositis on muscle biopsy, and elevated creatine phosphokinase (CPK) and aldolase?

Dermatomyositis

What is vitiligo?

Partial or complete loss of melanocytes within the epidermis

Vitiligo is most commonly associated with what conditions?

Thyroid disease; pernicious anemia; Addison disease; diabetes mellitus type 1

What are some clinical manifestations of type I hypersensitivity reactions?

Anaphylaxis; urticaria; exanthema; angioedema

Urticaria is what type of hypersensitivity reaction?

Immunoglobin E (IgE)-mediated, type I hypersensitivity reaction

Autoantibodies to desmosomes and desmogleins, the intercellular junctions of epidermal cells, are found in which disease?

Pemphigus vulgaris

Pemphigus vulgaris is associated with which type of autoantibody?

IgG

What are the clinical findings of pemphigus vulgaris?

Patients with pemphigus vulgaris present with multiple, large, often open bullae involving the oral mucosa and skin, especially the scalp, face, axilla, groin, and trunk. They are at high risk of mortality due to secondary infection of open bullae.

Patients with pemphigus vulgaris have an increased incidence of which haplotypes?

HLA-DR4; HLA-DRw6

Touching normal-appearing skin with a sliding motion and having upper portions of the epidermis separate from the basal layer of the epidermis is what physical examination finding?

Nikolsky sign—and is positive (meaning that the layers separate) in pemphigus vulgaris

What are the clinical findings of bullous pemphigoid?

Patients with bullous pemphigoid present with multiple, variously sized, tense (unopened) bullae on erythematous skin distributed over inner thighs, flexor surfaces of the forearm, axillae, groin, and lower abdomen.

What do the autoantibodies in bullous pemphigoid target?

BP1 (bullous pemphigoid peptide 1) and BP2 (bullous pemphigoid peptide 2) in the basement membrane of the epidermis

Bullous pemphigoid is an autoimmune disorder that rarely affects which part of the body (in contrast to pemphigus vulgaris, which affects it frequently)?

Oral mucosa

Dermatitis herpetiformis is often associated with what condition?

Gluten-sensitive enteropathy (eg, Celiac disease)

Mantoux (PPD or TB) skin test, transplant rejection, and contact dermatitis are what type of hypersensitivity reaction?

Delayed hypersensitivity reaction, type IV

Infectious

Viral Exanthems

Describe the rash associated with herpes simplex type I:

Small recurrent painful vesicles involving oral mucosa; recurrent events may appear to be related to stressful life events or periods of other illness.

Describe the rash associated with herpes simplex type II:

Small recurrent painful papules and/or vesicles involving genital mucosa; primary infection may also be associated with fever, headache, vaginal or meatal discharge, and painful urination.

Which test can be used to assist in the diagnosis of herpes virus infection?

Tzanck smear

What is the treatment for herpes simplex?

Topical or oral acyclovir

What infection causes unilateral, painful vesicles along a dermatome of the face or trunk?

Shingles (herpes zoster)—reactivation of a latent varicella zoster virus (VZV) infection that is otherwise dormant in dorsal root ganglia

Which disease of childhood presents with acute vesicular eruptions that occur in successive crops, so that the rash typically consists of vesicles at different stages of resolution?

Primary varicella zoster virus (VZV) infection, also known as chicken pox

What is the classic description of a chicken pox vesicle?

"Dewdrop on a rose petal"

What are the classic six childhood exanthemas?

1. Measles (first disease)
2. Scarlet fever (second disease)
3. Rubella (third disease)
4. Duke disease (fourth disease)—term rarely used today, is controversial if this is truly a separate entity
5. Erythema infectiosum (fifth disease) or more commonly "slapped cheek disease"
6. Roseola (sixth disease)

What childhood exanthema is referred to as "first disease" and how does this present?

Measles—caused by infection with measles virus (paramyxovirus); presents with rash, cough, conjunctivitis, and coryza and Koplik spots on buccal mucosa. The rash is classically red-brown *morbilliform* (maculopapular) rash that spread from head to toe.

What ribonucleic acid (RNA) virus, spread by respiratory droplets, is also called rubeola?

Measles

What are Koplik spots?

Ulcerated lesions on the oral mucosa seen in measles

What childhood exanthema is referred to as "second disease" and how does this present?

Scarlet fever—caused by infection with *Streptococcus pyogenes* (group A beta-hemolytic), presents with sore throat and an erythematous popular rash involving face and trunk that spreads downward

What childhood exanthema is referred to as "third disease" and how does this present?	Rubella (aka German measles)—caused by infection with rubella virus (togavirus), presents with fever and an erythematous maculopapular rash that spreads from head to toe and may become confluent
What are the findings of congenital rubella?	Deafness, glaucoma, cataracts, congenital heart disease, and mental retardation
What childhood exanthema is referred to as "fifth disease" and how does this present?	Erythema infectiosum—caused by infection with parvovirus B19, presents with a lacy erythematous rash over the cheeks ("slapped cheek disease") that may then spread to trunk, arms, and legs
What are the other complications of fifth disease?	Nonimmune fetal hydrops (virus infects and destroys fetal red blood cells); more severe anemia in patients with other types of chronic anemia (like aplastic crisis in a sickle cell patient)
What childhood exanthema is referred to as "sixth disease" and how does this present?	Roseola (exanthema subitum)—caused by infection with human herpes virus-6 (HHV-6) or HHV-7, presents with fever, possibly diarrhea, and rash after defervescence of the fever. The rash is erythematous, maculopapular, and initially distributed over trunk and neck.
What is the causative agent of verruca vulgaris?	Human papillomavirus (HPV)
What HPV serotypes cause the common wart?	• HPV-1—planter/palmer warts • HPV-2—common warts, some forms of plantar warts • HPV-3—flat warts
How does molluscum contagiosum appear clinically?	Flesh-colored umbilicated papules
How does molluscum contagiosum appear microscopically?	Epidermal hyperplasia producing a basin with molluscum bodies (Henderson-Patterson bodies)
What type of virus causes molluscum contagiosum?	Pox virus
What agent causes hand-foot-and-mouth disease?	Coxsackie virus type A16

What are the signs and symptoms of hand-foot-and-mouth disease?	Fever and malaise with small oval vesicles along creases of palms, soles, and lips
Which diseases cause rashes distributed on the hands and feet?	Syphilis; hand-foot-and-mouth disease; Rocky Mountain spotted fever
What is the etiologic agent for mononucleosis?	Epstein-Barr virus (EBV)
What are the classic laboratory criteria for diagnosing mononucleosis?	Lymphocytosis, presence of at least 10% atypical lymphocytes on peripheral smear, and a positive serologic test for EBV
What causes milker nodules?	Paravaccinia virus
What disease may follow paravaccinia infection?	Bullous pemphigoid

Bacterial

What condition is described as having thin-walled vesicles or pustules that rupture to form golden-yellow crusts (honey-colored crusts)?	Impetigo
What is the most common bacterial infection of the skin in children?	Impetigo
What bacteria cause impetigo?	*Staphylococcus aureus* or *Streptococcus pyogenes*
What test is helpful to determine the organism involved in impetigo?	Culture of vesicle or pustule fluid contents and catalase tests (*Staphylococcus* is catalase positive, *Streptococcus* is catalase negative)
What is the infectious agent that causes scalded skin syndrome?	*Staphylococcus aureus*
What is erysipelas ("St. Anthony's fire") and what is the causative organism?	Infection of the dermis by streptococcal species, most commonly *Streptococcus pyogenes*
How do patient with erysipelas present?	With a rapidly enlarging erythematous, swollen, warm, indurated, skin lesion, typically with a sharply demarcated raised boarder. Patients may also have fever.

What is cellulitis and what are the common causative organisms?	Inflammation and often infection of the subcutaneous connective tissue; most commonly caused by *Staphylococcus* or *Streptococcus* species
What is the rapid developing infection of the skin and fascia that may lead to death if not treated quickly?	Necrotizing fasciitis
What are the organisms responsible for necrotizing fasciitis?	Group A streptococci or *Clostridium perfringens*
What is erythrasma and which bacteria are associated with this condition?	A chronic bacterial infection of overlapping skin folds, generally appearing as red-brown patches with sharp borders; usually caused by *Corynebacterium*
What is the most common type of bacterial infection in burn victims?	*Pseudomonas aeruginosa* infections
What is the typical primary syphilis skin manifestation?	Painless indurated genital or lip ulcer (chancre)
What are the typical secondary syphilis skin manifestations?	There are several possible forms, including maculopapular lesions distributed on palms and soles, warts (condylomata lata) involving the anogenital region, symmetric non-pruritic erythematous rash involving the trunk and extremities, or alopecia.
Name the three stages of Lyme disease:	Stage 1: tick bite, erythema migrans Stage 2: disseminated infection—fever, chills, arthritis, meningitis, and so forth Stage 3: persistent infection—usually nervous system damage like encephalitis or peripheral neuropathy
What type of rash is seen in spotted fever?	An inward or centripetal spreading rash
What is the vector for Rocky Mountain spotted fever (*Rickettsia rickettsii*)?	*Dermacentor* tick
What is used to test for typhus and Rocky Mountain spotted fever?	A positive Weil-Felix reaction—tests for cross-reaction of antirickettsial antibodies with *Proteus* antigen
What is the treatment for Rocky Mountain spotted fever?	Tetracyclines or chloramphenicol

What disease does *Rickettsia prowazekii* cause?	Typhus
What is the vector of *R. prowazekii*?	Human body louse
What type of rash is seen in typhus?	An outward or centrifugal-spreading rash
How do the rickettsiae cause severe tissue damage?	Organisms infect endothelial cells and cause vascular leakage, which results in hypovolemic shock, pulmonary edema, renal failure, and central nervous system (CNS) damage.
What does *Rickettsia akari* cause?	Rickettsialpox—papule at the site of a mouse bite degenerates into an eschar, then chills, fever, eventually papulovesicular rash
What is special about Q-fever?	It is the only rickettsial infection transmitted by aerosol; there is no arthropod vector and no rash.
Which type of plague causes painful enlargement of inguinal nodes (buboes)?	Bubonic plague
What is the plague native to the United States that lives in squirrels and prairie dogs?	Sylvatic plague
What are the cutaneous manifestations in Whipple disease?	Hyperpigmentation of scars and sun-exposed skin (melanoderma)

Fungal

What is the easiest and quickest way to determine if the etiology of a skin rash is a fungus?	KOH preparation—will see fungal forms on microscopy
What are the cutaneous mycoses?	A group of skin infections caused by organisms including *Malassezia furfur*, *Cladosporium werneckii*, and dermatophytes. Infections manifest differently according to distribution on the body. Members of this group include: tinea versicolor, tinea pedis, tinea capitis, tinea barbae, and tinea cruris.
Dermatophytes include members of which genera?	*Trichophyton*; *Microsporum*; *Epidermophyton*

What organism is responsible for tinea versicolor?	*Malassezia furfur*
Which form of *M. furfur* generally causes disease?	Hyphal form
What does the rash of tinea versicolor look like?	Groups of variably sized, either hypo- or hyperpigmented, macules with a fine peripheral scale
What is used to treat tinea versicolor?	Topical miconazole; selenium sulfide
Describe the rash of tinea pedis:	Primary infection features erythematous and scaling skin, primarily confined to the web spaces between digits.
What is the treatment for tinea pedis ("athlete's foot")?	Topical or oral antifungals
Describe the rash of tinea capitis:	Usually in children, can present on the scalp with hair loss, erythema, and scale or may be asymptomatic hair loss
What is the most likely etiologic organism of tinea capitis?	*Trichophyton tonsurans*
What is the treatment for tinea capitis?	Griseofulvin; terbinafine
What does disseminated disease of coccidioidomycosis manifests as on the skin?	Verrucous plaques (usually on face); subcutaneous abscesses; pustular lesions

Neoplastic

Skin carcinogenesis is primarily thought to be caused by the accumulation of mutations in which tumor suppressor gene?	p53
What is the most common type of skin cancer?	Basal cell carcinoma
What is the neoplasm that is often described as a pearly, red macule, papule, or nodule that is found on sun-exposed areas of the head or neck?	Basal cell carcinoma
What skin cancer is microscopically characterized by nests of basophilic cells ringed by palisading basophilic cells?	Basal cell carcinoma

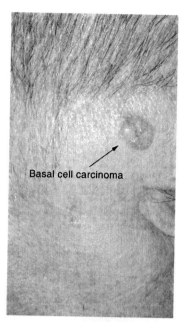

Figure 13.2 Basal cell carcinoma located on the right temple. (Reproduced, with permission, from Wettach T, et al: *Road Map Pathology*, New York: McGraw-Hill, 2009; fig. 3-6.)

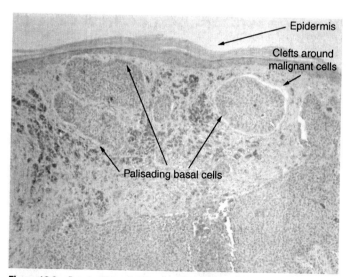

Figure 13.3 Basal cell carcinoma spreading under attenuated epidermis. Note borders of palisading, basaloid cells, and clefting around clusters of malignant cells. (Reproduced, with permission, from OHSU.)

Which neoplasm is often described as a red papule, nodule, or plaque that may be hyperkeratotic or ulcerated on sun-exposed skin?	Squamous cell carcinoma
Arsenic exposure is associated with which type of skin cancer?	Squamous cell carcinoma
Which neoplasm is microscopically characterized by nests of atypical squamous epithelial cells and keratin pearls?	Squamous cell carcinoma
Actinic keratosis lesions may transform into what type of skin cancer if left untreated?	Squamous cell carcinoma
What are some risk factors for squamous cell carcinoma?	Sun exposure; ionizing radiation; actinic keratosis; immunosuppression; arsenic; industrial carcinogens
What are tan/brown plaques or papules that have a "stuck on" appearance and may be found anywhere on the body of adults, except the palms and soles?	Seborrheic keratosis
From what cell type does melanoma arise?	Melanocytes
Large (>20 cm) congenital nevi and dysplastic nevi may be precursor lesions for what type of cancer?	Melanoma
Which clinical criteria are used to help diagnose melanomas?	Asymmetry; Border irregularity; Color variation; Diameter *ABCDs of melanoma
How is dysplastic nevus syndrome inherited?	Autosomal dominant inheritance
On which chromosome is the gene associated with dysplastic nevus syndrome located?	Chromosome 1
What is the peak age range for incident melanoma?	40 to 70 years of age
What are the risk factors for melanoma?	Sunburns; chronic sun exposure; fair skin; dysplastic nevi

What is the most common subtype of melanoma?	Superficial spreading melanoma
Which type of melanoma has the best prognosis?	Lentigo maligna melanoma
Which type of melanoma has the worst prognosis?	Nodular melanoma
What is the most common type of melanoma in dark-skinned individuals?	Acral-lentiginous melanoma
What is the most important prognostic parameter for melanoma?	Depth (Breslow thickness)
In what condition would you find cytoplasmic Birbeck granules through electron microscopy?	Langerhans cell histiocytosis (formerly Histiocytosis X)
In Langerhans cell histiocytosis, proliferation of which cell type is usually found in the epidermis?	Langerhans cells (macrophages)
What are the histologic findings in cutaneous T-cell lymphoma (CTCL) (aka mycosis fungoides)?	Epidermotropic lymphocytes (Sézary-Lutzner cells) and Pautrier microabscesses
What is CTCL called when there is blood involvement?	Sézary syndrome
What type of cutaneous neuroendocrine carcinoma microscopically resembles metastatic small cell carcinoma from the lung?	Merkel cell carcinoma
Which HPV serotypes cause condyloma acuminatum?	HPV 6 and HPV 11
Which autosomal recessive disease is characterized by defective DNA repair and photosensitivity?	Xeroderma pigmentosa
Patients with xeroderma pigmentosa usually develop which skin lesions?	Basal cell carcinoma; squamous cell carcinoma; actinic keratosis; melanoma in childhood
Exposure to ultraviolet (UV) light causes what type of dimers in epidermal cells?	Thymine-thymine dimers

Traumatic/Degenerative

What is the most common type of collagen in a keloid?	Type III collagen
What are the risk factors for keloid formation?	African American race, <30 years of age, and increased skin tension in a wound
Single or multiple bright red papules measuring a few millimeters in diameter that occur predominantly on the trunks and limbs of patients over 40 years are what type of lesions?	Cherry angiomas (senile angiomas)
What skin condition is described as dark, rough-looking, or velvety skin in the axilla or on the back of the neck?	Acanthosis nigricans
What may be associated with acanthosis nigricans?	Long-standing hyperglycemia, some underlying lymphoproliferative disorders
What is the most common cause of burns in children?	Scalds from hot liquids
What is the most common cause of burns in adults?	Accidents with flammable liquids
Which kind of burn affects only the epidermis?	First-degree burn
Which kind of burn usually blisters and affects the dermis and adnexal structures?	Second-degree burn
Which type of burn involves the entire thickness of the skin, including variable amount of underlying fat and causes loss of sensation in affected areas?	Third-degree burn
The scar that follows a deep second- and third-degree burn is composed of what?	Hyalinized collagen

Drugs/Toxins

Which drugs cause erythema multiforme or "target" lesions?

Aspirin; penicillin; sulfonamides; phenytoin; corticosteroids; cimetidine; allopurinol; oral contraceptives

Which drugs cause Stevens-Johnson syndrome?

Sulfa drugs; carbamazepine; phenytoin; valproic acid; phenobarbital; quinolones; cephalosporins; allopurinol; corticosteroids; aminopenicillins

What is Stevens-Johnson syndrome?

A systemic form of erythema multiforme that often occurs with fever, erosions, and hemorrhagic crusts of lesions involving the lips and oral mucosa, may also involve the urethra and genital and perianal areas

What are patients with Stevens-Johnson syndrome more susceptible to due to the rash?

Secondary infection of skin which may result in life-threatening sepsis

Which drugs may induce acne?

Lithium; steroids; androgens; oral contraceptive pills

Which marker is associated with a genetic susceptibility to fixed-drug reactions?

HLA-B22

What do you call a symmetrical, hyperpigmented lesion of the forehead and cheeks that occurs in women who are on oral contraceptives or pregnant?

Melasma

What are some common drugs that are associated with hyperpigmentation?

Bleomycin; minocycline; amiodarone; chloroquine; gold; chlorpromazine; 5-fluorouracil (FU); daunorubicin; busulfan

Which groups of patients have an increased risk of an adverse drug reaction?

Women; patients with Sjögren syndrome; AIDS patients

Which drug causes *red man syndrome* usually during rapid intravenous infusion?

Vancomycin

Metabolism

What is the most likely vitamin deficiency that manifests as petechiae, ecchymoses, abnormal hair growth, bleeding gums, and poor wound healing?

Vitamin C (scurvy)

Which vitamin deficiencies have cutaneous manifestations?

Vitamin C; Vitamin A; Nicotinic acid; Riboflavin; Pyridoxine

What are some skin manifestations of kwashiorkor?

Dry skin; patches of hypopigmentation; skin peeling; peripheral edema; thin hair shafts

Patients with carcinoid syndrome may have which skin manifestation?

Episodes of flushing of the head, neck, and sometimes trunk

What are the metabolic causes of hyperpigmentation?

Porphyria cutanea tarda; hemochromatosis; Vitamin B_{12} deficiency; folic acid deficiency; pellagra; malabsorption; Whipple disease

CLINICAL VIGNETTES

An 8-month-old presents with large, easily ruptured flaccid bullae, with large areas of desquamation of skin and a positive Nikolsky sign. What is the most likely diagnosis?

Staphylococcal scalded skin syndrome

A sexually active 23-year-old patient presents with painful vesicles on his penis and a slight fever. He refers to having the same type of vesicles multiple times a year. Multinucleated giant cells and ballooning of nuclei are seen microscopically. What is the likely diagnosis?

Herpes simplex infection

A 16-year-old presents with multiple dome-shaped, umbilicated, waxy papules on the face and chest. What is the most likely diagnosis?

Molluscum contagiosum

A 35-year-old patient with acquired immunodeficiency syndrome (AIDS) presents with multiple brownish/purplish macules on the trunk and lower extremities. What is the likely diagnosis?

Kaposi sarcoma (human herpes virus 8 [HHV 8])

A 7-year-old presents with multiple hard, rough-surfaced papules on his fingers and elbows. What is the most likely diagnosis?

Verruca vulgaris (common wart)

A 24-year-old man from the Northeast, visits the physician because of a centrifugally spreading, erythematous lesion on his right leg. The patient noticed the rash after he went hiking. What is the most likely diagnosis?

Erythema chronicum migrans (Lyme disease)

A mother brings her 5-year-old son to the physician because she noted her son scratching a pinkish lesion on his neck. Upon examination, the physician notes a ring-shaped scaling plaque with central clearing and elevated borders. What is the most likely diagnosis?

Tinea corporis

A 22-year-old man presents with a rash that first appeared on his palms and soles, and then spread to his face and trunk. The rash initially appeared about 6 days after a camping trip in North Carolina. What is the most likely diagnosis?

Rocky Mountain spotted fever

A 26-year-old woman from Texas complains of small hypopigmented spots on her upper back that usually disappear in the winter months. What is the likely diagnosis?

Tinea versicolor (*Malassezia furfur*)

A 25-year-old sexually active man presents with a painful, nonindurated genital ulcer, and tender regional lymphadenopathy. What is the most likely diagnosis?

Chancroid

A 35-year-old homeless woman visits a shelter physician because of multiple, extremely pruritic papules in her axilla, groin, and finger webs. The patient indicates her husband also has the same lesions. What is the most likely diagnosis?

Scabies

A 15-year-old boy on the school swim team visits the dermatologist because of itchiness on both his feet. He states he is not on any medication and has not had it before. Upon inspection, the physician notes erythematous, dry scaling lesions on both feet. What is the most likely diagnosis?

Tinea pedis

A 67–year-old woman visits her dermatologist because of small reddish papules/pustules predominantly on her cheeks, nose, chin, and forehead. She states that her face becomes worse if she uses hot water or is in warm weather. What is the most likely diagnosis?

Rosacea

A 12-year-old boy visits his physician because of a "slap-like" red mark on his cheek and a rash on his arms that appeared 1 day after the cheek rash. Upon physical examination, the physician notes malar erythema and a maculopapular rash on his extremities. What is the most likely diagnosis?

Fifth disease (erythema infectiosum) caused by Parvovirus B19

A 16-year-old girl is given ampicillin for complaints of fatigue, fever, sore throat, and lymphadenopathy. Two days later, she returns with a cutaneous rash on her face. What is the most likely underlying diagnosis in this patient?

Mononucleosis

A 23-year-old farmhand presents to the dermatologist with multiple red-violaceous nodules on the hand, fever, and history of diarrhea. During the examination, the patient states he is in charge of the cows on the farm. What is the most likely diagnosis?

Milker nodules

A 45-year-old rancher visits a dermatologist because of a black 2-cm lesion on his hand. He states that the lesion was itchy and had a reddish color a day or two ago. What is the most likely diagnosis?

Anthrax (*Bacillus anthracis*)

A 36-year-old migrant worker from Mexico visits the physician because of small disfiguring nodules forming on his ears and hands. The patient also states that he is losing sensation in the affected areas. What is the most likely diagnosis?

Leprosy (*Mycobacterium leprae*)

An inner-city child is brought to the physician because of patches of hair loss. His mother states that he has had this problem for at least a month. The lesions are painless and have some scaling. What is the most likely diagnosis?

Tinea capitis

A 54-year-old man visits the dermatologist because of a dark brown-black 5-mm freckle in between his third and fourth toe. The patient stated that he noticed the freckle about a year and a half ago. The dermatologist biopsies the lesion and under the microscope, the pathologist sees atypical confluent melanocytes with asymmetrical proliferation. What is the most likely diagnosis?

Melanoma

A 40-year-old man has a rash of scaly red patches on his trunk, face, and extremities. A biopsy is taken and superficial dermal infiltrates of T lymphocytes and a collection of atypical lymphocytes are seen within the epidermis. What is the most likely diagnosis?

Cutaneous T-cell lymphoma (Mycosis fungoides)

A 59-year-old man visits his family physician because of loss of appetite, weight loss, and fatigue. During the physical examination, the physician notes dark, rough-looking skin in the axilla region. What should the physician suspect?

An endocrine disorder or a visceral malignancy

A 39-year-old man comes to the physician because he has noted a bluish-black color on his ears, nose, and sclera. The patient also states that his urine is sometimes very dark. What is the most likely diagnosis?

Alkaptonuria

A 45-year-old patient presents with intense skin hyperpigmentation, areas of epithelial desquamation, diarrhea, and confusion. What is the most likely deficient vitamin?

Niacin (nicotinic acid)

A 35-year-old woman visits her physician because she recently noticed multiple small nodules on the back of her ankle. The patient's vital signs are normal and she has no prior clinical illnesses. A blood test is taken with the following results—sodium 142, glucose 100, creatinine 1.0, blood urea nitrogen (BUN) 17, cholesterol 310, triglycerides 412. What do the small nodules likely represent?

Xanthomata

A mother brings her 7-year-old son to the physician because of two small masses on his right chest. The mother states that the child is adopted and does not know the child's family medical history. On examination, 3- and 4-cm masses are palpated overlying his right pectoralis muscle, small tan lesions are seen on his back and right arm, and a small growth is seen on his iris. What is the most likely diagnosis?

Neurofibromatosis (NF) 1

A 16-year-old boy with a clinical history of acne visits his family physician because he has a red rash on his face and various exposed parts. During the examination, he states the rash occurred after he spent a couple of hours outside playing football. What medication is he most likely taking?

Tetracyclines

A 75-year-old woman patient with history of heart problems visits her dermatologist because her skin has begun to turn a light blue color. She is embarrassed to go in public because children say she looks like a "smurf." What medication did her cardiologist most likely give her?

Amiodarone

A 24-year-old woman presents to the dermatologist because of target-like lesions on her right arm. The patient states she is taking some type of antibiotic for a urinary tract infection (UTI). What drug class most likely caused the lesions?

Sulfonamides

A 32-year-old woman visits her family physician because of rapid weight gain, profuse sweating, sudden abnormal hair growth, and easy bruising. Upon physical examination, the physician notes purplish striae on the abdomen, telangiectasia, thin skin, and an increase of fatty tissue on her back at the level of C6. What is the most likely diagnosis?

Cushing syndrome

A 3-year-old boy presents to the physician with a photosensitive rash, cerebellar ataxia, mental disturbances, and aminoaciduria. Niacin levels are within normal range. What is the most likely diagnosis?

Hartnup disease

CHAPTER 14

Musculoskeletal Pathology

EMBRYOLOGY

From what embryologic tissue type are muscle, bone, and connective tissue derived?	Mesoderm
What are the two embryologic processes by which bone may be formed?	1. Endochondral ossification—bones are formed by ossification of a cartilaginous matrix 2. Membranous ossification—bones are formed from connective tissues (eg, the skull)
Describe the process of endochondral ossification:	Primitive mesenchyme differentiates into chondrocytes which create a cartilaginous matrix at what will be the base of an articular surface. Osteoclasts remodel and mineralize this matrix creating bone tissue. Osteoblasts and blood vessels migrate into the newly forming bone.
Which stage of bone formation present in endochondral ossification is missing in membranous ossification?	Cartilaginous stage—in membranous ossification, mesenchyme differentiates directly into fibrous tissue containing osteoblasts.

ANATOMY

What are the three general types of bones in the human body?	1. Long bones 2. Flat bones 3. Short, tubular bones The skeleton can also be classified as axial (central) or appendicular (appendage related).

What are the anatomic portions of long bones?	Epiphysis, metaphysis, diaphysis, and physis (the growth plate)
What are the four tendons that comprise the rotator cuff?	1. Supraspinatus 2. Subscapularis 3. Infraspinatus 4. Teres minor
What are the four major ligaments of the knee?	1. Anterior cruciate ligament 2. Posterior cruciate ligament 3. Medial collateral ligament 4. Lateral collateral ligament
What is the functional difference between a ligament and a tendon?	Ligaments connect bone to bone while tendons connect muscle to bone.
What system innervates smooth muscle?	Autonomic nervous system

HISTOLOGY

In cross-section of the diaphysis, what are the layers observed in bone?	From external to internal: periosteum, cortex, and medullary space
Name the two types of vascular channels found in compact bone:	1. Haversian (longitudinal) canals 2. Volkmann (transverse) canals
What are the main cell types found in bone?	Osteoblasts, osteoclasts, osteocytes, progenitor cells
What are osteoblasts?	Cells derived from osteoprogenitor cells that produce osteoid, hormones for local activity, alkaline phosphatase, and many other matrix proteins
What is osteoid?	A protein material produced by osteoblasts which will mineralize to become bone
What are osteocytes?	Mature osteoblasts that line areas of mineralized bone
What are osteoclasts?	Cells derived from monocytes that are responsible for bone resorption and remodeling
What cell type is responsible for creating calcified columns into which osteoblasts will migrate?	Chondrocytes

What is found in the medullary cavity of long bones?

Trabecular bone, bone marrow, blood vessels

What is the histologic composition of tendons?

Fibroblasts arranged in parallel rows, proteoglycan matrix, and type I collagen fibrils

What are the histologic differences between ligaments and tendons?

These structures are very similar histologically except that ligaments have slightly less collagen and more proteoglycan matrix.

Describe the histologic appearance of smooth muscle tissue:

Smooth muscle consists of spindle shaped cells of variable size each with one centrally placed nucleus.

Describe the histologic appearance of skeletal muscle tissue:

Skeletal muscle consists of tubular shaped cells (myocytes) with abundant red striated cytoplasm and peripherally located nuclei.

What is a sarcomere?

The smallest contractile unit in skeletal muscle. Regions of the sarcomere that are visible histologically, include I-band, A-band, H-band, Z-line, and M-line.

What is the "I-band" in a sarcomere?

A region of only actin filaments—this region becomes smaller during contraction.

What is the "H-band" in a sarcomere?

A region of only myosin filaments within the A-band—this region becomes smaller during contraction

What is the "A-band" in a sarcomere?

Represents the length of the myosin filaments, both ends of which overlap with actin filaments. The A-band stays the same length during contraction.

What molecular events occur during contraction of skeletal muscle?

Calcium enters the myocyte which binds troponin C causing a conformational change that results in release of tropomyosin from the myosin binding region on the actin filaments. In an ATP-dependent reaction, myosin binds the now exposed binding region on the actin filament. Contraction occurs when myosin relaxes back to its resting conformation causing movement of the actin and myosin filaments relative to each other.

| How is the smooth muscle contractile apparatus different from the skeletal muscle contractile apparatus? | The smooth muscle apparatus utilizes calmodulin instead of troponins. |

PATHOLOGY

Congenital

What is the condition in which patients experience failure of longitudinal bone growth resulting in short limbs but normal skull, facial bones, and axial skeleton development?	Achondroplasia
What is the condition associated with a genetic abnormality of type I collagen and susceptibility to bone fractures?	Osteogenesis imperfecta
What is the inheritance pattern of osteogenesis imperfecta (OI)?	Autosomal dominant—but sporadic cases are also possible
What are the abnormalities of type I collagen in OI?	There are eight types of OI, each with different clinical and genetic features. In all cases, there is either a qualitative (abnormal function) or quantitative (abnormal production) defect of type I collagen.
What eye abnormality is classically associated with OI?	Blue-colored sclera—sclera is thinner in OI patients due to collagen defect
What is Ehlers-Danlos syndrome (EDS)?	EDS is actually a group of inherited connective tissue disorders caused by a defect in type III collagen function or production. There are six types of EDS, each with different clinical and genetic features.
What are the usual major signs and symptoms of EDS?	Highly flexible joints which are prone to injury, hyperextension of joints, easy bruising and fragile blood vessels, "stretchy" skin, and abnormal wound healing and scar formation
What is muscular dystrophy?	A group of many inherited muscle disorders that are characterized by progressive skeletal muscle weakness, defective muscle proteins, and ultimately death of myocytes and muscle tissue

What is the most common form of childhood muscular dystrophy?	Duchenne muscular dystrophy
What gene is affected in Duchenne muscular dystrophy (DMD)?	Dystrophin gene—which normally encodes for a protein that is part of a complex which anchors myocytes to the surrounding connective tissue framework. In DMD, this protein is nonfunctional.
What is the inheritance pattern of DMD?	X-linked recessive—predominately affects males, while carrier females have a milder phenotype; sporadic mutations account for one-third of cases
What is Becker muscular dystrophy (BMD)?	Clinically, BMD is a less severe form of DMD. Whereas patients with DMD usually die in the twenties or thirties, patients with BMD may survive much longer.
What gene is affected in BMD?	Dystrophin gene—unlike DMD, in BMD the dystrophin protein is truncated but partially functional. Inheritance is also X-linked recessive.

Anatomic

What is osteopetrosis?	A condition resulting from the failure of normal bone resorption which results in thickened, dense bones
What cell type is defective in osteopetrosis?	Osteoclasts
With what other clinical features may patients with osteopetrosis present?	Anemia, thrombocytopenia, leukopenia—due to decreased marrow space
What is osteitis fibrosa cystica?	Associated with hyperparathyroidism, this condition is characterized by cystic spaces lined by osteoclasts that are filled with fibrous stroma and sometimes blood.
What pattern of serum calcium, phosphorous, and alkaline phosphatase is expected in osteitis fibrosa cystic patients?	Elevated serum calcium, low serum phosphorous, and high alkaline phosphatase

What is osteomalacia? How is this different from rickets?	Defective bone mineralization due to vitamin D deficiency and subsequent decreased serum calcium. This process is called osteomalacia when it occurs in adults and called rickets when it occurs in children.
What is thoracic outlet syndrome?	A syndrome of clinical features resulting from compression of the subclavian artery, subclavian vein, or structures in the brachial plexus as they pass through the superior thoracic outlet
What are some common causes of thoracic outlet syndrome?	Fibrous bands; cervical ribs; hypertrophied muscles

Traumatic

What name is given to a fracture of the distal radius caused by falling onto an outstretched hand?	Colles fracture
What is the most common carpal bone fracture?	Scaphoid fracture
Where is the pain located in scaphoid fractures?	Anatomical snuffbox
What is the injury that results in jersey finger?	Avulsion of flexor digitorum profundus
What causes de Quervain tenosynovitis?	Repetitive movements (like washing, hammering, or skiing) causing inflammation in the tendons of abductor pollicis longus and extensor pollicis brevis which control thumb movements
What nerve is entrapped in carpal tunnel syndrome?	The median nerve as it passes through the carpal tunnel at the wrist
What are some clinical conditions commonly associated with carpal tunnel syndrome?	Diabetes; hypothyroidism; renal failure; heart failure; pregnancy; amyloidosis

Degenerative

What disease is characterized by pain in weight-bearing joints, is worse after use, has crepitation with motion, no signs of inflammation, and is seen in the middle-aged population?	Osteoarthritis, aka degenerative joint disease (DJD)
What are the signs of DJD on x-ray?	Joint space narrowing, osteophytes
What are Heberden nodules?	Palpable distal interphalangeal (DIP) joints with osteophytes
What are Bouchard nodules?	Palpable proximal interphalangeal (PIP) joints with osteophytes
What are some treatments of DJD?	Nonsteroidal anti-inflammatory drugs (NSAIDs) and weight reduction to reduce strain on joints
What is osteoporosis?	Most often, an age-related reduction in bone density and mass
What are the two dominate clinical patterns of osteoporosis?	1. Postmenopausal 2. Senile
Name two fractures that are common among osteoporotic patients:	1. Vertebral crush fractures 2. Distal radius fractures

Inflammatory/Autoimmune

What is podagra?	Gout of the metatarsophalangeal (MTP) joint of the big toe
What is gout?	A condition in which monosodium urate crystals precipitate in joint spaces due to hyperuricemia
What other findings should be looked for in a patient with gout?	Tophi, subcutaneous deposits of uric acid crystals
How do tophi appear on x-ray?	As "punched out" lesions
What lab tests help to diagnose gout?	Uric acid level; joint fluid aspiration of needle-shaped crystals with negative birefringence

What other historical findings are associated with gout?

Thiazide diuretic use; Lesch-Nyhan syndrome; diets with high protein and alcohol

What is the treatment for gout?

Acute—colchicine, NSAIDs; maintenance—allopurinol

What are the notable differences between gout and pseudogout?

Pseudogout is clinically similar to gout except that it affects predominately large joints (eg, knee), is the result of deposition of calcium pyrophosphate crystals, and has no effective treatment options.

What other conditions are associated with pseudogout?

Hyperparathyroidism; hemochromatosis

How are the crystals of pseudogout different from the crystals of gout?

Calcium pyrophosphate (pseudogout) instead of monosodium urate (gout) and weakly positively birefringent (pseudogout) instead of negatively birefringent (gout)

Which joints are most commonly involved in rheumatoid arthritis (RA)?

Wrists, PIP, and metacarpophalangeal (MCP)—generally presenting with morning stiffness, symmetric distribution, and other systemic symptoms

What are some other findings with RA?

Fever; malaise; pericarditis; pleural effusions; uveitis; subcutaneous nodules

Which lab test should you order when you suspect RA?

Rheumatoid factor (RF)

What is rheumatoid factor (RF)?

An immunoglobin M (IgM) antibody to the Fc (fragment crystallizable) portion of IgG

What is the name given to the chronically inflamed cartilage found in RA?

Pannus

What disease would be expected in a young woman that suffers with RA-like symptoms (polyarthritis), leukopenia, leg ulcers, and splenomegaly?

Felty syndrome

What disease is similar to RA (bilateral joint pain, fever) but is seen in children, along with rash and hepatosplenomegaly?

Still disease (juvenile RA)

What is different about juvenile RA compared to adult RA?	It is often RF negative.
A 5-year-old child with juvenile RA presents with complaints in only two joints. Which subtype of juvenile RA is this?	Pauciarticular juvenile RA
What is a child with pauciarticular RA at risk for?	Iritis (requires slit lamp examination to diagnose)
What is Reiter syndrome?	Considered a seronegative spondyloarthropathy, Reiter syndrome is a form of arthritis associated with anterior uveitis or conjunctivitis and urethritis. There is a strong association with HLA-B27 and a male predominance.
What does "seronegative" refer to when discussing spondyloarthropathy?	Patients are seronegative for rheumatoid factor.
Previous exposure to which bacteria can precipitate Reiter syndrome?	*Chlamydia trachomatis*; GI infections including: Shigella, *Salmonella, Campylobacter,* or *Yersinia species*
Name two other types of seronegative spondyloarthropathy:	1. Ankylosing spondylitis 2. Psoriatic arthritis
What is ankylosing spondylitis?	A seronegative spondyloarthropathy involving chronic inflammation of the spine and sacroiliac joints and is also associated with uveitis, aortic regurgitation, and HLA-B27.
What clinical test should be performed in the office if considering a diagnosis of ankylosing spondylitis?	Schober test—decreased angle of anterior flexion of the back, eliciting pain
What is the classic sign on radiograph for ankylosing spondylitis?	Bamboo spine
What is the most common distribution of psoriatic arthritis?	Asymmetric arthritis in fingers or toes
What other symptoms are common with psoriasis?	Nail pitting; psoriatic arthritis with sausage digits
What is the phenomenon that describes the development of a psoriatic plaque in an area of previous trauma?	Koebner phenomenon

What is the name of the sign that occurs when a small amount of scale is removed from a psoriatic plaque, leaving small bleeding points behind?

Auspitz sign

What HLA type is associated with psoriatic arthritis?

HLA-B27

What are the official criteria for the diagnosis of SLE?

Oral ulcers; Renal disorder; Photosensitivity; Hematologic (anemias, cytopenias); Arthritis (nonerosive synovitis); Neurologic (seizures, psychosis); Serositis; Malar rash; Antinuclear antibody; Immunologic (anti-DNA, anti-Smith [anti-Sm], false positive rapid plasma reagin/Venereal Disease Research Laboratory (RPR/VDRL); Discoid rash

*The ORPHANS' MAID has lupus

*4 of 11 criteria are needed for diagnosis

In which sex and race is SLE most common and severe?

African American females

What cardiac lesion is associated with SLE in the adult and consists of nonbacterial verrucous valvular vegetations?

Libman-Sacks endocarditis

What are some other causes for chest pain in a patient with SLE?

Pleuritis; pericarditis

Which antibody system is associated with drug-induced lupus?

Antihistone antibodies

What are wire-loop lesions in the kidney and what do they represent?

Thickening of the capillary wall found in diffuse proliferative glomerulonephritis (GN); indicate a poor prognosis with SLE

Which neoplasm is associated with SLE and myasthenia gravis?

Thymoma

Which antibody is sensitive but not specific for the diagnosis of SLE?

Antinuclear antibody

Which two antibodies are very specific for SLE?

1. Anti-Smith antibody
2. Anti-double-stranded DNA antibody

Which two HLA types is SLE linked to?	1. HLA-DR2 2. HLA-DR3
What is sarcoidosis?	A multisystem inflammatory disease characterized by the presence of noncaseating granulomas often found in the lungs and lymph nodes but can be present in any organ system. Presenting symptoms are often vague but may include arthralgias, muscle pains, and skin rash.
What electrolyte abnormality is common with sarcoidosis?	Hypercalcemia
On biopsy of affected tissue, what is the classic finding?	Noncaseating granulomas
What skin findings are associated with sarcoidosis?	Erythema nodosum; lupus pernio (chronic, indurated, often violaceous skin lesion which may appear on the face, fingers, and ears)
What is scleroderma (systemic sclerosis)?	A condition of excessive fibrosis and collagen deposition throughout the body usually involving the skin and also heart, GI tract, and kidneys
What is the autoantibody that is most closely associated with this disease?	Anti-DNA topoisomerase I (anti-Scl-70) antibody
What are the two types of scleroderma?	1. Diffuse scleroderma 2. CREST syndrome
What are the characteristics of CREST syndrome?	Calcinosis (subcutaneous); Raynaud phenomenon; esophageal dysfunction; sclerodactyly; telangiectasia
What antibodies are most closely associated with CREST syndrome?	Anti-centromere antibody
What is the difference in clinical behavior between diffuse scleroderma and CREST syndrome?	Diffuse scleroderma has widespread skin involvement and rapid progression to involvement of visceral organs. CREST syndrome has a more benign clinical course with skin involvement often limited to the face and fingers.

What are the classic symptoms of Sjögren disease?

Xerostomia (dry mouth) and xerophthalmia (dry eyes)—(this combination is known as Sicca symptoms), secondary to autoimmune destruction of exocrine glands

What other symptoms are commonly associated with Sjögren disease?

Constipation, pancreatic insufficiency, parotid gland enlargement, vaginal dryness

How is Sjögren disease diagnosed?

Lip biopsy—looking for fibrosis and collagen deposition; Schirmer test (showing decreased lacrimation)

What autoantibodies are associated with Sjögren disease?

Anti-nuclear antibody (ANA) (nonspecific) and antinucleoprotein antibodies (SS-A [Ro] and SS-B)

What are patients with Sjögren disease at risk for developing?

Lymphoma

What is polymyositis?

A chronic inflammatory myopathy which may present with proximal muscle weakness. The etiology is not clearly known.

What lab findings support the diagnosis of polymyositis?

Increased ESR; increased creatine phosphokinase (CPK); increased aldolase; increased lactate dehydrogenase (LDH); antinuclear antibody (ANA) may be positive; abnormal electromyography

What is the only specific test that provides a definitive diagnosis of polymyositis?

Muscle biopsy showing lymphoid inflammation

What disease is characterized by symptoms and lab values similar to polymyositis, but also has a lilac edematous rash on the eyelids?

Dermatomyositis

What is the name of the rash on the eyelids found in dermatomyositis?

Heliotrope rash

What is the treatment for dermatomyositis and polymyositis?	High-dose steroids
What is polymyalgia rheumatic?	A syndrome associated with aching and stiffness in the neck, shoulders, and pelvic girdle of older adults. The etiology is not known.
What lab value would be abnormal in polymyalgia rheumatica?	Elevated ESR
With what other disease is polymyalgia rheumatica associated?	Temporal arteritis
What is fibromyalgia?	A chronic syndrome involving diffuse pains affecting the entire body and areas of tenderness in joints, muscles, and other soft tissues
What lab values should be evaluated in fibromyalgia?	CBC—normal; ESR—normal
How should a patient with fibromyalgia be treated?	Nonsteroidal anti-inflammatory drugs (NSAIDs) and antidepressants

Vascular

What is Buerger disease (aka thromboangiitis obliterans)?	A condition of segmental, thrombosing inflammation of medium to small peripheral arteries and veins, often seen in smokers
What are the signs and symptoms of Buerger disease?	Intermittent claudication of small vessels; Raynaud phenomenon; nodular phlebitis
What HLA types are increased in these patients?	HLA-A9 and HLA-B5
What is the treatment for Buerger disease?	Stop smoking
What is Takayasu arteritis?	A chronic inflammatory process affecting medium to large vessels producing a granulomatous thickening of vessel walls, often affecting the aortic arch and proximal great vessels

What lab test is usually abnormal in Takayasu arteritis?	ESR (elevated)
What imaging test should be done?	Angiogram—revealing thickening of the aortic arch and proximal vessels
What are some complications of Takayasu arteritis?	Pulmonary hypertension; stroke
What is Kawasaki disease?	An acute, self-limiting inflammatory process resulting in necrotizing vasculitis of small to medium vessels occurring in infants and children
What are the criteria for a diagnosis of Kawasaki disease?	Fever >5 days; lymphadenopathy; bilateral conjunctival injection; mucosal changes (fissuring, injection, strawberry tongue, erythema); extremity changes (edema, erythema); rash (truncal, may be desquamative); arthritis (may be present)
What are the major complications of this disease?	Coronary artery aneurysms and myocardial infarction
What autoantibodies are found in Kawasaki disease?	Antiendothelial antibodies
Which vessels does Kawasaki disease typically affect?	Medium and small arteries
What should be done if the disease is suspected?	Treat with aspirin and IV immunoglobulin
Why is Kawasaki disease one of the only indications for using aspirin in children?	The risk of developing Reye syndrome limits the use of aspirin in children, a notable exception is in the treatment of Kawasaki disease.
What is Churg-Strauss syndrome?	A systemic vasculitis affecting small to medium vessels causing necrosis of the vessel wall; mainly involving vessels of the lungs, GI tract, and peripheral nerves
How does Churg-Strauss syndrome clinically present?	Often as new-onset or worsening of existing allergies and/or asthma
What are some laboratory findings of Churg-Strauss syndrome?	Blood eosinophilia; increased IgE

Churg-Strauss syndrome may appear clinically similar to which other inflammatory condition?

Polyarteritis nodosa (PAN)

Which autoantibody groups are associated with Churg-Strauss?

Antineutrophil cytoplasmic antibody (ANCA), antimyeloperoxidase antibody

What is temporal cell arteritis?

Also known as giant cell arteritis, it is a vasculitis affecting medium to large arteries, primarily of the head, but can involve other large vessels such as the aorta.

What should be done immediately when this disease is strongly suspected?

Start high-dose steroids

What is the major complication of temporal arteritis that prompt administration of steroids prevents?

Blindness

What is the diagnostic test that confirms temporal arteritis?

Temporal artery biopsy

What would the biopsy show?

Granulomatous arteritis

What is Wegener granulomatosis?

A small to medium vessel vasculitis affecting vessels of respiratory tract and kidneys, often presenting with kidney dysfunction, hemoptysis and pulmonary hemorrhage, and arthritis

Which antibody is found in Wegener granulomatosis?

Classical antineutrophil cytoplasmic antibody (c-ANCA), predominantly antiproteinase 3

What facial deformity is associated with Wegener granulomatosis?

Saddle nose deformity

What is the other disease that involves both the respiratory tract (hemoptysis) and kidney (renal failure)?

Goodpasture syndrome

What is the antibody associated with Goodpasture syndrome?

Antiglomerular basement membrane antibody

What does immunofluorescence (IF) of the biopsy of affected tissue show?

Linear deposits of IgG and C3 in the glomerular basement membrane (GBM)

What is polyarteritis nodosa (PAN)?	A medium vessel vasculitis which can produce ischemic damage via vessel destruction often involving the skin, heart, nervous system, and kidneys
How is the diagnosis made?	Tissue biopsy showing transmural necrotizing arteritis of medium-sized arteries
What is the treatment for PAN?	Steroids and cyclophosphamide
What is the disease that is a variation of polyarteritis nodosa, which affects smaller arterioles, capillaries, and venules rather than the larger vessels?	Microscopic polyangiitis
What clinical symptoms do patients with microscopic polyangiitis have?	Hemoptysis; hematuria; abdominal pain/blood in stool; skin findings (purpura)
Which antibody is microscopic polyangiitis most closely associated with?	Protoplasmic (perinuclear) anti-neutrophil cytoplasmic antibody (p-ANCA)
How is the diagnosis made?	Skin biopsy showing infiltration of dermal capillaries
What is Henoch-Schönlein purpura?	A systemic vasculitis typically occurring in children, which is characterized by the deposition of IgA immune complexes in small vessels of the skin and kidneys.
What are two common clinical histories associated with Henoch-Schönlein purpura?	1. Poststreptococcal infection or upper respiratory infection (URI)—may have an etiologic role 2. Use of a new medication—drug reaction may have an etiologic role
What types of immune complexes are found in tissue biopsy?	IgA dominant
What musculoskeletal pathology is associated with Henoch-Schönlein purpura?	The classic presenting triad includes purpura, arthritis, and abdominal pain. Arthritis classically affects the ankles, knees, elbows, and is nonerosive.

Neoplastic

What is the most common primary benign tumor of bone?	Osteochondroma
What benign tumor of bone has a characteristic "double bubble" appearance on x-ray?	Giant cell tumor of bone
What is an enchondroma?	A benign cartilaginous neoplasm usually found in distal extremities
What is the "most common primary malignant tumor of bone?"	Multiple myeloma—which is actually of hematopoietic origin
What is the most common primary malignant tumor derived from bone (not bone marrow elements)?	Osteosarcoma
In which portion of long bones does osteosarcoma typically present?	The metaphysis
What are some predisposing factors of osteosarcoma?	Previous radiation; previous diagnosis of Paget disease; retinoblastoma
What neoplasm of bone is associated with translocation 11;22?	Ewing sarcoma
In which gender and age group is Ewing sarcoma most common?	Males, less than 15 years old
What neoplasm of bone presents as an expansile mass within the medullary cavity?	Chondrosarcoma

Infectious

What are the presenting features of septic arthritis?	Erythema, warmth, joint pain, and swelling of any joint, but usually knee, hip, shoulder, or spine
How can you make a diagnosis of septic joint?	Arthrocentesis with high white blood cell (WBC) count and Gram stain
What is the most common causative organism?	*Staphylococcus aureus*
What are some common organisms that are found uniquely in the joints of infants and young children?	Group B streptococci; *Haemophilus influenzae*

What are some common organisms associated with implantable devices and prosthetics?

Staphylococcus epidermidis; S. aureus; Gram-negative bacilli

If a patient presents with clinical features of a septic joint, is sexually active, and has symptoms of urethritis, what organism is likely responsible?

Neisseria gonorrhea

How can the diagnosis be made in a patient who is suspected of having *N. gonorrhea* infection?

Urethral swab and culture

How do you treat gonorrhea?

Ceftriaxone

Which organism should be suspected in a patient with diabetes and osteomyelitis?

Pseudomonas aeruginosa

Which organism should be suspected in a sickle cell patient with osteomyelitis?

Salmonella

What is rheumatic fever?

An inflammatory disease that usually occurs 2 to 3 weeks after an acute infection with group A *Streptococcus*. The disease is presumed to be mediated by antibody cross reactivity.

What is antibody cross-reactivity in the context of rheumatic fever?

Host B cells make antibodies against bacterial "M proteins" during the acute infection. After the infection these antibodies begin to attack cells of the host myocardium and joints.

What are the Jones criteria of rheumatic fever?

Fever; Erythema marginatum; Verrucous valvular vegetations; Erythrocyte sedimentation rate (ESR) increase; ARthritis; Subcutaneous nodules; Chorea (Sydenham); Preceded by *Streptococcus* infection

FEVERS and Chorea preceded by a *Streptococcus* infection

What is the distinctive inflammatory heart lesion associated with rheumatic fever?

Aschoff bodies—enlarged eosinophilic collagen surrounded by lymphocytes and macrophages

Which titers are elevated with rheumatic fever?

Antistreptolysin O (ASO) titer; ESR

What type of musculoskeletal pathology is associated with Lyme disease?

The initial presentation of Lyme disease generally includes fever, headache, fatigue, and annular or "bull's eye" skin rash (erythema migrans). If left untreated, patients may also develop nerve palsies, radiculoneuritis, or polyneuropathy.

What causes Lyme disease?

Infection with *Borrelia burgdorferi*, which is transmitted by *Ixodes* tick bites

What cardiac complications are possible with Lyme disease?

First-degree AV-block

At what stage does syphilis infection cause musculoskeletal pathology?

Rarely arthritis can be associated with secondary syphilis. Untreated tertiary syphilis can result in neuropathic joint disease due to degeneration of articular surfaces due to loss of sensation and proprioceptive sense.

What is the best way to diagnose syphilis in the primary stage?

Darkfield microscopic examination

Which serologic test detects syphilis earliest, is the most specific, and stays positive even after treatment?

Fluorescent treponemal antibody absorption test (FTA-ABS)

Which serologic tests are used for a presumptive diagnosis of syphilis?

VDRL and RPR

What are the treatment options for syphilis in primary and secondary stages?

Intramuscular penicillin G

What is the classic reaction occurring hours after treatment that involves shaking chills, sore throat, myalgia, and malaise?

Jarisch-Herxheimer reaction

What is the mechanism by which this reaction occurs?

The reaction is due to release of large quantities of bacterial toxin into the body as a result of antibiotic therapy which overwhelm the body's normal clearance mechanisms.

CLINICAL VIGNETTES

A 14-year-old football player is seen by his PCP for finger pain that began when while in the process of catching a football there was violent hyperextension of his distal interphalangeal (DIP). The patient is able to extend at the joint, but is unable to flex it. What common injury is this?

Jersey finger

A basketball player presents with pain in his finger that began when the basketball struck his rigid finger on the distal tip causing forceful hyperflexion at the DIP. Now the patient is able to flex normally, but there is a decrease in extension. What common injury is this?

Mallet finger

A 45-year-old tennis player presents complaining of pain with extension of the wrist when the elbow is extended. What injury is this?

Lateral epicondylitis (tennis elbow)

A 45-year-old man complains of pain with flexion of his wrist and repetitive contraction of his forearm during golf games. What is the injury?

Medial epicondylitis (golfer's or pitcher's elbow)

A 55-year-old woman housekeeper complains of pain in her thumb, near the radial styloid. The pain is reproduced with ulnar deviation of the fist formed when the thumb is folded across the palm and fingers are flexed over thumb (positive Finkelstein test). What is this injury?

De Quervain tenosynovitis (washer woman's strain)

A 40-year-old woman secretary presents with bilateral numbness and tingling in her hands. She recalls that it is usually after a long day of typing and it is the worst around her thumbs. What is the most likely injury?

Median nerve compression in the carpal tunnel

A 40-year-old woman presents with tingling and numbness over her little finger and part of her ring finger. What is the most likely diagnosis?

Ulnar tunnel syndrome

A 12-lb baby is delivered by a medical student. After the delivery, the baby is found to have medial shoulder rotation and forearm pronation of the left arm. What is the most likely injury?

Erb-Duchenne paralysis (waiter's tip hand)—upper trunk of brachial plexus injury

A 35-year-old man is admitted for a stab wound to the anterior chest just lateral to the midaxillary line. The patient has a winged scapula on physical examination. Which nerve was damaged?

Long thoracic nerve

A 14-year-old boy presents to the ER with a fracture of the humerus in the distal one-third. On physical examination, the boy exhibits wrist drop. What nerve injury is likely to cause this symptom?

Injury to the radial nerve which lies in the spiral groove of the humerus

A 13-year-old girl presents to the ER after a fall and is found to have a fracture of the medial epicondyle. On physical examination, she has a claw hand. Which nerve was damaged by the fall?

Ulnar nerve

A 56-year-old man complains of thickening and contracture of his palms causing his fingers to constantly be in a fist. What is the injury?

Dupuytren contracture (idiopathic palmar fascia contracture)

A 3-year-old child presents to the ER with an injured arm that he refuses to move. The child's mother reports that the injury occurred when she grabbed his arm as he was about to run into the street. The child looks anxious, but is not crying. What injury is likely?

Nursemaids' elbow (slippage of the head of the radius under the annular ligament)

A crying 2-year-old child is brought to the ER by his teenage mother. The mother says that the child fell off the couch and broke his arm. X-ray reveals a spiral fracture and multiple other rib fractures in various stages of healing. What is the most likely diagnosis?

Child abuse

A 35-year-old writer presents with posterior elbow pain and swelling over the olecranon. There is no decrease in the range of motion. What is the injury?

Olecranon bursitis (from chronically resting elbows on desk or from acute trauma to elbow)

A 24-year-old pitcher complains of pain in his shoulder with abduction and elevation of his right arm. What is the most likely diagnosis?

Rotator cuff injury

A 28-year-old bodybuilder presents with pain and numbness in his medial arm that extends to his forearm and little finger. The pain occasionally wakes him up at night. What is the most likely diagnosis?

Thoracic outlet syndrome (impingement on the brachial plexus)

A 23-year-old football player presents with a painful, rigid, flexed neck that is rotated to one side. A prominent sternocleidomastoid is observed. He reports prior neck injury 2 months earlier. What is the most likely diagnosis?

Torticollis

An 85-year-old woman presents to the ER after a fall. She complains of pain in her groin and is unable to rotate her hip. What is the most likely injury?

Femoral neck fracture

What is a major complication of this injury?

Avascular necrosis of the femoral neck

A 13-year-old boy presents with left knee pain that is reproducible with squatting or extending knee against resistance. There is edema over the anterior tibial tuberosity. What is the diagnosis?

Osgood-Schlatter (traction apophysitis)
*SchlaTTer has two Ts for Tibial Tuberosity

A 7-year-old white boy presents to clinic with a limp and some mild groin pain. Imaging shows that there is avascular necrosis of the femoral head. What is the most likely diagnosis?

Legg-Calvé-Perthes disease

A 12-year-old obese African American boy presents with pain in his knee and groin with walking. X-ray shows a wide epiphysis and osteopenia. What is the diagnosis?

Slipped capital femoral epiphysis
*Obese kids are more likely to Slip

A 7-year-old girl presents with fever and a swollen, erythematous knee. Joint fluid is cloudy with gram-positive bacteria and many polymorphonuclear neutrophils (PMNs). What is the most likely diagnosis?

Septic arthritis

A 14-year-old boy presents with bone pain, swelling, and tenderness in his right distal femur. He has decreased range of motion. X-ray shows elevation of the periosteum and a "sunburst pattern." What is the most likely diagnosis?

Osteosarcoma

A 7-year-old boy presents with leg pain. There is a characteristic bone appearance of "onion skinning." The biopsy reveals sheets of small uniform round cells. What is the diagnosis?

Ewing sarcoma

A housekeeper complains of pain anterior to the patella after kneeling repeatedly while scrubbing floors. What is the diagnosis?

Prepatellar bursitis (housemaid's knee)

A 55-year-old with a history of osteoarthritis presents with swelling and pain in the midline of the posterior knee. What is the most likely cause?

Baker cyst

A 19-year-old woman presents after "twisting her ankle." It is determined to be an inversion sprain. What is the ligament that is most likely injured?

Anterior talofibular part of the lateral ligament

A 29-year-old man is admitted to the ER after a motor vehicle accident (MVA). He sustained a crush injury to his lower leg and is in pain. On physical examination, the leg is pale, pulseless, and cold. What is the diagnosis?

Compartment syndrome
*Five Ps—pain, pallor, paralyzed, pulseless, poikilothermal

What is the immediate treatment indicated in compartment syndrome?

Fasciotomy

A 4-year-old boy presents with arthralgias, soft hyperextensible skin, corneal and scleral abnormalities, joint laxity, and easy bruising. What is the most likely diagnosis?

Ehlers-Danlos syndrome

A 32-year-old woman presents to your office complaining of morning stiffness for greater than 1 hour, pain in joints bilaterally, with fatigue and hand deformations over time. What disease should you suspect?

Rheumatoid arthritis (RA)

A patient presents with urethritis, conjunctivitis, arthritis, and happens to be human leukocyte antigen-B27 (HLA-B27) positive; what disease should be suspected?

Reiter disease
*Can't pee, can't see, can't climb a tree

A 43-year-old man presents to your clinic with a history of falling on his knee 2 days ago. Since then, the knee has become red, swollen, and warm. What is the diagnosis?

Septic joint

A 65-year-old man presents to clinic with a 2-hour history of sudden onset of extreme pain in his great toe. What disease should be suspected in this patient?

Gout

A 12-year-old girl presents with migratory polyarthritis, rash, fever, and general malaise. She recalls having a sore throat about 3 weeks ago but did not get treatment. What is the most likely diagnosis?

Acute rheumatic fever

A 35-year-old man presents with diffuse red/purple plaques with silver scale on extensor surfaces and scalp. What disease is suspected?

Psoriasis

A 22-year-old man presents with avascular necrosis of the femoral head. Which hematologic disease should be considered in this patient?

Sickle cell anemia

A 28-year-old African American woman presents to the clinic with new onset of fatigue, weight loss, joint pain, and Raynaud phenomenon. On examination, she is found to have a malar rash. What disease is suspected?

Systemic lupus erythematosus (SLE)

A 30-year-old man presents with new onset of SLE-like symptoms. Which drugs can cause these?

*H*ydralazine; *I*NH; *P*rocainamide; *P*henytoin
*You won't be *HIPP* with drug-induced lupus

A woman with SLE delivered an infant with bradycardia, which is later found to have arteriovenous (AV)-block. What autoantibody could have caused this congenital heart block?

Anti-Ro antibodies which cross the placenta

An 18-year-old woman patient presents with a 5-week history of arthritis, fever, 15-lb weight loss, and diarrhea. What diseases should be considered?

Inflammatory bowel disease (IBD)—Crohn disease or ulcerative colitis

A 33-year-old man complains of joint pain. He mentions that he has noticed an increase in pigmentation along with frequent urination and a strange tendency to set off metal detectors. What is the diagnosis?

Hemochromatosis

A 65-year-old woman presents with increasing headache, vision changes, scalp pain, and jaw pain. She also complains of a few previous months of aching joints and muscles. What should immediately be suspected?

Temporal (giant cell) arteritis

An 18-year-old football player complains of joint pain, bruising, and somewhat limited range of motion. He reports that he has always been a "free bleeder". What is the diagnosis?

Hemarthroses associated with hemophilia

A 15-year-old Boy Scout complains of a 2-week history of flu-like illness and joint pain which started in his left knee, and now is in his right knee. It all began after a camping trip in Connecticut. What is the most likely diagnosis?

Lyme disease

The Boy Scout recalls a strange *bull's eye* rash that appeared and then disappeared before he could get an appointment. What is the rash called?

Erythema chronicum migrans

A 34-year-old abstinent Asian patient presents with a several-year history of arthritis, recurrent genital and oral ulcers, and a painful rash over the pretibial areas. What is the most likely diagnosis?

Behçet disease

An 18-year-old man presents with migratory arthritis, currently in his ankle, a rash, and pain with urination. A Gram stain of urethral discharge shows gram-negative cocci. What is the most likely diagnosis?

Gonococcal arthritis

A 28-year-old man presents with a 2-week history of joint pain, fever, malaise, as well as a new rash all over his body including his palms and soles. What is the probable diagnosis?

Secondary (disseminated) syphilis

A 20-year-old man presents with a 1-month history of worsening back pain that is worse in the morning and improves with exercise. What is the suspected diagnosis?

Ankylosing spondylitis

A 45-year-old smoker complains of cold sensitivity and pain in his fingers. Some fingers have signs of gangrene. What is he suffering from?

Buerger disease (smoking and thromboangiitis obliterans)

A 22-year-old Asian woman presents to your office with arthritis, fevers, night sweats, change in vision, and skin nodules. On physical examination, she is found to have weak and uneven pulses in the upper extremities. What disease should be ruled out?

Takayasu arteritis (pulselessness disease)

A 4-year-old Japanese girl presents to the ER with a 5-day history of fever above 102°F, arthritis, bright red lips, swollen hands and feet, and swollen lymph nodes. What is the most likely diagnosis?

Kawasaki disease (mucocutaneous lymph node syndrome)

A 7-year-old boy presents with arthritis, lower extremity palpable purpura, abdominal pain, and blood in the stool and urine. What is the most likely diagnosis?

Henoch-Schönlein purpura

A young man presents with arthritis, asthma, allergy, weight loss, fever, and vasculitis. What disease is suspected?

Churg-Strauss syndrome

A 42-year-old man presents with chronic sinusitis, hemoptysis, necrotizing granulomas of the nose and palate, and a previous diagnosis of crescentic glomerulitis. What is the diagnosis?

Wegener granulomatosis

A 40-year-old African American woman presents with increasing shortness of breath, polyarthritis, change in vision, fevers, and malaise. On chest x-ray, there is bilateral hilar lymphadenopathy. What is the most likely diagnosis?

Sarcoidosis

A 26-year-old man presents with malaise, fever, weight loss, hypertension, abdominal pain, and melena. He has a history of hepatitis B and drug use. What disease is suspected?

Polyarteritis nodosa (PAN)

A 50-year-old man presents with fever, arthralgias, and palpable purpura on the lower extremities after starting several new medications. What is the most likely diagnosis?

Hypersensitivity angiitis

A 55-year-old woman presents with polyarthritis, dysphagia and reflux esophagitis, pulmonary fibrosis, and hypertension. On physical examination, her face appears tight and masklike and she has swelling of the hands and thickening of the skin. What is the most likely diagnosis?

Scleroderma (systemic sclerosis)

A 50-year-old woman presents with very dry mouth (xerostomia) and dry eyes (keratoconjunctivitis sicca). She reports that she had several dental caries filled recently. What is the most likely diagnosis?

Sjögren disease

A 55-year-old woman presents with 1-month history of proximal muscle weakness and pain, increasing fatigue, and malaise. What disease should be ruled out?

Polymyositis

A 55-year-old woman complains of 3 months of neck stiffness, pelvic and pectoral girdle weakness, and pain, fatigue, and malaise. What is the most likely diagnosis?

Polymyalgia rheumatica

A 45-year-old woman presents with a 2-month history of decreased sleep and several (>11) very tender points on her anterior and posterior torso and neck that produce extreme pain with palpation. She has a history of an anxiety disorder and depression. What is the most likely diagnosis?

Fibromyalgia

CHAPTER 15

Pediatric Pathology

CARDIOVASCULAR

What are the characteristics of Tetralogy of Fallot (TOF)?

Pulmonary valve stenosis; Right ventricular hypertrophy; Overriding aorta; Ventricular septal defect (VSD)

*You have to PROVe TOF with an echo

What is the treatment for TOF?

Surgical repair

How does the anatomy differ from normal in transposition of the great arteries (TGA)?

The aorta arises anteriorly from the right ventricle, while the pulmonary artery (PA) arises from the left ventricle. The aorta is posterior to the PA in a normal heart. This condition may also be referred to as transposition of the great vessels (TGV) by some sources.

Is TGA compatible with life?

No, unless there is a shunt (patent ductus arteriosus [PDA], VSD, patent foramen ovale [PFO], etc) present to allow mixing of the blood

What are the five congenital heart diseases that cause cyanosis (right-to-left shunt) early in postnatal life?

1. Truncus arteriosus
2. TGA
3. Tricuspid atresia
4. Tetralogy of Fallot
5. Total anomalous pulmonary venous connection (five words)

*5Ts—count them out on your hand

Why does right-to-left shunting cause cyanosis?

Right-to-left shunting means that deoxygenated blood from the right side of the heart passes into the left side of the heart and is pumped to the systemic circulation. This bypasses the lungs, resulting in circulation of deoxygenated blood which does not meet the oxygen demand of peripheral tissues, resulting in cyanosis.

382 Deja Review: Pathology

What is the murmur associated with a patent ductus arteriosus (PDA)?

Continuous machinery-like murmur

At birth, what is used to close a PDA?

Indomethacin

What is used to keep a PDA open?

Prostaglandin E (PGE)

What is the most common congenital cardiac anomaly?

VSD

What are the different types of VSD?

Membranous (most common); infundibular; muscular (multiple: Swiss-cheese septum)

What are the three congenital heart diseases that cause a left-to-right shunt and late cyanosis?

1. PDA
2. VSD
3. Atrial septal defect (ASD)

*All are three-letter acronyms containing a D

Why does late cyanosis occur?

With persistent left-to-right shunting, pulmonary resistance increases, leading to pulmonary hypertension. Eventually a left-to-right shunt becomes a right-to-left shunt, causing cyanosis.

What is the name for the situation when a left-to-right shunt becomes a right-to-left shunt?

Eisenmenger syndrome

What are the different types of ASDs?

Primum (septum primum fails to fuse with endocardial cushions); *Secundum* (most common due to inadequate development of the septum secundum)

What are endocardial cushion defects?

A spectrum of malformations including VSD, foramen primum, cleft anterior leaflet of the mitral valve, and atrioventricular canal defects

What cardiac defect is associated with Turner syndrome?

Coarctation of the aorta

What are the two types of coarctation of the aorta?

1. Infantile type—aortic stenosis is proximal to the insertion of the ductus arteriosus (DA)
2. Adult type—aortic stenosis is distal to the insertion of DA

What are the clinical and radiographic characteristics of coarctation of the aorta?

Higher blood pressure in the upper extremities when compared to the lower; notching of the ribs

RESPIRATORY

What are the risk factors for infantile respiratory distress syndrome (IRDS)?

Prematurity, male gender, maternal diabetes, and delivery by cesarean section

What is the etiology of IRDS?

Insufficient pulmonary surfactant

What does the chest x-ray of an infant with RDS show?

Uniform, minute reticulogranular densities producing a diffuse "ground-glass" appearance

What are the microscopic features of RDS?

Collapsed air spaces, expanded respiratory bronchioles, and alveolar ducts lined by eosinophilic hyaline membranes

What is the treatment of IRDS?

Surfactant replacement therapy and oxygen

What is the treatment given to the mother to prevent IRDS?

Steroids (glucocorticoids)

What is the classic presentation of cystic fibrosis (CF)?

History of meconium ileus; recurrent sinusitis, bronchitis; foul smelling stools

How is the diagnosis of cystic fibrosis confirmed?

Sweat test shows increased sweat chloride concentration

What is the genetic defect in cystic fibrosis?

Autosomal recessive mutation of the cystic fibrosis transmembrane conductance regulator (CFTR) gene on chromosome 7

What is the pathogenesis of cystic fibrosis?

The defective chloride channel causes secretion of abnormally viscid mucus that plugs the liver, pancreas, and lungs. This leads to impaired food digestion and absorption and increased susceptibility to pulmonary infections leading ultimately to chronic infection and subsequent respiratory failure.

What organisms infect and may subsequently colonize the lungs of individuals with cystic fibrosis?

Pseudomonas aeruginosa; Staphylococcus aureus; Hemophilus influenza; Burkholderia cepacia

What is the treatment for cystic fibrosis?

There is no curative treatment. Symptomatic treatment with N-acetylcysteine can loosen mucous plugs. Antimicrobials are given for pulmonary infections. Ultimately, lung transplant may be necessary. Pancreatic enzyme replacement is also typically needed.

What clinical feature of cystic fibrosis is unique in males?

Congenital bilateral absence of the vas deferens, azoospermia, and infertility

What is the number one cause of death in infants age 1 month to 1 year?

Sudden infant death syndrome (SIDS)

What preventative measure has been shown to reduce the incidence of SIDS?

"Back to bed"

GASTROINTESTINAL

What congenital malformation typically presents with immediate regurgitation upon feeding?

Tracheoesophageal fistula (TEF)

What are the defects associated with tracheoesophageal fistula?

Vertebral; Anal; Cardiac; Tracheal; Esophageal; Renal; Limb
*The VACTERL anomalies

What is the most common type of tracheoesophageal fistula?

~85% of cases are a blind upper esophageal atresia with a distal fistula between the lower esophagus and trachea (Type C).

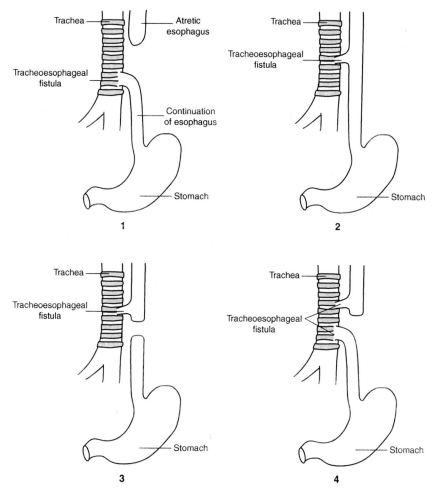

Figure 15.1   Types of tracheoesophageal fistulas. **1.** Type C—esophageal atresia with distal TEF, most common type, ~85% of cases. **2.** H type—TEF without atresia, about ~5% of cases. **3.** Type B—esophageal atresia with proximal TEF. **4.** Type D—esophageal atresia with both proximal and distal TEF. (Type A is not shown, but is esophageal atresia without TEF.)

How does pyloric stenosis typically present?	Projectile, nonbilious vomiting in a 2- to 4-week-old, classically firstborn male, infant
What is the pathogenesis of pyloric stenosis?	Hypertrophy and possibly hyperplasia of the muscularis propria in the pylorus. Inflammation and edema may also contribute to further narrowing of the pyloric outlet.

What is the treatment of pyloric stenosis?

Pyloromyotomy (surgical muscle splitting)

What malformation is associated with projectile, bilious vomiting, and bloating in a new born?

Annular pancreas

How does an annular pancreas form?

A band of pancreatic tissue (from a bifid ventral pancreatic bud) surrounds the duodenum

What congenital malformation is associated with Down syndrome and presents with bilious emesis within the first day of life?

Duodenal atresia

What is the radiographic finding/sign associated with duodenal atresia?

The *double bubble* sign (air bubbles in the stomach and duodenum)

What is the treatment for duodenal atresia?

Surgical repair

What is a Meckel diverticulum?

Persistence of the vitelline duct, which connects the developing gut to the yolk sac

What are the characteristics of Meckel diverticulum?

- 2% of the general population have a Meckel diverticulum
- 2% of Meckel diverticula are symptomatic
- Symptoms occur in patients 2 years old or younger, typically
- They arise 2 ft from the ileocecal valve
- They are 2 in (3-5 cm) in length
- There are 2 types of commonly associated ectopic tissue—gastric and pancreatic

*Follow the rule of 2s and try not 2 miss it!

What is the classic presentation of intussusception?

Severe episodic abdominal pain, often patients will curl into the fetal position, sometimes accompanied by nausea, vomiting, and bloody stools

What is the pathophysiology of intussusception?

Proximal portion of the gastrointestinal (GI) tract telescopes into the adjacent portion; proximal portion, or leading point, may be a Meckel diverticulum, polyp, or tumor

What is the treatment for an intussusception?

Air contrast enema to increase intraluminal pressure and facilitate reduction of the intussusception

What are the clinical characteristics of Hirschsprung disease?

Delayed passage of meconium, constipation, and abdominal distention

What is the next step in diagnosis?

Rectal biopsy showing lack of ganglion cells is confirmatory.

The biopsy of the intestine reveals a lack of ganglion cells (in Auerbach and Meissner plexuses) in the muscle wall. What is the mechanism of this defect?

Failure of neural crest cell migration. These neural crest cells eventually become ganglion cells.

What is the treatment of Hirschsprung disease?

Colostomy prior to corrective surgery allows for pelvic growth and normalization of dilated bowel.

An infant is born with the abdominal contents outside the body, yet contained in a midline sac of peritoneum. What is the diagnosis?

Omphalocele

*The "O" reminds you of the belly button which is midline and covered (by skin)

What other abnormalities are associated with omphalocele?

GI and cardiac defects

An infant is born with the abdominal contents outside of the body lateral to the umbilicus and not covered by peritoneum. What is the most likely diagnosis?

Gastroschisis

What are the classic features of appendicitis?

Right lower quadrant abdominal pain (often initially periumbilical), fever, vomiting

What is the treatment of appendicitis?

Appendectomy

Which side of the body is more common for a congenital diaphragmatic hernia?

Left

What is the pathogenesis of congenital diaphragmatic hernia?

Abnormal formation of one of the pleuroperitoneal membranes or a defect in the fusion of pleuroperitoneal membrane with the septum transversum and mesentery of the esophagus

What is the treatment of congenital diaphragmatic hernia?	Surgical repair
What is the most common complication/cause of death in congenital diaphragmatic hernia?	Respiratory distress secondary to pulmonary hypoplasia
What is necrotizing enterocolitis (NEC)?	Severe gastrointestinal disease of neonates of currently unclear etiology that is characterized by necrosis of the mucosa of the intestine. Premature infants are at particularly high risk of developing NEC.

MUSCULOSKELETAL

What is the genetic defect in Duchenne muscular dystrophy?	X-linked (Xp21.2) deletion of the dystrophin gene
Why are the calf muscles large in Duchenne muscular dystrophy?	Pseudohypertrophy of calf muscle due to fibrofatty replacement of muscle
How do you diagnose Duchenne muscular dystrophy?	Muscle biopsy and elevated creatine phosphokinase (CPK)
What is the typical clinical course of Duchenne muscular dystrophy?	Progressive muscular atrophy requiring wheelchair use by 12 to 15 years of age and eventual death from respiratory complications typically in the patient's twenties
What is a milder form of myopathy that also contains a mutated dystrophin gene?	Becker muscular dystrophy
What is the clinical presentation of osteogenesis imperfecta?	Multiple bone fractures ("brittle bones"), which may be initially suspicious for child abuse, and blue sclerae
What is the pathogenesis of osteogenesis imperfecta?	Deficiencies in the synthesis of type I collagen
What is the inheritance pattern and gene mutation of osteogenesis imperfecta?	Autosomal dominant mutation of the COL1A1 gene

What is achondroplasia?

The most common form of dwarfism, resulting in shortened limbs with relative preservation of trunk length. Other features include macrocephaly, frontal bossing, and "trident" hand appearance.

What is the inheritance pattern and gene mutation of achondroplasia?

Autosomal dominant inheritance of FGFR3 mutation on the short arm of chromosome 4

What is the classic presentation of osteosarcoma?

Teenage or young adult male with leg pain (there may be swelling if the tumor is large enough), classically located in the distal femur

What are the histological features of Ewing sarcoma?

Sheets of uniform, small, round, blue cells; scant, clear cytoplasm; Homer Wright rosettes

What is the genetic defect associated with Ewing sarcoma?

Translocation of 11;22

What is the treatment for Ewing sarcoma?

Chemotherapy and surgical excision with or without radiation

What are the other *small round blue cell tumors* which may occur in children?

Lymphoma; Neuroblastoma; Rhabdomyosarcoma; Ewing sarcoma; Wilms tumor

*Remember *Lyn Rhew* knew tumors

What is the most common soft tissue tumor of childhood and adolescence?

Rhabdomyosarcoma

What are the three histologic variants of rhabdomyosarcoma?

1. Embryonal—sheets of blue cells and diagnostic rhabdomyoblasts
2. Alveolar
3. Pleomorphic

NEUROLOGIC

During a newborn examination in the nursery, you note a tuft of hair over the base of the spine. What is the most likely diagnosis?

Spina bifida occulta

What neural tube defect causes meninges to herniate through a spinal canal defect producing a cystic swelling at the base of the spine?

Meningocele

What neural tube defect causes meninges and the spinal cord to herniate through a spinal canal defect?

Meningomyelocele

What diet supplement has been shown to reduce the incidence of neural tube defects?

Folic acid

What clinically characterizes an absence seizure?

Short (5-10 second) intervals of unresponsiveness, where the patient "stares off into space"

How do you diagnose absence seizures?

Electroencephalogram (EEG) will show the classic 3-Hz spike-and-wave pattern

What is the treatment for absence seizures?

Ethosuximide

What is the classic presentation of infantile spasm?

4- to 6-month-old infant with onset of tonic seizures occurring in clusters of 5 to 10 spasms (but may be as many as 100). Clusters may occur 10 to 12 times a day. Spasms tend to occur upon awakening and feeding. Often patients will also have evidence of developmental delay.

What is the characteristic finding on EEG for infantile spasms?

Hypsarrhythmia—abnormal interictal high amplitude waves and background of irregular spikes

What is the treatment for infantile spasms?

Adrenocorticotropic hormone (ACTH)—primarily short-term therapy

How does neurofibromatosis type 2 (NF2) differ from neurofibromatosis type 1 (NF1)?

NF2 is characterized by bilateral acoustic neuromas, meningiomas, gliomas, schwannomas, neurofibromas which are unlikely to undergo malignant transformation, and juvenile cataracts.

NF1 is characterized by prominent cutaneous findings (café au lait spots, axillary and inguinal freckles), neurofibromas which are more likely to undergo malignant transformation, optic gliomas, and Lisch nodules.

*Remember all of the -omas in type II

What is the genetic association with NF1 and NF2?

- NF1—chromosome 17q
- NF2—chromosome 22q

What are the characteristic findings of Sturge-Weber syndrome seen on CT?

Calcifications in the cerebral cortex in a railroad-track pattern

What is responsible for the clinical symptoms observed in tuberous sclerosis?

Symptoms are secondary to small benign tumors (tubers) that grow on the face, eyes, brain, kidney, and other organs.

What is the genetic defect in VHL disease?

Deletion of *VHL* gene on chromosome 3

*Three letters for chromosome 3

What is the treatment for hereditary hemorrhagic telangiectasia (Osler-Weber-Rendu) syndrome?

Iron and folate supplementation for anemia (due to blood loss) along with surgical excision of enlarging or symptomatic arteriovenous malformations

What is the most common brain tumor in children?

Medulloblastoma

What are the clinical characteristics of medulloblastoma?

The tumor may compress the fourth ventricle causing an increase in intracranial pressure and hydrocephalus.

What are the histologic characteristics of medulloblastoma?

Hypercellular small round blue cell tumor; rosettes or perivascular pseudorosettes

What is the classic histologic characteristic associated with astrocytoma?

Rosenthal fibers

Table 15.1 Lysosomal Storage Diseases

Disorder	Inheritance Pattern	Lysosomal Deficiency	Deposited Substance
Gaucher	AR	β-Glucocerebroside	Glucocerebroside
Tay-Sachs	AR	Hexosaminidase A	GM2 gangliosides
Niemann-Pick	AR	Sphingomyelinase	Sphingomyelin
Krabbe	AR	Galactosylceramide β-galactosidase	Galactocerebroside
Fabry	X-linked recessive	α-Galactosidase A	Neutral glycosphingolipids
Hunter	X-linked recessive	Iduronate sulfate	Heparan and dermatan sulfate
Hurler	AR	α-L-iduronidase	Heparan and dermatan sulfate

SYNDROMES

For more on genetic syndromes, please refer to Chapter 3, "Genetic Pathology."

What are the clinical features of Pierre Robin sequence?	Micrognathia, glossoptosis, upper airway obstruction, and cleft lip/palate
What are the clinical features of Treacher Collins syndrome?	Micrognathia, small zygoma, malformed or absence external ears (with resultant conductive hearing loss), lower eyelid colobomas, down slanting eyes, dropping lower eyelids
What is the developmental defect in DiGeorge syndrome?	Failure of the third and fourth pharyngeal pouches to differentiate
What are the clinical features of fetal alcohol syndrome?	Delayed/poor growth, dysmorphic facies (smooth philtrum, thin lips, and small palpebral fissures), mental retardation, and other CNS manifestations
What effects can alcohol have on fetal cellular development?	Alcohol can cause inhibition of cell migration, disruption of cellular differentiation and growth, and disruption of DNA and protein synthesis.
How does the fetus metabolize alcohol?	Fetal alcohol dehydrogenase activity is less than 10% of that observed in the adult liver, so the fetus is dependent primarily on maternal hepatic metabolism.

CLINICAL VIGNETTES

A 4-month-old girl has a history of cyanosis while feeding. She has an x-ray that reveals a boot-shaped heart. What is the most likely diagnosis?

Tetralogy of Fallot (TOF)

A 4-year-old boy presents for a well-child checkup. On examination, you note a continuous machinery-like murmur. What should you suspect?

Patent ductus arteriosus (PDA)

A 2-year-old girl presents with a flat, hypoplastic face, prominent epicanthal skin folds, small, low-set ears, stubby fingers, a transverse palmar crease, and mental retardation. What is the diagnosis and what cardiac malformation do you suspect?

Trisomy 21 (Down syndrome) with an endocardial cushion defect

A mother brings her 15-year-old daughter to your clinic because she does not show any signs of breast development. The girl is 4 ft 10 in tall, with a webbed neck, pigeon chest, and delayed sexual development. What do you suspect?

Turner syndrome

A newborn, born at 28 weeks gestational age, begins gasping for air. She shows signs of cyanosis and retraction of the sternum. What is the most likely diagnosis?

Infantile respiratory distress syndrome (IRDS) (aka hyaline membrane disease)

An infant, born at 42 weeks gestational age, develops respiratory distress. His birth was complicated by fetal distress and the amniotic fluid was stained with meconium. What is the most likely cause of distress?

Meconium aspiration (chemical pneumonitis)

A 5-year-old white boy presents with a history of a meconium ileus at birth, recurrent sinusitis, and foul-smelling stools. What diagnosis should you consider?

Cystic fibrosis

The parents of a 4-month-old boy present to the ED after finding their son lifeless in his crib. The autopsy, examination of death scene, and review of the case history are negative. What is the probable cause of death?

Sudden infant death syndrome (SIDS)

A 2-day-old girl is evaluated in the newborn nursery with immediate regurgitation when feeding is attempted. What is the most likely diagnosis?

Tracheoesophageal fistula

A 3-week-old boy presents to your ED with projectile, nonbilious vomiting. He has a palpable abdominal "olive" on examination. What is the most likely diagnosis?

Hypertrophic pyloric stenosis

A 2-week-old newborn presents with forceful, bilious vomiting, and abdominal distention. What do you suspect?

Annular pancreas

An 18-month-old presents to your office with painless, rectal bleeding. She has a history of intestinal obstruction with a volvulus at birth. What is the most likely diagnosis?

Meckel diverticulum

A 13-month-old girl presents with intense, episodic abdominal pain and currant-jelly stools. On examination, you palpate a sausage-like mass in the right upper quadrant. What do you suspect?

Intussusception

A 4-day-old infant with a patent anus has not passed a bowel movement and is developing abdominal distention. An abdominal x-ray after a barium enema reveals a dilated megacolon. What do you suspect?

Hirschsprung disease

A 17-year-old boy presents with lower abdominal cramping and bloody diarrhea. Colonoscopy reveals mucosal damage extending from the rectum proximally in a continuous fashion. What do you suspect?

Ulcerative colitis

A 13-year-old boy presents with watery diarrhea and a 10-lb weight loss over the past 2 months. On examination, you find perianal fissures and a fistula. What is the most likely diagnosis?

Crohn disease

An 8-year-old girl presents to the ER with abdominal pain, fever, and vomiting. She states the pain began around her belly button and now she has right lower quadrant pain and rebound tenderness. What is the most likely diagnosis?

Appendicitis

An infant, born at 25 weeks gestational age with birth weight of 1450 g, begins to develop bloody stools, abdominal distention, and circulatory collapse. Abdominal x-ray reveals gas in the intestinal wall. What do you suspect?

Necrotizing enterocolitis (NEC)

A 3-year-old girl presents with hematuria and abdominal pain after falling off her tricycle. On physical examination, you palpate a mass in her abdomen. What is the most likely diagnosis?

Wilms tumor (WT)

A 7-year-old boy presents with tea-colored urine. His mother reports that he had a sore throat 2 weeks ago. What is the most likely diagnosis?

Poststreptococcal glomerulonephritis

A 24-year-old woman has a stillbirth. There is a history of severe oligohydramnios throughout pregnancy. What is a potential cause of the stillbirth?

Bilateral renal agenesis

At autopsy, an infant with bilateral renal agenesis is also found to have pulmonary hypoplasia and limb and facial deformities. What is the associated syndrome?

Potter syndrome

A 40-week gestation infant is seen in the newborn nursery with underdevelopment of the mandible, glossoptosis, and a cleft palate. What do you suspect?

Pierre Robin syndrome

Another infant presents with underdevelopment of the zygomatic bones, mandibular hypoplasia, lower lid colobomas, and malformed external ears. What is the most likely diagnosis?

Treacher Collins syndrome

A 3-month-old girl is taken for surgical aortic arch repair. During the operation, the surgeon cannot find the thymus. You note that she also suffers from hypocalcemia, a cleft palate, and low-set ears. What is the most likely diagnosis?

DiGeorge syndrome

A 14-year-old girl presents with intermittent draining from a midline swelling in her anterior neck. She reports that it often moves with her tongue. What is the most likely diagnosis?

Thyroglossal duct cyst

A 13-year-old girl presents with a left-sided anterior neck swelling. What is the most likely diagnosis?

Branchial cleft cyst

You are making rounds in the neonatal intensive care unit. One infant has rocker-bottom feet, low-set ears, micrognathia, a prominent occiput, and clenched hands. What is the name and cause of the most likely diagnosis?

Edwards syndrome—caused by Trisomy 18

Another child in the unit presents with microcephaly, microphthalmia, cleft lip/palate, abnormal forebrain structures, and polydactyly. What is the name and cause of the most likely diagnosis?

Patau syndrome—caused by Trisomy 13

A 35-week gestation infant is born with intrauterine growth retardation, indistinct philtrum, shortened palpebral fissures, and microcephaly. The mother is a known alcoholic. What is the most likely diagnosis?

Fetal alcohol syndrome

A mother brings in her 13-month-old daughter because she is concerned that she is not sitting up, crawling, or saying any words. You note the child has microcephaly, a moonlike face, and a high-pitched cry. What is the name and cause of the most likely diagnosis?

Cri du chat syndrome—caused by a macrodeletion of the short arm of chromosome 5 (5p-)

A 7-year-old boy presents with his mother who states she cannot control his appetite. She catches him eating food out of the trash cans and she had to put a lock on the pantry. He has small extremities, mental retardation, and microphallus. What is the name and cause of the most likely diagnosis?

Prader-Willi syndrome—Paternal 15q11-13

A 9-year-old girl presents to the clinic with inappropriate laughter, hypopigmentation of the irises, ataxia, tongue protrusion, and seizures. What is the name and cause of the most likely diagnosis?

Angelman syndrome—Maternal 15q11-13

A 4-year-old boy with abnormally large calves presents to your office. You watch as he rises from the floor putting his hands on his thighs to help him stand. What is this called and what is the diagnosis?

Gowers maneuver—Duchenne muscular dystrophy

A 5-year-old boy presents to your office with his sixth fracture. On careful examination, you note he has blue sclerae. What is the most likely diagnosis?

Osteogenesis imperfecta type I (brittle bone disease)

A 2-year-old girl presents for her well-child check-up. You note she is short in stature, has shortened limbs, frontal bossing, and slight midface deficiency. What do you suspect?

Achondroplasia

An 18-month-old presents for an abnormal gait. The parents report he has bowing of the legs and lumbar lordosis. You also note craniotabes and a pigeon breast deformity. What do you suspect?

Rickets (Vitamin D deficiency)

A 14-year-old boy presents with left knee pain and swelling that has increased over the month. On examination, you palpate a mass over the tibia with warmth, tenderness, and decreased range of motion in the knee. What is the most likely diagnosis?

Osteosarcoma, the most common primary malignant tumor of the bone in children

A 12-year-old boy presents with a painful mass on his thigh. You note the area is tender, warm, and swollen. An x-ray shows a destructive lytic tumor with surrounding bone in an "onion-skin" appearance. What is the most likely diagnosis?

Ewing sarcoma

A 4-year-old girl presents with high, spiking fevers for 3 weeks. She also has a rash, body aches, and refuses to stand. You find she has lymphadenopathy and joint swelling. What do you suspect?

Juvenile rheumatoid arthritis (JRA)

An 8-year-old girl previously diagnosed with attention-deficit/hyperactivity disorder presents with continued attention problems. Her mother states that several times a day, her daughter will stare off into space for 5 to 10 seconds, become unresponsive, and have eye fluttering. What do you suspect?

Absence seizures

A 7-month-old boy with developmental delay presents to your office with a history of tonic seizures occurring daily for the past week. His mother states the seizures involve both arms and occur in clusters of 5 to 10 spasms. What is the likely diagnosis?

Infantile spasms (West syndrome)

A 2-month-old presents to your office with unusual skin lesions. On examination, you count 10 café au lait spots, note freckling in the axilla, and pigmented iris hamartomas (Lisch nodules). What do you suspect?

Neurofibromatosis 1 (NF1) (von Recklinghausen disease)

A 5-year-old girl presents with recurrent nausea, vomiting, and headaches. She has an ataxic gait, retinoblastoma, and hemangioblastomas of the brain. What is the most likely diagnosis?

von Hippel-Lindau (VHL) disease

A 3-year-old boy with a history of infantile spasms presents to your office for evaluation. On examination, you note an *ash-leaf* lesion on his back, sebaceous adenomas on his face, and retinal phakomas. What is the likely diagnosis?

Tuberous sclerosis

A 4-year-old girl presents to your office with a large port-wine stain over her face, encephalofacial angiomatosis, mental retardation, and epilepsy. What do you suspect?

Sturge-Weber syndrome

A 6-year-old boy presents with recurrent epistaxis, hepatomegaly with right upper quadrant pain, telangiectasias, and a family history of similar symptoms. What do you suspect?

Hereditary hemorrhagic telangiectasia (HHT) (aka Osler-Weber-Rendu syndrome)

A 13-year-old boy from England presents with fatigue, easy bruising, bone pain, and hepatosplenomegaly. A peripheral blood smear reveals pancytopenia without leukemic cells. What do you suspect?

Gaucher disease (Type 1), the most common lysosomal storage disease

A 2-month-old girl presents to your office with decreased eye contact, increased startle response, seizures, and a cherry-red spot on the macula. What do you suspect?

Tay-Sachs disease

A 12-month-old presents with failure to thrive, organomegaly, seizures, and discolored skin. What do you suspect?

Niemann-Pick disease

A 6-month-old girl presents with optic atrophy, spasticity, and dies within 1 month. What is the most likely cause of death?

Krabbe disease

A 6-year-old boy presents in a pain crisis with angiokeratomas, hypohidrosis, and corneal opacities. What is the most likely diagnosis?

Fabry disease

A 14-month-old boy presents with coarse facies, mild mental retardation, gingival hyperplasia, organomegaly, but no corneal clouding. What do you suspect?

Hunter syndrome

An 8-month-old girl presents with coarse facies, severe mental retardation, gingival hyperplasia, organomegaly, and corneal clouding. What is the most likely diagnosis?

Hurler syndrome

A 7-year-old girl presents with persistent headaches over the past month and recent onset of left-sided facial paralysis. What might you suspect?

Astrocytoma

A 5-year-old boy presents limping into your office with petechiae on his face and chest. He has a temperature of 100.5°F and hepatomegaly. What do you suspect?

Acute lymphoblastic leukemia (ALL)

A 3-year-old girl presents with a mediastinal mass and immature T cells. What do you suspect?

Lymphoblastic lymphoma

CHAPTER 16

Radiology & Pathology Correlation

GENERAL PRINCIPLES

What are x-rays?

Electromagnetic waves that interact with matter and are absorbed, scattered, or transmitted

How are plain radiographs produced?

By passing an x-ray beam through the patient and producing an x-ray shadow on film

What are the five basic densities on a radiograph, from least to most dense?

1. Air—least dense
2. Fat
3. Water (blood and soft tissue)
4. Bone
5. Metal—most dense

How do the different densities appear on film?

Air does not absorb much radiation and appears black (radiolucent). Fat is generally gray and darker than muscle or blood. Bone and calcium appear white (radiopaque), as do metals and contrast agents, which absorb significant amounts of radiation.

Why are frontal and lateral views necessary when assessing plain radiographs?

Each view is a two-dimensional representation of a three-dimensional structure, and therefore two views are necessary to capture all three dimensions and to perform a complete evaluation.

What do the terms posteroanterior (PA) or anteroposterior (AP) indicate?

The direction in which the x-ray beam traverses the patient on its way to the film

What are decubitus films?

Films taken with the patient lying directly on his or her side

Why is patient position important when evaluating a radiograph?

It can affect apparent organ size (eg, magnification of heart size), organ position, and blood flow.

What is the advantage of using contrast agents in radiography?

It allows better visualization of anatomic structures that are normally obscured by surrounding structures of similar densities.

What is computed tomography (CT)?

A diagnostic imaging method in which x-ray measurements from many angles are combined into a single image which is typically presented as a series of axial body slices

What is the relative radiation exposure per chest CT scan in comparison to a plain chest x-ray?

100 fold increase in radiation

What is the main advantage of CT over plain radiography?

CT produces higher quality and more detailed images.

Why should you NOT use intravenous (IV) contrast when doing a CT on a patient with a new head injury?

IV contrast can be confused with fresh blood in the brain.

What is ultrasonography?

A technique using high-frequency sound waves to make images

What else can be evaluated using these sound waves?

The direction and magnitude of moving blood (Doppler analysis)

What makes the technology used in ultrasonography attractive?

It does not use ionizing radiation and is relatively inexpensive.

What is nuclear imaging?

A noninvasive imaging technique that creates a picture by measuring the radiation emitted from a patient's body after a radioactive material has been injected and allowed to distribute within the body.

What is magnetic resonance imaging (MRI)?

A diagnostic procedure that uses a combination of a large magnet, radio frequencies, and a computer to produce detailed images of the soft tissues of the body

What are the two basic types of images in magnetic resonance (MR)?	1. T1-weighted images 2. T2-weighted images
How does a T1-weighted image show fat and water?	Fat is seen as a bright signal (white) and water as a dark signal (black)
How does a T2-weighted image show fat and water?	Fat is seen as a dark signal (black) and water as a bright signal (white)
What are some advantages of MR?	Can produce detailed images of the central nervous system (CNS) and stationary soft tissues; does not use ionizing radiation
What are the disadvantages of MR?	Artifact is produced if the patient moves; inability to bring ferrous objects near the magnet; high cost and time intensive
What are the contraindications to having an MR scan?	Cardiac pacemakers, defibrillators, spinal cord stimulators, most aneurysm clips, and a patient's inability to stay still (ie, children, claustrophobia)

HEAD AND NECK

What two modalities provide definitive imaging of the skull and brain?	1. CT 2. MRI
When is CT the procedure of choice?	When there is trauma (possible loss of bone integrity, penetrating injury, or hemorrhage) or the possibility of hemorrhagic stroke
When is imaging indicated in a patient with a headache?	Trauma, severe headache (ie, worse headache of the patient's life), headache with neurologic findings
What does a *thunderclap headache* or a sudden onset of the "worst headache of one's life" indicate?	Subarachnoid hemorrhage
What should one suspect if there is a fracture over the middle meningeal artery area?	Epidural hematoma
What are the signs of a basilar skull fracture?	Hemotympanum, periorbital ecchymoses (*raccoon eye*), cerebrospinal fluid rhinorrhea or otorrhea, and Battle sign

What is a Battle sign?

Ecchymosis over the skin of the mastoid region of the skull

What does a noncontrast CT scan show when there is acute brain hemorrhage?

An area of increased density

What additional findings can you have with an intracranial bleed?

Mass effect leading to compression of the ventricles or midline shift

What are the two types of stroke?

1. Ischemic
2. Hemorrhagic

Which patients tend to get hemorrhagic strokes?

Hypertensive or anticoagulated patients

What imaging technique is most appropriate for visualization of an acute hemorrhagic stroke?

A noncontrast CT scan because the fresh blood is very dense and appears white

Can the diagnosis of stroke be excluded with a normal CT scan?

No, a scan within 12 hours of the event may not yet show changes on CT.

What is the best way to visualize an ischemic stroke?

MRI. An ischemic stroke is difficult to visualize on a CT scan unless there is mass effect whereas edema due to ischemia can be identified as a bright area on MR T2-weighted images.

What is the best initial way to visualize an intracranial aneurysm?

CT-Angiography or MRI

Where do most intracranial aneurysms occur?

Anterior communicating artery

What is the imaging method of choice for most CNS neoplasms?

MRI

Are meningomas considered intracranial or extracranial tumors?

Extracranial—they arises from arachnoid cells external to the brain parenchyma.

Where is the majority of adult and pediatric primary brain tumors located, respectively?

Adult—supratentorial; pediatrics—infratentorial

On imaging, a pediatric patient has a suprasellar (supratentorial) mass with calcifications, what is the likely diagnosis?

Craniopharyngioma

What is the imaging study of choice for a patient with suspected multiple sclerosis (MS)?

An MRI of the brain and spinal cord because it will show demyelination plaques

Does the workup of vertigo involve imaging procedures?

No, unless patients do not respond to initial conservative measures

When vertigo is accompanied by sensorineural hearing loss, what type of study is suggested?

MRI of the brain

When vertigo is accompanied by conductive hearing loss, what type of study is recommended?

CT scan of the petrous bone

What is the best technique used to image intracranial infections?

MRI

What is the imaging procedure of choice for a patient with seizures?

MRI

Who requires imaging as part of a seizure workup?

Patients with new-onset seizures; epileptics with poor therapeutic response to medicines; seizure patients with new neurologic deficits

What is the initial imaging procedure of choice for a facial fracture?

Plain radiography

What is the best imaging technique for diagnosing upper airway obstruction?

Lateral soft tissue view of the neck

What is seen on lateral film when a patient presents with epiglottitis?

The affected epiglottis looks like a thumb rather than its normal curved shape ("thumb" sign)

What is seen on lateral film when a patient presents with a retropharyngeal abscess?

Prevertebral soft tissue swelling with or without air inside the tissue

What type of imaging should be done on a patient who presents with hyperthyroidism and an enlarged gland?

Radioactive iodine uptake scan, a type of nuclear medicine thyroid scan

What type of imaging should be done on a solitary thyroid nodule or a multinodular goiter?

Ultrasound with FNA (fine needle aspiration) of suspicious solid or calcified nodules

CHEST

When should an expiratory film be ordered in addition to the routine inspiratory film?

Suspected pneumothorax; suspected postobstructive atelectasis with foreign body aspiration

Is chest radiography routinely ordered for uncomplicated asthma attacks?

No, unless aspiration of foreign object needs to be excluded

What are the complications of an acute asthma attack, seen on a plain film?

Pneumomediastinum and pneumothorax

What is bronchiectasis?

Dilatation of the bronchi, either diffuse or focal, often as a result of chronic infection and subsequent cartilage damage

What is seen on chest radiograph in a patient with bronchiectasis?

Involvement of the medial aspects of both the right and left lower lobes with associated pleural thickening and honeycombing

What is seen on the chest x-ray of a patient with chronic bronchitis?

Increased or indistinct bronchovascular markings at the lung bases and bronchial wall thickening

When are chest radiographs indicated for patients with chronic obstructive pulmonary disease (COPD)?

Only with acute exacerbation, a suspected pneumonia, or history of weight loss

What is atelectasis?

Collapse of a small area of lung with resorption of air from the alveoli

What conditions cause atelectasis?

Obstructing bronchial lesion; extrinsic compression; fibrosis; loss of surface tension in the alveoli; shallow inspiration or decreased mobility

What commonly causes the collapse of an entire lung segment?

Obstruction—for example, a mucous plug, tumor, or foreign body such as malposition of an endotracheal tube

On chest x-ray (CXR), what is a consolidation and what does it represent?

An area of increased density (whiteness), that represents alveolar spaces filled with some material other than air, for example, pus, blood, fluid, or cells.

What is an air bronchogram?

Increased visibility of a bronchus secondary to a change (increase) in the surrounding density. For example, water or edema in the lungs makes the surrounding lung more dense on CXR, highlighting the contrast between the now water-filled lung parenchyma and air-filled bronchus (an air bronchogram).

How is pneumonia diagnosed?

Correlation of signs and symptoms (clinical features) with confirmatory evidence of CXR

What does bacterial pneumonia look like on chest x-ray?

Typically, a dense consolidation that may involve patches of lung, a segment, or the entire lobe

In general, how would atypical PNA appear on CXR?

Bilateral, often diffuse ground glass consolidations

What does primary tuberculosis look like on chest x-ray?

Focal consolidation of the middle or lower lobe with lymphadenopathy and pleural effusion

What does reactivation tuberculosis look like?

Consolidation or cavitary nodule of either the posterior segment of the upper lobe or the superior segment of the lower lobe without lymphadenopathy

What are the complications of tuberculosis?

Death, miliary tuberculosis, abscess, empyema, secondary infection

What does healed tuberculosis look like on chest radiography?

Affected lung parenchyma undergoes fibrosis (especially in apices), often with areas of calcification (Ghon complex)

What does miliary tuberculosis look like on chest radiography?

A diffuse bilateral process with multiple very small nodules scattered throughout both lungs (named after the appearance of millet seeds)

What causes lung abscesses?

Necrotic pneumonias or superinfection of cavitary lesions

What is the typical appearance of a lung abscess?

A nodule or large mass with central cavitation that may have an air-fluid level and a thick wall ("rind")

What is the differential diagnosis of a thick-walled cavitary lesion in the lung?

Either a lung abscess or a cavitating neoplasm, usually squamous cell carcinoma

What is the next step in the diagnosis of a lung abscess?

Bronchoscopy or CT-directed needle biopsy

What are Kerley B lines?

Linear opacities on chest x-ray that represent interlobular lymphatics which have been distended by fluid or tissue. They are an indication of increased pulmonary venous pressure.

What conditions are associated with Kerley B lines?

Left ventricular failure (CHF) and mitral stenosis

What are the findings of CHF on chest radiography?

Cardiomegaly, pulmonary vascular congestion and edema, Kerley B lines, and bilateral pleural effusions

What is the differential diagnosis for a solitary pulmonary nodule?

Granuloma; primary lung cancer; metastatic lesion; septic embolus; arteriovenous malformation; hamartoma; small area of atelectasis

What are the characteristics of a benign nodule?

Well-defined, round with dense central calcifications

What is the most important tool for characterizing a solitary pulmonary nodule?

Comparison of the patient's current chest radiograph to an old chest radiograph

What lung cancers more commonly arise centrally (near the hilum)?

Squamous cell and small cell carcinomas

What are the peripherally located lung cancers?

Adenocarcinomas and large cell lung carcinoma

What is the most valuable imaging method for staging lung cancers?

CT scan

Where do lung cancers commonly metastasize?

Lymph nodes, liver, bones, brain, and adrenal glands

What does lymphoma classically look like on chest x-ray?

Large anterior mediastinal mass with hilar adenopathy

What is the most common cancer found in the lung?

Metastatic carcinoma

What is a *spontaneous* pneumothorax (PTX)?

An accumulation of air in the pleural space that results in lung collapse, often from rupture of an apical bleb

What is a *tension* pneumothorax?

A tension PTX is accumulating air in the pleural space, secondary to trauma, leading to creation of a one way valve that leads to continual increase of air in the pleural space and therefore increasing intrathoracic pressure. This results in a mediastinal shift with depression of the hemidiaphragm and displacement of the heart and trachea away from the side of the pneumothorax.

What is the negative outcome of increased intrathoracic pressure?

This is a medical emergency! The increase intrathoracic pressure decreases venous return and ultimately can lead to death.

How large does a pleural effusion need to be in order to be seen on a routine upright chest radiograph?

At least 250 mL

What is an empyema?

Pus within the pleural space usually as a result of a primary infectious process or postsurgical/posttraumatic circumstances

What are the most common etiologies of anterior mediastinal masses?

Thymoma, ectopic Thyroid, Teratomas, and Terrible lymphomas

*Four Ts

What are the most common etiologies of middle mediastinal masses?

Lymphadenopathy (lymphoma, sarcoid), duplication cysts, teratoma, fat pad, diaphragmatic hernia, extension of esophageal or bronchogenic carcinoma

What are the most common etiologies of posterior mediastinal masses?

Neurogenic tumors, including neurofibromas, schwannomas, or ganglioneuromas; other lesions include hernias, lymphadenopathy (lymphoma), aortic aneurysm, hematomas, or extramedullary hematopoiesis

On what side do most ruptures of the diaphragm occur?

On the left side because the liver usually protects the right side from damage

CARDIOVASCULAR SYSTEM

What causes cardiomegaly or an enlarged cardiac silhouette?

Valvular disease, cardiomyopathy, congenital heart disease, pericardial effusion, and mass lesions

In general, how can one differentiate between the multiple causes of cardiomegaly on plain film?

Cardiomyopathies and pericardial effusions generally lead to symmetric enlargement, whereas valvular disease and congenital heart disease often have specific chamber enlargement.

What are some causes of dilated cardiomyopathy?

Ischemia, alcohol, infections, metabolic disorders, collagen vascular disease, and toxic agents such as chemotherapeutic drugs

What does acute enlargement of the cardiac silhouette most likely represent?

Pericardial effusion

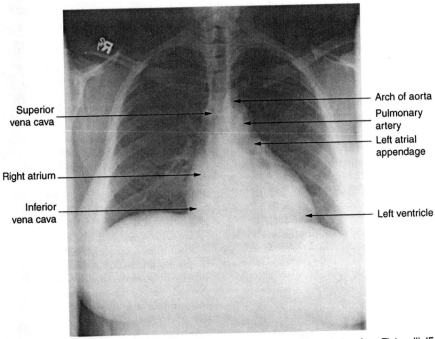

Figure 16.1   Normal CXR—Mediastinal silhouette. (Reproduced, with permission, from Tintanalli JE, Kelen GD, Stapczynski JS: *Tintinalli's Emergency Medicine: A Comprehensive Study Guide*, 6th ed, New York: McGraw Hill; fig 61-1.)

What does cardiac enlargement secondary to pericardial effusion look like?

The heart is pendulous and is much wider at the base giving it the appearance of a water bag.

What is the imaging procedure of choice if a pericardial effusion is suspected?

Echocardiography

What imaging studies provide the best quantitative evaluation of cardiac ejection fraction?

Nuclear medicine gated blood pool or multiple gated acquisition (MUGA) studies; echocardiography

What is the normal left ventricular ejection fraction?

65% to 75%

At what point does a patient require an angiogram?

Only if ejection fraction is less than 35% or if exercise treadmill, nuclear medicine, or echocardiography results are positive

What causes isolated left atrial enlargement?

Mitral stenosis

What is seen on a frontal chest radiograph of a patient with mitral stenosis?

Prominence of the left atrial appendage and the widening of the inferior carinal angle (greater than 75°)

What are the clinical signs of constrictive pericarditis?

These include signs of right cardiac failure such as hepatomegaly, distended neck veins, ascites, and peripheral edema.

What is the best study for constrictive pericarditis?

Echocardiogram

What are the three most common causes of pulmonary artery enlargement?

1. Pulmonary stenosis
2. Pulmonary hypertension
3. Patent ductus arteriosus (PDA) or atrial septal defect (ASD) (due to increased flow through the pulmonary artery)

What is found on chest x-ray if a patient has tetralogy of Fallot?

Decreased pulmonary vascularity and a boot-shaped heart with an uplifted apex and a concavity along the left cardiac border

What is the differential diagnosis for cardiomegaly with an enlarged right atrium?

Ebstein anomaly/malformation, tricuspid atresia, and pulmonary atresia

Which causes of cyanotic heart disease have increased pulmonary vascularity?

All have increased vascular markings except tetralogy of Fallot.

What are the causes of acyanotic heart disease with normal pulmonary vascularity?

Aortic stenosis, pulmonary stenosis, coarctation, and interruption of the aortic arch

What should one look for in the case of acyanotic heart disease with increased pulmonary vascularity?

Left atrial enlargement and a possible PDA or VSD

How is coarctation of the aorta diagnosed?

Coarctation is suspected clinically with asymmetric pulses and/or blood pressures (classically, with hypertension in the right upper extremity, hypotension in the lower extremities, and diminished femoral and peripheral pulses). The diagnosis is confirmed with imaging, MRI, CT, or ECHO.

What is a characteristic x-ray finding of coarctation?

Notching of the inferior aspect of the ribs due to erosion by tortuous and dilated intercostal arteries that form secondary to necessary collateral flow given the restricted aortic blood flow

What are the chest x-ray findings in a patient with PE?

Most commonly there are NO findings on chest x-ray! If the PE is large enough to cause pulmonary infarction then a wedge-shaped consolidation (Hampton hump) and/or pulmonary vascular asymmetry (Westermark sign) may be apparent.

What is the most sensitive and specific study to evaluate for suspected PE?

CT angiogram (CTA) is the gold standard

What are the signs of a PE on an angiogram?

Signs include an abrupt termination of a vessel or an intraluminal filling defect

If a patient cannot tolerate a CTA (eg, in patients with renal failure) or in some subsets of patients including otherwise healthy nonsmokers or pregnant women, what other study can be obtained to evaluate for possible PE and minimize radiation exposure?

Ventilation-perfusion scan (V/Q scan)

What kind of defect does a PE cause on a V/Q scan?

A defect on the perfusion scan that is not seen on the ventilation scan (mismatched defect)

V/Q scans are of little value in what type of emboli?

Septic or fat emboli

What is the most common source of a PE?

Lower extremity DVT

What is the initial imaging test of choice for a patient with suspected DVT?

Duplex ultrasonography

What is seen on ultrasound when a DVT is suspected?

With pressure, the femoral vein usually compresses, but when there is a clot within the vein, echoes are seen within the lumen and no compression is identified.

A patient gets a nuclear medicine study to evaluate his coronary artery disease (CAD). How is a defect seen on both stress and rest images different from a defect seen only on stress images?

A defect seen on both stress and rest images likely represents a scar, whereas a defect seen only on stress images implies ischemia.

How are individual coronary arteries visualized and localized?

Coronary angiography

What does calcification of the aortic arch on chest x-ray suggest?

This clearly demonstrates that the patient has atherosclerosis, implying that they may also have underlying coronary artery disease (CAD) and/or peripheral artery disease (PAD).

What yields the most definitive evaluation of normal and anomalous aortic anatomy?

Injection of contrast material directly into the aorta (contrast angiography)

What is the most common cause of aortic tears?

Traumatic disruption secondary to motor vehicle accidents

What are the signs of a tear on an AP chest radiograph?

Increased mediastinal density and width at or above the level of the aortic arch; apical pleural density caused by blood above the left apical portion of the lung; deviation of the trachea to the right and depression of the left mainstem bronchus

What is the initial test of choice to exclude aortic injury?

CT scan

What causes aneurysms of the aortic arch and the descending thoracic aorta?

The most common cause is atherosclerosis, but they can also result from fibromuscular dysplasia and cystic medial necrosis.

What causes aneurysms of the ascending aorta?

Historically, aneurysms of the ascending aorta were due to syphilis. At present, Marfan syndrome is the more likely cause.

What is an aortic dissection?	Separation of the layers of the wall of the aorta secondary to intimal tearing that allows for the creation of a false lumen where blood flow can occur
Which patients have an increased risk of developing an aortic dissection?	Hypertensive patients with atherosclerosis
What is a characteristic finding of aortic dissection on chest x-ray?	Dilated aorta with a widened and dense mediastinum and cardiomegaly
What other imaging technique can be used to diagnose dissection?	CT scan
What is the best way to evaluate an abdominal aortic aneurysm?	Abdominal ultrasonography
When is surgery an appropriate treatment option for patients with abdominal aortic aneurysms?	When the abdominal aortic diameter exceeds 5 cm
What is the gold standard for the evaluation of peripheral arteries?	Contrast angiography

BREAST

What is the study of choice for breast imaging in women >40 years?	Mammography
What is the primary purpose of screening mammography?	To detect small breast cancers in asymptomatic patients early enough to intervene and improve survival
What are the two views that mammograms are obtained in?	1. Craniocaudal 2. Axillary oblique views
How do the breasts of young women differ from those of older females?	Young women have extremely dense breast tissue, whereas older women have more fatty tissue and atrophy of the breast parenchyma.
Why are mammograms not recommended for women under the age of 30?	Cancer is not easily detected by mammography in dense tissue.
What imaging technique is used to assess cancer in high-risk young women?	Ultrasonography

What factors are associated with an increased risk of breast cancer?

Female gender; advancing age; early menarche/late menopause (estrogen effect); nulliparity; first pregnancy after age 30; first-degree relative with breast cancer; history of invasive or in-situ breast cancer; history of atypical epithelial proliferations (atypical ductal hyperplasia or atypical lobular hyperplasia); history of certain benign proliferative lesions (RR 1.5-2.0)

What are the primary mammographic signs of breast cancer?

Tumor (mass/density), often stellate appearance; clustered microcalcifications; asymmetric additional densities

What are the secondary mammographic signs of breast cancer?

Nipple retraction; skin thickening or dimpling; asymmetry of ductal or vascular markings; fixation of the skin overlying the abnormality; enlarged axillary lymph nodes

Are all calcifications a sign of cancer?

No, some calcifications can be entirely benign

What are the examples of benign breast calcifications?

Calcifications that are rounded in appearance and greater than 2 mm in size; serpiginous calcifications which are seen within blood vessel walls (linear pattern) in women over 60 years

What happens after an abnormality is detected on mammography?

Further investigations, including magnified mammogram, ultrasound examination, or a biopsy

An ultrasound examination of the breast is useful for distinguishing what types of lesions?

Solid lesions from cystic ones

Where are most breast tumors located?

Upper outer quadrant of the breast

GASTROINTESTINAL

What is the most common imaging study of the abdomen?

A plain film of the abdomen (aka KUB [kidneys, ureter, bladder])

What are the things one should look for on a plain abdominal film (KUB)?

Gas pattern, organ shapes and sizes, calcifications, basilar lung abnormalities, and skeletal abnormalities

What is the imaging study of choice used to examine nonintestinal abdominal pathology?

CT scan

What is the role of ultrasonography in abdominal imaging?

It is used primarily to image the liver, kidneys, gallbladder, and common bile duct.

What is the easiest way to identify small amounts of free air in the peritoneal cavity?

Upright chest x-ray or KUB. Free air in the abdomen will rise and be visible under the diaphragm.

What is a Rigler sign?

A Rigler sign is visualization of the bowel wall due to normal air within bowel loops (intraluminal air) on one side of the bowel wall and abnormal free air within the abdominal cavity on the other side of the bowel wall.

What radiographic study is used to assess esophageal motility and morphology?

An esophagogram or fluoroscopic study of the esophagus

What are important esophageal abnormalities often found by esophagogram?

Esophageal varices, tumors of the esophagus, esophageal strictures, and diverticula. Motility disorders such as scleroderma and achalasia can also be assessed.

Under what condition would you order an upper gastrointestinal (GI) series?

For radiographic evaluation of the esophagus, stomach, duodenum, and/or the proximal small bowel

What are some of the more common entities diagnosed by an upper GI series?

Hiatal hernias, peptic ulcers, and carcinomas of the stomach (linitis plastica)

What is a small bowel series?

Serial films of the abdomen that are obtained as contrast agent (usually barium) progresses through the small bowel. It is usually done in conjunction with an upper GI series.

When is a small bowel series usually ordered?

Usually when the jejunum or ileum are the location of suspected pathology. It is particularly useful when patients are suspected of having malabsorption (sprue), regional enteritis (Crohn disease), or a small bowel obstruction.

A barium study is indicated for the diagnosis of what conditions?

Carcinoma of the colon; colonic polyps; diverticulosis/diverticulitis; inflammatory bowel disease; large bowel obstruction

What are the two imaging modalities that are often used to evaluate the appendix?

1. Ultrasound (especially in children)
2. CT scan

What imaging studies are used to evaluate diverticulitis?

CT scan is used to confirm the diagnosis of acute diverticulitis. A contrast enema and/or endoscopy can be used later on, but have no role in acute presentation due to an increased risk of bowel perforation.

What are the classic clinical and radiographic signs of UC?

Pseudopolyps, lead-pipe colon on barium study, and toxic megacolon

What are the classic clinical and radiographic signs of Crohn disease?

Fistulas/abscesses, cobblestoning, and string sign on barium study

What is ischemic colitis?

Inflammation and injury to the bowel secondary to diminished blood flow which can occur secondary to thrombosis in the superior or inferior mesenteric artery, hypercoagulable states, small vessel disease, or obstruction of the colon

What will a plain abdominal film reveal in a patient with ischemic colitis?

It may reveal free air or *thumb printing* from mucosal edema/intramural hemorrhage.

True or false? About 90% of polyps are hyperplastic or only show low-grade dysplasia (and are essentially benign):

True

What would an ultrasound study reveal in a patient with acute cholecystitis?

Sonographic Murphy sign (RUQ pain with pressure from the US probe); thickening of the gallbladder wall; stones in the gallbladder (cholelithiasis); fluid around the gallbladder

What other test is useful in assessing gallbladder function (evaluate for biliary dyskinesia), especially when ultrasound fails to confirm a diagnosis of cholecystis?

A nuclear medicine hepatobiliary iminodiacetic acid (HIDA) scan

What are the complications of acute pancreatitis and the study of choice to rule out these complications?

Possible complications include pseudocyst and abscess formation, which typically present 4 to 6 weeks after the original bout of pancreatitis. A CT scan is the imaging modality of choice.

What are the two most common imaging techniques used to evaluate the biliary system?

1. Ultrasonography
2. Endoscopy

What imaging procedure can also be used for therapy?

Endoscopy with cannulation can be used for biliary drainage

What causes biliary obstruction?

Common duct stone; carcinoma of the head of the pancreas; carcinoma arising from the common duct ampulla (Ampulla of Vater); carcinoma of the small bowel involving the ampulla

GENITOURINARY SYSTEM

What is the initial imaging study for the urinary system?

A plain film of the abdomen (KUB)

What classically can a KUB evaluate for?

"Stones, bones, gases, and masses"

What should one look for when examining the kidneys?

Size, shape, position, and axis

What is the simplest, noninvasive method of evaluating the kidneys?

Renal ultrasonography

Renal ultrasonography is the preferred imaging technique used to study patients who have a high risk of reacting to contrast material. Who are these patients?

Pregnant women; patients with impaired renal function (creatinine >2 mg/dL); patients with proteinuria; diabetics; patients with CHF; patients with a prior contrast reaction

What is the most utilized imaging modality for the urinary tract and what is it used to evaluate?

CT scan:
- Noncontrast studies—stone disease (including ureteral stones), other calcifications, overview of anatomy
- Contrast studies—masses and cysts, staging of neoplasms, trauma, infection, vessels

What precaution should be taken in patients who are receiving metformin therapy?

Metformin should be withheld for 48 hours after administration of a contrast agent because there is an increased risk of lactic acidosis. Given this risk, most hospitals hold metformin administration throughout the patient's hospitalization.

A patient presents with adult polycystic renal disease that is confirmed by a CT scan which shows kidneys with multiple ill-defined cysts. Where else are cysts usually identified?

Liver and pancreas

What is the most common clinical presentation of renal stone disease?

Intense unilateral flank pain with hematuria

What percent of urinary tract calculi (renal stones) are radiopaque?

~90%

What percent of renal stones are detected on KUB?

Evidence suggests at best 40% to 60% of stones are detected on KUB. Detection is limited when stones are small, overlapping bones are present, overlapping stool or air is obscuring the stone, and when other calcifications are present.

What is the most sensitive imaging modality for detecting renal stones?

CT scan

What unusual form of acute pyelonephritis are patients with diabetes prone to?

Emphysematous pyelonephritis caused by bacteria generating gas within the renal parenchyma

How do you treat emphysematous pyelonephritis?

It is a medical emergency requiring decompression.

What is the differential diagnosis for bilaterally enlarged kidneys?

Ureteral obstruction, leukemia, glycogen storage diseases, lymphoma, and polycystic disease

When should significant kidney trauma be suspected?

After blunt trauma that results in a fracture of the twelfth rib or fractures of the transverse processes of the lumbar vertebrae

Where do metastases from renal cell carcinoma (RCC) tend to go?

Local lymph nodes, lung, or bone

What imaging studies are indicated even in asymptomatic patients with RCC?

Periodic chest x-ray examinations and CT scans are indicated for periodic follow-up

What is the best imaging study for the evaluation of hydronephrosis or obstruction of the renal collecting system?

Ultrasonography

How can you differentiate between a flaccid collecting system and an obstructed one?

Order a nuclear medicine Lasix (furosemide) renogram. Rapid clearance of activity from the kidney and renal pelvis is indicative of a flaccid system rather than an obstructed one.

What is the differential diagnosis for a dilated ureter?

Obstruction by stone or mass, vesicoureteral reflux, infection, and congenital megaureter

What are the primary imaging techniques used to evaluate the bladder?

Cystograms and CT scans

What is a cystogram?

A radiograph of the bladder

What type of imaging study is needed when there is penetrating trauma to the lower abdomen or pelvis with suspected urinary system involvement?

A retrograde cystogram or a CT scan

What type of study is needed when there is pelvic trauma that results in injury to the urethra?

A retrograde urethrogram

A male patient comes to the ER with pelvic trauma and blood in the urethral meatus. What must be done before catheterization of the bladder can take place?

A retrograde urethrogram must be done to avoid enlarging a small initial tear upon catheter entry.

What is the treatment of emphysematous cystitis?

Antibiotic therapy

The majority of bladder tumors have what type of histology?

95% of them are transitional cell carcinomas

Enlargement of the prostate results from what two common entities?

1. Benign prostatic hypertrophy (BPH)
2. Prostate cancer

What should the initial investigation of an enlarged prostate consist of?

A digital rectal examination and a prostate-specific antigen (PSA) level

Can PSA levels be used as a screening tool for men with possible prostate cancer?

Given that PSA is neither sensitive nor specific, it is NOT an optimal screening test. However, it is useful for checking overall trends in PSA levels and following PSA levels posttreatment for prostate cancer.

What are the most common lesions of the male external genitalia that require imaging?

Epididymitis, testicular torsion (a medical emergency!), hematoma, hydrocele, and testicular tumors

What is the best study to differentiate between epididymitis and testicular torsion?

Radionuclide testicular scan

What other study can be done to evaluate testicular torsion?

Doppler ultrasound to evaluate the degree of occlusion of blood flow to the testis

What study should be ordered when evaluating the testicle for either a hydrocele or a tumor?

Testicular ultrasound

What kind of tumors makeup the majority of solid testicular masses?

Germ cell tumors, most commonly seminoma

What makes a testicular mass likely to be benign?

Location outside the testicle but within the scrotum

What makes a testicular mass likely to be malignant?

Location within the testicle and the presence of microcalcifications

What is the most common imaging technique used to evaluate the female pelvis?

Ultrasonography

What is the best imaging technique to evaluate the patency of the fallopian tubes?

Hysterosalpingogram

What is the imaging method of choice to evaluate the status of a pregnancy?

Ultrasonography

What are commonly used diagnostic techniques after physical examination for evaluating PID?	Ultrasound, CT scan, and laparoscopy
What kind of imaging is done for suspected pelvic malignancies to determine size, involvement of pelvic side walls, and ureteral obstruction?	CT scan
What is the imaging study of choice for suspected adrenal pathology?	CT scan
What is the only practical way to assess patients for retroperitoneal adenopathy?	CT scan

SKELETAL SYSTEM

What is the most common utility of plain films of the skeletal system?	To evaluate for fracture
What is the role of CT scanning in the evaluation of the skeletal system?	It is useful for the evaluation of fine bone structure, particularly of the skull, spine, and pelvis.
What is the role of MRI in the evaluation of the skeletal system?	It is used mostly for the evaluation of the soft tissues—muscles, ligaments, cartilage, spinal cord, and marrow spaces.
What is the role of nuclear medicine in the evaluation of the skeletal system?	It is used to evaluate the skeleton for bone metastases and to evaluate for possible osteomyelitis.
What are the most common sites of injury to the spine?	C1-C2, C5-C7, and T9-L2
What is a hangman's fracture?	A fracture of the posterior elements of C2 that occurs as a result of hyperextension with compression of the upper cervical spine
What typically causes fractures of the thoracic spine?	Motor vehicle accidents or osteoporosis
What is spondylolysis?	A term used to describe a break in the pars interarticularis of the vertebral body

What is spondylolisthesis?	A term used to describe bilateral spondylolysis, when the vertebral body slips forward on the vertebral body immediately below it
What is typically observed in a patient with degenerative changes of the spine?	Narrowing of the disk spaces with sclerosis of the vertebral body end plates; spurring of the anterior, lateral, and posterior margins of the vertebral bodies
What are the three most common degenerative findings in the thoracic spine?	1. Hypertrophic osteophytes 2. Calcification along the anterior spinal ligament 3. Calcification of an intervertebral disk
What are the common degenerative changes that occur in the lower lumbar spine?	Herniated and protruded disks
What is the most common neoplasm involving the spine?	Metastasis
What kind of primary tumors result in lytic (osteoclastic) metastatic lesions?	Multiple myeloma, lung, renal, and breast cancers
What kind of primary tumors result in sclerotic (osteoblastic) metastatic lesions?	Prostate cancer and some breast cancers
Do metastases begin in the bone cortex or in the bone marrow?	They begin in the bone marrow which filters tumor cells out of the circulating blood (hematogenous spread).
What is seen on lateral plain radiography in patients with ankylosing spondylitis?	Calcium bridges across the disk spaces that is commonly referred to as *bamboo spine*
What is primary osteoporosis?	An age-related disorder characterized by decreased bone mass and increased susceptibility to fractures
What are the two types of primary osteoporosis?	1. Type I or postmenopausal osteoporosis which is related to estrogen deprivation 2. Type II or senile osteoporosis which occurs secondary to aging
What are some of the causes of secondary osteoporosis?	Hyperparathyroidism; osteomalacia; malabsorption; multiple myeloma; diffuse metastases; glucocorticoid therapy/excess

What is the current technique used to evaluate bone mineral density?

The dual energy x-ray absorptiometry (DEXA) scan

What is a periosteal reaction?

A thickening of the bone that arises from both benign and malignant lesions. It is commonly seen about a healing fracture, but can also be secondary to infection (osteomyelitis) or a neoplasm.

In 5- to 20-year-old patients, a periosteal reaction in the midportion or diaphysis of a long bone is suggestive of what kind of tumor?

Ewing sarcoma

How does Ewing sarcoma appear radiographically?

A long permeative, lytic lesion in the middiaphysis of a long bone with a large mass extending into the surrounding soft tissues

What does subperiosteal, reactive new bone in Ewing sarcoma look like on radiography?

It looks like an "onion skin."

If the periosteal reaction is located around a joint like the knee, what kind of tumor should be suspected?

Osteosarcoma

What kind of periosteal reaction pattern is worrisome for malignancy?

A sunburst-type or radiating pattern should raise concern for a malignancy

What is reflex sympathetic dystrophy (RSD)?

Localized burning (neuropathic) pain, swelling, and/or temperature changes associated with vascular vasodilation, that persist for months/years after trauma or surgery

What are the radiographic manifestations of RSD?

Focal osteoporosis and a coarsened trabecular pattern in an articular and periarticular distribution

What is myositis ossificans?

Calcification of the soft tissues usually secondary to trauma with subsequent bleeding

Where do most clavicular fractures occur?

Midportion or the distal third of the clavicle

The majority of shoulder dislocations occur with anterior dislocation of the humeral head relative to the glenoid. Is this the same or different from the hip?

It is different since the vast majority of femoral head dislocations are posterior

What is a Hill-Sachs deformity?

A deformity of the superolateral portion of the humeral head caused by its repeated interaction with the inferior edge of the glenoid as a result of chronic trauma

What is the most common fracture of the elbow seen in adults?

Fracture of the radial head

What causes olecranon fractures?

Falling directly on the elbow when it is flexed

What are the three classic forearm fractures requiring a forearm x-ray?

1. Nightstick fracture
2. Monteggia fracture
3. Galeazzi fracture

Describe each of the three classic forearm fractures requiring x-ray:

- Nightstick fracture—a single fracture through the midportion of the ulna
- Monteggia fracture—a fracture of the proximal ulna with dislocation of the radial head
- Galeazzi fracture—a fracture of the distal radius with dislocation of the ulnar head from the wrist joint

What is carpal tunnel syndrome?

A compression neuropathy of the medial nerve at the wrist (carpal tunnel) that can result in numbness/paresthesias of the hand, hand and wrist pain (especially with repetitive movements), hand/grip weakness, and in severe cases atrophy of the thenar eminence

What is a Colles fracture?

A fracture of the distal radius with dorsal angulation of the distal fragment and an associated fracture of the ulnar styloid

When do Colles fractures commonly occur?

After falling on an outstretched hand with the palm facing down

What is the most common fracture of the carpal bones?

A fracture of the midportion of the carpal navicular

Why is a scaphoid fracture important to recognize?

The scaphoid has a tenuous blood supply, and a fracture could cause disruption of blood flow resulting in aseptic necrosis of the bone.

What is a boxer's fracture?

Fracture of the distal fifth metacarpal

What is a gamekeeper's thumb?

An avulsion fracture of the base of the proximal phalanx

A patient complains of recently needing to buy larger-sized hats for his slowly expanding head. What disease do you suspect?

Paget disease of the bone

What is Paget disease of the bone?

A disease characterized by abnormal bone architecture/matrix where bone is broken down and regenerated often simultaneously (high turnover rate). It typically involves the pelvis and the skull, and occurs in people over age 40.

What are patients who have Paget disease at risk of?

Osteosarcoma in the affected bones

Where do the majority of hip fractures occur?

90% occur in the femoral neck and in the intertrochanteric region

What types of deformities are associated with femoral neck and intertrochanteric hip fractures?

Fractures of the femoral neck usually result in little deformity. Intertrochanteric fractures often result in a shortened leg with internal rotation.

What is fibrous dysplasia?

A skeletal developmental defect of the bone forming mesenchyme that results in medullary bone being replaced by fibrous tissue, which results in a lytic lesion (radiographically what appears to be a hole in the bone).

How does fibrous dysplasia typically present?

Most common symptom is pain; fibrous dysplasia can be associated with cutaneous pigmentation/café au lait spots and associated with McCune Albright syndrome. There are four disease patterns:
- Single lesion (monostotic)—most common
- Multiple areas (polyostotic)
- Craniofacial form
- Cherubism—rare

What age-group is typically affected by fibrous dysplastic lesions?

Children and young adults

What is a bone infarct?

An area of bone which has become necrotic secondary to loss of its arterial blood supply

How does a bone infarct look on gross dissection?	Scattered calcifications projecting within the marrow space
What patients are at risk of developing bone infarcts?	Sickle cell patients and divers with decompression sickness
What is a chondrosarcoma?	A malignancy arising from the cartilage; it is the third most common adult primary bone tumor (after multiple myeloma and osteosarcoma)
Where do chondrosarcomas tend to occur?	They most commonly arise from the axial skeleton, including the pelvis, femur, humerus, ribs, scapula, sternum, or spine.
At what age do chondrosarcomas typically present?	The mean age for occurrence is 40 to 45 years.
What is an osteochondroma?	A benign outgrowth of the bone that typically occurs in the lower extremity. The cortex of the bone sticks out on a stalk and ends with a bulbous cartilage cap.
What is an osteoid osteoma?	A neoplastic proliferation of the osteoid and fibrous tissue which most commonly occurs at the ends of the diaphysis of the long bones of the appendicular skeleton. It most commonly presents with focal pain, often occurring at night and relieved by aspirin or other NSAIDs.
True or False? Most fractures of the ankle involve either the medial or the lateral malleolus:	True
What are growth arrest lines?	Radiographic evidence of a time when there was some interference with the normal longitudinal growth process of the bone
What causes growth arrest lines?	Illness or the ingestion of heavy metals like lead
What is a march fracture?	Classic fracture of the metatarsals that commonly occurs in army recruits who are not used to but are made to march long distances
What is the usual location of a march fracture?	The distal third of the second, third, or fourth metatarsal

What is a Köhler-Freiberg infarction?

A form of aseptic/avascular necrosis that involves the head of the second metatarsal

What is Legg-Calvé-Perthes disease?

Idiopathic (likely avascular) necrosis of the epiphysis of the femoral head in children

What are the clinical and radiographic findings of Legg-Calvé-Perthes disease?

Clinical findings include a limp and pain with limitation of motion in the hip. Radiographic findings include irregularity, sclerosis, and fragmentation of the epiphysis.

What is Osgood-Schlatter disease?

A type of juvenile traction osteochondritis of the tibia that occurs in late childhood or early adolescence, and is more common in boys

What is the mechanism of injury in Osgood-Schlatter disease?

It may represent an "overuse injury," as the condition occurs at a time when increasing demands are made on a still immature skeleton

What are the radiographic findings of Osgood-Schlatter disease?

Radiographs will not be helpful if injury occurs during the preossification phase of bone growth. Once the ossification center develops, radiographs will reveal radiodense fragments separated from the tibial tuberosity.

What is slipped capital femoral epiphysis (SCFE)?

Posterior and inferior slippage of the proximal femoral epiphysis on the metaphysis (femoral neck), occurring through the physeal plate during the early adolescent growth spurt

SCFE occurs more frequently in what patient population?

Obese children

What are the radiographic findings of SCFE?

Minimal posterior step-off at the anterior epiphyseal-metaphyseal junction on lateral radiograph. The AP view will be normal since the initial slippage is usually posterior.

What are the two most common soft tissue injuries of the knee?

1. Injuries that involve the cruciate ligaments
2. The menisci

PEDIATRICS

What are the most common conditions in children that require imaging?

Infections, trauma, and congenital abnormalities

What type of imaging is done when evaluating the fetal and infant brain?

Ultrasonography, as long as the fontanelles remain open

What structures are normally visualized on ultrasound?

Lateral ventricles, choroid plexus, thalamus, temporal lobes, and posterior fossa

What are the two most common indications for ultrasound imaging?

1. Evaluation of ventricular enlargement (hydrocephalus)
2. Assessment of suspected brain hemorrhage

How are brain tumors in children evaluated?

CT scan or MRI

What are the most common brain tumors in children?

Astrocytoma, medulloblastomas, craniopharyngiomas, and ependymomas

When is imaging recommended for pediatric seizures?

It is limited to children with new-onset seizures who have experienced head trauma, and those who have an abnormal neurologic examination or encephalogram.

What imaging is usually done?

MRI is the study of choice (to avoid radiation exposure, which increases the risk of malignancy later in life); although noncontrast CT is used initially if intracranial hemorrhage or recent trauma is suspected.

What kind of imaging is done in cases of suspected croup or epiglottitis?

A lateral soft tissue view of the neck

What is seen on lateral soft tissue view of the neck in acute epiglottitis?

A thickened epiglottis, often appearing bulbous and in the shape of a "thumb." Other findings include ballooning of the hypopharynx and subglottic edema.

The *steeple sign* is a common radiographic finding in children with croup. What does it represent?

Narrowing of the upper portion of the trachea caused by subglottic edema

What is the major difference (besides size) between the chest x-ray of an adult or child and that of a neonate?

The presence of the thymus, which is routinely identified on chest films from birth to approximately 2 years of age

What does the thymus look like on chest x-ray?

It can overlie parts of the lungs giving it a sail-like appearance (sail sign).

What airway diseases cause hyperinflation in children?

Pneumonia, bronchiolitis, or reactive airways disease (asthma)

What sort of film should one request if aspiration of a foreign object is suspected?

Both an inspiratory and expiratory film to evaluate for a ball-valve phenomenon

What will you see on expiratory film if there is aspiration of a foreign object?

Air will be trapped on the affected side, while the unaffected lung will decrease in volume.

What causes respiratory distress in the newborn period?

Transient tachypnea of the newborn (birth-2 days); hyaline membrane disease/infant respiratory distress syndrome (birth-7 days); congenital diaphragmatic hernia; meconium aspiration

What lung findings will accompany meconium aspiration on chest x-ray?

Coarse, patchy infiltrates and hyperinflation of the lungs which clears in about 3 to 5 days

What are the lung findings seen on chest x-ray in transient tachypnea of the newborn?

Lung volumes may be larger than normal, and there may be linear or streaky opacities that clear within 2 days.

Newborn infants born by cesarean section are at risk of what lung complication during the first hours of life?

Transient tachypnea of the newborn

What is hyaline membrane disease (HMD/IRDS)?

A disease caused by surfactant deficiency, often associated with prematurity that results in increased surface tension and alveolar collapse. On CXR, low lung volumes with granular or "ground-glass" opacities of both lungs are seen.

What are the lung findings seen on chest x-ray in a patient with neonatal pneumonia?

The affected lung may be low in volume, normal, or hyperinflated. Lung opacities are typically granular and the time course is variable.

What causes neonatal pneumonia?	TORCH organisms or perineal flora acquired as a result of premature rupture of membranes
What feature of pregnancy should be suspect when a newborn is identified with a tracheoesophageal fistula (TEF)?	Polyhydramnios
What are the clinical symptoms of a TEF?	Excessive salivation with aspiration, coughing, and choking
How is the diagnosis of TEF made?	By passing a small, soft feeding tube down the esophagus to the blind end and taking a lateral radiograph
What is VATER syndrome?	It describes the association between vertebral anomalies (hemivertebra), anal atresia, TEF, and radial limb dysplasia.
What are the characteristic signs of an adynamic ileus?	All bowel loops are distended equally and a disorganized bowel gas pattern is observed on plain film.
What are the characteristic signs of a bowel obstruction?	Dilated loops proximal to the obstruction with normal to small loops distally. There is an organized bowel gas pattern seen on plain film.
What are the common causes of bowel obstruction by age-group?	• Newborn to 1 month—congenital obstruction • 4 to 6 weeks—hypertrophic pyloric stenosis • 6 weeks to 6 months—incarcerated hernias • 6 months to 3 years—intussusception • Older than 3 years—perforated appendix
What is Hirschsprung disease?	Also called congenital aganglionic megacolon, it is the result of the absence of enteric ganglion cells (neurons) within the myenteric and submucosal plexuses of the rectum and/or segments of the colon.
How do children present with Hirschsprung?	Children typically present with obstruction or constipation in the first 6 weeks of life and have a history of not passing meconium within the first 24 hours of life.

What is seen on radiography after barium enema in Hirschsprung disease?

A narrowed (aganglionic) segment may be identified

How is intussusception diagnosed and treated?

Usually with a water-soluble contrast enema; however, most radiologists prefer to reduce an intussusception with air. If reduction fails, then surgery is necessary.

What is the earliest radiographic sign of necrotizing enterocolitis (NEC)?

Air within the wall of the bowel (pneumatosis). Another early finding is small bowel dilation due to an adynamic ileus.

What is a common complication of NEC and a certain indication for surgery?

Free air within the peritoneal cavity (perforation)

What is the imaging study of choice for a Meckel diverticulum?

A nuclear medicine scan done with technetium 99-m pertechnetate

Why is technetium 99-m used?

Technetium 99-m concentrates in the normal and ectopic gastric mucosa, and allows rapid identification of the Meckel diverticulum.

What conditions cause painful, dark rectal bleeding in children?

Volvulus, mesenteric thrombosis, and Meckel diverticulum

What conditions cause painless, bright rectal bleeding in children?

Polyps, neoplasm, colitis, or sigmoid intussusception

What conditions cause painful, bright rectal bleeding in children?

Anal fissure, hemorrhoids, or rectal prolapse

What are the two most common urinary problems in children?

1. Hydronephrosis
2. Vesicoureteral reflux

What is the initial imaging test of choice for evaluating hydronephrosis?

Abdominal ultrasound

What is vesicoureteral reflux?

The intermittent reversal of normal antegrade flow of urine due to the maldevelopment of ureteral valves, and less commonly, to the ectopic insertion of a ureter

What is the most common imaging study done to evaluate reflux?

A voiding cystourethrogram

How can you differentiate Wilms tumor from neuroblastoma?

- Wilms tumor—most common renal malignancy in children; rarely calcifies
- Neuroblastoma—most common tumor of the adrenal medulla in children; often calcifies

What imaging modality is used to distinguish between the two masses?

CT scan

What chromosome abnormality is associated with Wilms tumor?

A deletion of the short arm of chromosome 11

What is the WAGR complex?

Wilms tumor, aniridia, genitourinary malformations, and mental-motor retardation

How are skeletal injuries of child abuse best documented?

They are best documented by doing a radiographic skeletal survey.

What are the common midshaft fractures that occur in both children and adults?

Transverse, oblique, spiral, and comminuted fractures

What is a buckle or torus fracture?

A simple fracture through the metaphyseal region of a long bone that produces a kink or bump along one or both cortical surfaces

What is a greenstick fracture?

A break in only one side of the cortex that occurs when the duration of stress is shorter than would be required for a complete fracture

What is a bending or bowing fracture?

A fracture that shows no cortical break on x-ray, but pathologically has numerous microfractures along the outer surface of the bent bone

What are epiphyseal-metaphyseal fractures?

Fractures produced by a shearing force applied to the end of a long bone that affects the zone of provisional calcification at the growth plate

Why do periosteal hematomas frequently occur in children?

The periosteum is very vascular and separates easily from the cortex in children. The Sharpey fibers which bind the periosteum to the shaft in adults are sparse and short in children, making separation relatively easy.

What is traumatic cortical hyperostosis?

The residual thickening of the cortex that occurs after a hematoma has been resorbed

CLINICAL VIGNETTES

A 65-year-old man with a recent stroke is being considered for anticoagulation therapy. What study is needed to exclude hemorrhage which is a contraindication to therapy?

Noncontrast CT scan

A patient complains of bloody diarrhea and abdominal distention. Pathology reports confirm inflammation of the rectum with mucosal involvement without skip lesions. What is the diagnosis and possible radiologic findings?

Ulcerative colitis (UC), pseudopolyps, lead-pipe colon on barium study, enlarged colon on abdominal imaging (toxin megacolon) may be seen

A patient presents with abdominal pain and states that he has not had a bowel movement in 4 days. He also states that he is unable to sit due to extreme pain in his anal region. What does this patient likely have and what is the classic radiographic finding on barium study?

Crohn disease, with possible anal fistula; may see a string sign on barium study. Crohn typically involves the distal ileum/proximal colon and causes transmural inflammatory changes. Its progression is typically irregular (skip lesions) and can involve the whole GI tract.

An obese 45-year-old woman presents to the ED shortly after eating a bucket of fried chicken, a side order of french fries, and a diet cola. She complains of intense right upper quadrant pain that is colicky in nature. She has involuntary guarding on examination. What is the likely diagnosis and the study indicated to evaluate the patient?

The patient likely has acute cholecystitis and requires ultrasonography for further evaluation.

A patient comes in with abdominal pain that is located midline, above the umbilicus. He states that about 4 weeks ago he had a bout of acute pancreatitis that landed him in the hospital for a few days. What is his likely diagnosis and how would you confirm it?

The patient likely has a pseudocyst or abscess which would be evaluated with a CT scan of abdomen/pelvis.

A 60-year-old patient came to the CT suite for follow-up evaluation of diverticular disease. Incidentally, two renal cysts were identified on his left kidney with well-defined margins and no septations. What do you tell this patient?

Renal cysts are quite common and their incidence increases with age. Because the two cysts identified had benign characteristics, they are likely simple cysts and require no further evaluation.

A 52-year-old woman presents with increasing abdominal girth. CT of her abdomen/ pelvis shows a solid mass of her left ovary, and study also caught the bases of her lungs which revealed a right pleural effusion. What is her diagnosis or what is needed to make a definitive diagnosis?

Possible ovarian malignancy versus Meigs syndrome; definitive diagnosis is needed through either cytology of pleural effusion or biopsy of ovarian mass. In Meigs syndrome the pleural effusion cytology would be benign and histology of the mass would show a fibroma.

A patient comes in complaining of pain in the lower extremity that is more intense at night and relieved by aspirin. On nuclear medicine bone scan, lesions along the cortex of the bone are found to be active. What is the suspected diagnosis?

Osteoid osteoma

A 2-year-old child presents to the ER with drooling, stridor, and difficulty breathing. He is NOT had any immunizations. What is the likely diagnosis and confirmatory radiographic findings?

Epiglottis; lateral neck x-ray would show thickened epiglottis, classically in the shape of a "thumb"

A 67-year-old patient presents with gross hematuria, flank pain, and a flank mass. What is the likely diagnosis?

Renal cell carcinoma (RCC)

A 14-year-old obese boy comes to your clinic complaining of knee pain. What should you include in your list of differential diagnoses and why?

Always consider SCFE because pain is often referred to other locations like the groin, thigh, or knee

A 3-year-old child presents to the ED with second-degree burns on the soles of his feet. Abuse is highly suspected. What are the other types of injuries that support the suspicion of child abuse?

Fractures and injuries not explained by history, multiple bruises at different stages of healing, multiple fractures of different ages, metaphyseal corner fractures with otherwise normal bones, rib fractures, and intracranial/visceral injuries

Index

Page numbers followed by *f* or *t* indicate figures or tables, respectively.

n be obtained

9 780071 627146